Antitrust Policy in Health Care Markets

Health care costs in the United States are much higher than in other countries. These cost differences can be explained, in part, by a lack of competition. Some markets, such as pharmaceuticals and medical equipment, have elements of monopoly. Other markets, such as health insurance, have elements of monopsony. Markets may also be subject to collusion on prices, such as generic drugs, or wages, such as the nurse labor market. Lawful monopoly and monopsony are beyond the reach of antitrust laws, but collusion is not. When appropriate, vigorous antitrust enforcement challenging anticompetitive conduct can aid in reducing health care costs. This book addresses monopoly, monopsony, cartels of sellers and buyers, horizontal and vertical mergers, and antitrust enforcement through private suits as well as the efforts of the antitrust Agencies. The authors demonstrate how enforcing the antitrust laws can ultimately promote competition and reduce health care costs.

TIRZA ANGERHOFER is Doctoral Fellow of Economics at Duke University.

ROGER D. BLAIR is Professor of Economics at the University of Florida.

CHRISTINE PIETTE DURRANCE is Associate Professor in the La Follette School of Public Affairs at the University of Wisconsin-Madison.

Antitrust Policy in Health Care Markets

TIRZA J. ANGERHOFER
Duke University

ROGER D. BLAIR
University of Florida

CHRISTINE PIETTE DURRANCE
University of Wisconsin–Madison

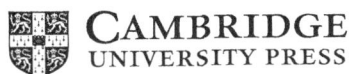

CAMBRIDGE
UNIVERSITY PRESS

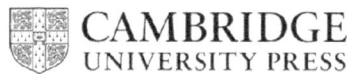
CAMBRIDGE
UNIVERSITY PRESS

Shaftesbury Road, Cambridge CB2 8EA, United Kingdom

One Liberty Plaza, 20th Floor, New York, NY 10006, USA

477 Williamstown Road, Port Melbourne, VIC 3207, Australia

314–321, 3rd Floor, Plot 3, Splendor Forum, Jasola District Centre,
New Delhi – 110025, India

103 Penang Road, #05–06/07, Visioncrest Commercial, Singapore 238467

Cambridge University Press is part of Cambridge University Press & Assessment,
a department of the University of Cambridge.

We share the University's mission to contribute to society through the pursuit of education,
learning and research at the highest international levels of excellence.

www.cambridge.org
Information on this title: www.cambridge.org/9781316515204

DOI: 10.1017/9781009099615

© Tirza J. Angerhofer, Roger D. Blair, and Christine Piette Durrance 2023

First published 2023

A catalogue record for this publication is available from the British Library.

Library of Congress Cataloging-in-Publication Data
Names: Angerhofer, Tirza J. author. | Blair, Roger D. author. | Durrance, Christine Piette,
   author.
Title: Antitrust policy in health care markets / Roger D. Blair, Christine Piette Durrance, Tirza
   J. Angerhofer.
Description: Cambridge, United Kingdom; New York, NY: Cambridge University Press, 2023. |
   Includes bibliographical references and index.
Identifiers: LCCN 2022009514 (print) | LCCN 2022009515 (ebook) | ISBN 9781316515204
   (hardback) | ISBN 9781009096492 (paperback) | ISBN 9781009099615 (epub)
Subjects: MESH: Health Care Sector–economics | Health Policy | Antitrust Laws–organization
   & administration | Marketing of Health Services–methods | United States
Classification: LCC RA410.56 (print) | LCC RA410.56 (ebook) | NLM W 74 `AA1| DDC
   362.1068/8–dc23/eng/20220328
LC record available at https://lccn.loc.gov/2022009514
LC ebook record available at https://lccn.loc.gov/2022009515

ISBN 978-1-316-51520-4 Hardback
ISBN 978-1-009-09649-2 Paperback

Additional resources for this publication at www.cambridge.org/9781316515204

To my parents, Alex and Nadia, for always believing in me and offering me their love and support.

TIRZA J. ANGERHOFER

To Chau and the rest of my family for their love, understanding, and support.

ROGER D. BLAIR

To my father, Michael, who inspired my love of economics and whose spirit I carry with me every day.

CHRISTINE PIETTE DURRANCE

Contents

Figures

Tables

Acknowledgments

In writing a book like this one, debts to others pile up quickly. It is extremely difficult to keep track of everyone who has made a positive contribution to our efforts. We hope that we have not missed anyone.

For prior collaboration, we thank Kristine Coffin, Thomas Cotter, Carlos Estrada, Jeffrey Harrison, Jill Herndon, the late David Kaserman, Thomas Knight, John Lopatka, William Page, and Richard Romano. Their influence on our reasoning and our understanding of the law and economics that we have employed is gratefully acknowledged. We have received more direct benefits from Sara Bensley, who was always ready to help with legal research. Devon Myers provided substantive input on several issues involving health care policy and details regarding pharmacy benefit managers and the insulin market. Herbert Hovenkamp contributed his wisdom on several antitrust issues. Last, but certainly far from least, we thank Lena Buonanno for her masterful editorial assistance. If not for her efforts, the book would be even less readable than it is.

None of these wonderful colleagues can be blamed for what follows. In a spirit of collegiality, we have agreed to blame one another for all errors of commission or omission that remain.

Table of Cases

I Health Care Markets and Competition Policy

In Economics 101, we learn that competition and competitive markets provide the biggest bang for the buck. In a perfectly competitive world, scarce resources are allocated in the most efficient way; the goods and services that are valued most highly are produced in the right quantities and are priced appropriately. Perfectly competitive markets, therefore, maximize social welfare, which is the sum of consumer surplus and producer surplus. Market imperfections can impede the competitive process and introduce inefficiencies that, in time, can reduce the well-being of society. These imperfections include externalities, asymmetric information, monopoly power, and public goods. The public policy response to these market failures is to promote and preserve competition. Concerns over market imperfections are also present in the US health care sector. Departures from competition can lead to poor-quality care and cause losses in the hundreds of billions of dollars.

1.1 THE MARKETPLACE OF HEALTH CARE SPENDING

Health care services are a vital component of a functioning economy since they ensure a healthy population capable of employment and consumption. Patients want access to physicians and hospitals for day-to-day care as well as to emergency rooms in cases of medical emergencies. Pharmaceutical drug companies manufacture prescription drugs that help patients manage or postpone ill health, and various medical device manufacturers produce prosthetic limbs and artificial joints, which restore mobility. Scientists and researchers in the health care industry discover new methods and products to promote health and cure disease. Health insurers, pharmaceutical benefit managers, and managed care organizations, among others, facilitate the transfer of these health services to patients. But such services come with costs.

The United States spent almost $4 trillion on health care in 2019, which accounts for about 18 percent of its gross domestic product (GDP).[1] This amounts to approximately $11,582 for every man, woman, and child in the United States. And spending continues to rise. In the United States, the majority of health care expenditures fall into three categories: (1) hospital care ($1.2 trillion), (2) physician or other professional services ($1 trillion), and (3) prescription drugs ($370 billion).[2]

A good deal of this spending is carried out by health insurers, who directly pay health care providers for the care offered to their policyholders. In contrast to other countries where health insurance is universal and heavily regulated by the government, the US health insurance system is fragmented, with individuals gaining access to health care coverage through private or government-sponsored insurance. In 2019, 91 percent of the US population was covered by private or government-sponsored health insurance (leaving approximately 30 million people uninsured). That same year, 50 percent of the population received private health insurance through an employer (i.e., employer-sponsored insurance), whereas 6 percent purchased private insurance in the individual market. Data suggest that private health insurers spend approximately $1.2 trillion on behalf of their policyholders. Meanwhile, government-supported Medicare and Medicaid insurance programs spend $800 billion and $614 billion, respectively. Medicare provides health care coverage to individuals over the age of 65 and those permanently disabled; Medicaid (a partnership between federal and state governments) provides health care coverage to low-income individuals who meet specific eligibility criteria. In 2019, Medicare covered 14 percent

---

[1] Centers for Medicare & Medicaid Services (2021b).
[2] Centers for Medicare & Medicaid Services (2021c).

of the population, whereas Medicaid covered 20 percent of the population.[3]

In 2019, the health care sector employed 22 million individuals (14 percent of total employment) in roles that range from licensed and advanced occupations working directly with patients, such as physicians and registered nurses, to those facilitating access to health care, such as hospital administrators or health insurance workers.[4] Moreover, each year approximately 36 million patients are admitted to and cared for in the approximately 6,000 hospitals in the United States, which together have a capacity of 924,000 beds.[5]

I.2 COMPETITIVE CONCERNS

In all markets, competition can be undermined on the selling side and the buying side. On the selling side, the profit-maximizing efforts of monopolists distort resource allocation and raise prices above the competitive level. Collusion among ostensible competitors to emulate the conduct of a monopolist imposes the same burden. On the buying side, a monopsonist distorts resource allocation by reducing the quantity of inputs that it buys in order to decrease the price that it pays. Somewhat counterintuitively, this leads to higher – not lower – prices for consumers. Collusion among buyers yields monopsonistic results that are equally undesirable.

The economic distortion by sellers and buyers can have enormous effects on the economy, especially in the health care sector where lives are at stake. If prices for health care services increase, insurance premiums may increase. Some patients may find themselves priced out of the health insurance market and must pay for health care on their own. Others may delay care, fail to take essential but expensive prescription drugs, or be unable to afford lifesaving treatment. The US government and, therefore, taxpayers are harmed as well through higher prices borne by Medicare and Medicaid. If, for

---

[3] Kaiser Family Foundation (2021).   [4] Laughlin et al. (2021).
[5] American Hospital Association (2021).

example, the price increases caused by market imperfections amounted to only 10 percent, correcting those imperfections would result in savings of $380 billion as well as increases in health care accessibility for patients.

1.3   ANTITRUST POLICY

In the United States, the public policy response to anticompetitive behavior is described in two antitrust statutes that provide the statutory foundation for antitrust policy. The Sherman Act of 1890 identifies both monopolizing and collusive behavior as violations of federal competition policy. The Clayton Act of 1914 prohibits specific business behavior – including tying, price discrimination, and mergers – that tends to limit competition. The Antitrust Division of the Department of Justice (DOJ) and the Federal Trade Commission (FTC) enforce these antitrust laws. In this role, the antitrust Agencies discipline businesses and individuals for anticompetitive business practices and mergers through the prosecution of those who they suspect have violated the antitrust laws. Public enforcement by the Agencies is enhanced by private enforcement, where competitors or classes of health care consumers may file antitrust litigation in pursuit of private damages. Given the size of the health care sector, efforts that protect the competitive process, even small efforts, could result in large monetary savings for health care consumers. For example, the State of California was awarded $575 million following litigation against Sutter Health, a large hospital organization that was prosecuted for anticompetitive behavior.[6]

The US health care system is quite different from the systems of other well-developed nations, many of which are controlled by their respective governments and therefore are not defined by competition. The US system is somewhat fragmented, with health insurance coverage originating from a variety of sources, including employers, the individual private market, and government-sponsored health

---

[6] Waters (2020). We discuss the Sutter Health case in more detail in Chapter 18.

insurance programs including Medicare and Medicaid. Although large-scale health reform has not been achieved in the United States, under the Obama administration, the Patient Protection and Affordable Care Act (ACA) became law in 2010 and made numerous changes affecting private and public aspects of the health care system, which substantially expanded health care access and consumer spending. First, the ACA expanded Medicaid, and despite court challenges,[7] 39 states (and the District of Columbia) have adopted Medicaid expansion for individuals with incomes below 138 percent of the federal poverty level.[8] Second, the ACA created state-based health insurance marketplaces where individuals could purchase health insurance in the individual market. Eligible consumers were offered sliding-scale subsidies on health insurance premiums; additionally, a subset of those eligible were also offered subsidies on cost sharing for out-of-pocket expenses.[9] Moreover, the ACA permits young adults to stay on their parents' health insurance plans through age 26. These efforts substantially expanded access and uptake of health insurance through public and private mechanisms, contributing to increases in health care spending.[10]

1.4   PLAN OF THE BOOK

The US health care system is complex and expensive. Between 2000 and 2019, health care spending increased by more than 170 percent, from $1.4 trillion to $3.8 trillion.[11] Moreover, private (family)

---

[7] *National Federation of Independent Business (NFIB)* v. *Sebelius*, 567 US 519 (2012).

[8] In 2021, the federal poverty level was $26,500 for a family of four (Centers for Medicare & Medicaid Services 2021a).

[9] Eligible consumers with incomes up to 400 percent of the federal poverty level were offered sliding-scale subsidies on health insurance premiums. Those individuals with incomes up to 250 percent of the federal poverty level were also offered subsidies on cost sharing for out-of-pocket expenses.

[10] In *National Federation of Independent Business (NFIB)* v. *Sebelius*, 567 US 519 (2012), the individual mandate (with penalty) was found to be constitutional, but in 2019, Congress set the penalty for failure to purchase insurance at $0, effectively repealing the mandate. Tax Cuts and Jobs Act, H.R. 1, 115th Congress (2019).

[11] Centers for Medicare & Medicaid Services (2021b).

health insurance premiums have increased from approximately $6,000 per year in 1999 to $19,000 per year in 2018, which greatly outpaces the rate of inflation.[12] To address concerns about access to and affordability of health care, there have been calls for large-scale health care reform and major modifications to our current health care system. Some have recommended replacing the current system with some form of universal health care, which is common in other countries. In this book, however, we focus on the concerns in our existing health care system that arise from failures of competition. Anticompetitive practices lead to higher prices, reduced service availability, and reduced quality. Protecting the competitive process can ensure lower prices and improved consumer welfare, with spillovers to the entire sector. Preserving competition can also increase innovation and improve accessibility of health care services. Competitive failures can be addressed with existing antitrust laws, which can provide immediate relief for the harms from anticompetitive conduct.

In this book, we focus on five areas of antitrust concern present in our health care system: monopoly, collusion among sellers, monopsony, collusion among buyers, and mergers.

Monopoly

We cover monopoly in Part I. A monopoly exists when there is a single seller of a good or service for which there are no close substitutes. For example, a rural hospital may have no close competition and, therefore, would be a monopolist in the provision of acute care hospital services. A profit-maximizing monopolist will decrease the quantity it sells below the competitive level in order to increase prices, which causes consumers to be overcharged for their purchases.[13] Monopoly may be objectionable from a social welfare perspective, but without

---

[12] Claxton et al. (2018).

[13] Patients are "overcharged" in the sense that the monopoly price exceeds the competitive price.

the presence of anticompetitive behavior that violates the antitrust laws, public policy cannot remedy this problem.

The major source of monopoly power in the pharmaceutical industry is derived from patents. A patent on a pharmaceutical drug provides exclusivity for a limited period of time, usually 20 years from when the patent application was filed. If there is ample demand for the drug and no reasonably close substitutes, then the patentee will have monopoly power that it can exercise freely. Note that a patent confers a legal monopoly, but not necessarily an economic monopoly. There can be other drugs that are different but are reasonable substitutes, or, if the drug has undesirable side effects, demand may be quite limited.

Prescription drugs that are economically successful in the marketplace can have very high prices during this period of exclusivity. For example, a drug that treats hepatitis C (Sovaldi) was first introduced in 2013 at a cost of $84,000 for a 12-week supply. At the same time, patent policy promotes innovation by preventing other companies from free riding on the innovative efforts of the patent holder during the patent exclusivity period. The patent, therefore, balances the need for innovation with affordability in the postpatent period. But patent policy does create tension with the antitrust laws since competition policy is designed to promote and protect competition by limiting the formation of monopolies and cartels. Prescription drug spending in the United States is considerable, and there are many public policy proposals under consideration that would reduce prescription drug spending for insurance companies and consumers. We discuss the merits of recent policy proposals in Chapter 3.

Moreover, there are some competitive concerns that arise beyond the tension between antitrust law and patent law. For example, the patent system may be manipulated through product hopping, where a patent holder can extend the legal monopoly over its patented drug by making a simple modification to the prescribed drug (perhaps altering the dose to improve efficacy, changing the absorption rate, or switching the medication form from tablets to capsules). The Agencies may not object to this practice if the modification confers real benefits to health care consumers. Product hopping, however, may be anticompetitive if the benefits to the patient from the simple modification are not greater than the harm to patients resulting from the delay in the entrance of cheaper generic alternatives on the market. The emergence of generic drugs after a patent expires typically leads to a reduction in prices through enhanced competition. In this way, product hopping may foreclose competition, resulting in higher prices and harm to consumers.

Another competitive concern for the Agencies involves bundled discounts. Multiproduct firms may offer bundled discounts where the amount of the discount depends on the purchase of multiple inputs. Firms that sell only a few inputs may be foreclosed if they are not able to compete with a discount that is spread over multiple products. If firms are foreclosed from the market, the remaining firms will have greater market power.

Collusion among Sellers

Collusion among sellers occurs when multiple sellers cooperate with one another to act as a single monopolist by raising prices and reducing output. In Part II, we outline the competitive consequences of collusive behavior among sellers and identify some examples where this kind of activity has occurred, including collusion among physicians and surgeons via staff privilege restrictions and collusion among pharmaceutical and medical device manufacturers. Each of these examples constitutes a violation of Section 1 of the Sherman Act.

When a seller cartel exists, consumers are harmed and social welfare decreases. We describe the harmful effects of collusion among sellers in the context of litigation alleging collusive price fixing among generic pharmaceutical manufacturers. There have also been allegations of anticompetitive agreements between generic and branded manufacturers. In attempting to keep prices high, branded drug manufacturers have colluded with generic manufacturers by using reverse payments (i.e., bribes) to delay generic entry.

We also discuss the rising costs of insulin and the allegations of a possible conspiracy among the three manufacturers of insulin in the United States. Despite the expiration of patents on branded insulin products, insulin prices have continued to rise, suggesting that competition is not present. Finally, we analyze occupational licensing within health care professions, where members of licensed professions have used their market power to displace competition.

Collusion among sellers is a violation of Section 1 of the Sherman Act. Enforcement of the antitrust laws has important consequences for the preservation of competitive prices and other benefits that flow from unrestricted competition.

Monopsony

We cover monopsony in Part III. Monopsony exists when there is only one buyer in the market. A monopsonist reduces the quantity of inputs that it buys below the competitive level in order to depress the prices it pays for those inputs. We review the monopsony model and identify the harms to social welfare. We then introduce countervailing power, whereby a monopsonist can check the power of a monopolist, resulting in better competitive outcomes than monopoly or monopsony alone. This market structure is known as a bilateral monopoly. We explore how countervailing power can offset the monopsony power health insurers have over physician groups. If physicians were permitted to collectively bargain with health insurers over reimbursement rates, this would transform a market of monopsony to one of bilateral monopoly and would improve social welfare.

Group purchasing organizations (GPOs) also wield monopsony power. In a GPO, hospitals consolidate their purchases of essential inputs to reduce prices and transaction costs. GPOs are quite pervasive, with over 98 percent of hospitals using GPOs for some purchases. But GPOs have been criticized for several anticompetitive concerns, including GPOs' revenue sources and possible competitive foreclosure from sole-sourced contracts. There has been some antitrust litigation in this space, and antitrust authorities will need to continue monitoring the contracting practices of GPOs.

Collusion among Buyers

In Part IV, we examine collusion among buyers in the health care setting. Collusion among buyers mirrors the anticompetitive consequences associated with the sole monopsonist. Buyers who collude can use their combined monopsony power to reduce input prices or wages below the level that would exist in the absence of the collusive behavior. We discuss three examples of collusive monopsony: First, we discuss collusion in the nurse labor market as one of many possible explanations for the persistent nurse shortage. Nurses have filed a series of class actions against hospitals that they allege have colluded in the hiring of nurses, resulting in nurse wage depression. Second, we highlight a recent class action involving collusion among the buyers of oocytes, which are eggs donated for use in assisted reproductive technology or in vitro fertilization. Collusion was accomplished through trade associations, where fertility clinics coordinated with one another to suppress compensation for egg donations. The class of donors was arguably paid less for their donated eggs than they would have been in the absence of the collusion. In both of these examples, sellers (i.e., nurses, donors) were undercompensated for their contributions (i.e., time, eggs). Finally, we examine no-poaching agreements, which have received so much attention in recent years that the Agencies issued formal guidelines in 2016 for human resource professionals to address agreements among employers to not hire another firm's employees. These agreements constitute illegal coordination among firms, even if they stop short of wage setting, and reduce wages by reducing competition for another firm's employees.

Mergers

In the final section of the book, we focus on horizontal and vertical mergers. The health care sector has been marked by ever-increasing consolidation through horizontal and vertical mergers in the past 20 years.[14],[15] This consolidation can lead to increased market power and anticompetitive harm. Depending on the specific market dynamics at play, mergers can be procompetitive, anticompetitive, or competitively neutral. The antitrust Agencies are tasked with evaluating large mergers before they are consummated to ensure that only procompetitive or competitively neutral mergers can proceed.

We first examine horizontal mergers and the procompetitive efficiencies that can result from these mergers. A horizontal merger occurs when two firms that were competitors in the same market consolidate to become one firm. Horizontal mergers necessarily decrease the number of firms in a market and thereby increase concentration and market power. Substantial consolidation can lead to anticompetitive outcomes, as was the case with Sutter Health, a hospital system that gained market power through mergers. We discuss the methodology antitrust Agencies use to evaluate horizontal mergers by considering specific instances of mergers among health insurers, physician groups, and pharmaceutical companies.

We also discuss vertical mergers, which occur when two firms at different levels of the supply chain consolidate to become one firm. In general, vertical mergers are less troubling than horizontal mergers because they can provide procompetitive benefits in the form of a reduction in transaction costs and elimination of double marginalization. These mergers, however, may increase a firm's market power, leading to the raising of rivals' costs or market foreclosure. It is up to the antitrust Agencies to determine whether a vertical merger will prove to be procompetitive on balance. We discuss vertical mergers in

---

[14] Irving Levin Associates (2017).

[15] We consider mergers to encompass mergers, acquisitions, and affiliations.

the biotechnology industry, within managed care, and between physician groups and hospitals to illustrate the difficult evaluation task assigned to the Agencies.

1.5   CONCLUDING REMARKS

Health care is vital to the health and well-being of the US population, and as such it should be protected by competition policy just like the markets for other goods and services. Enforcing the antitrust laws, publicly and privately, can protect the competitive process and thereby save health care consumers, health insurers, and government-funded health care programs billions of dollars. In Chapter 2, we introduce the US antitrust laws, which are the foundation for tackling the competitive concerns present in our health care system.

REFERENCES

American Hospital Association. (2021). *Fast Facts on US Hospitals.* www.aha.org/statistics/fast-facts-us-hospitals.

Centers for Medicare & Medicaid. (2021a). *Federal Poverty Level.* www.healthcare.gov/glossary/federal-poverty-level-FPL/.

Centers for Medicare & Medicaid Services. (2021b). *NHE Fact Sheet.* www.cms.gov/Research-Statistics-Data-and-Systems/Statistics-Trends-and-Reports/NationalHealthExpendData/NHE-Fact-Sheet.

Centers for Medicare & Medicaid Services. (2021c). *NHE Tables: Table 2: National Health Expenditures; Aggregate, Annual Percent Change, Percent Distribution and per Capita Amounts, by Type of Expenditure, 1960–2019.* www.cms.gov/files/zip/nhe-tables.zip.

Claxton, Gary, Matthew Rae, Michelle Long, Anthony Damico, and Heidi Whitmore. (2018). Health Benefits in 2018: Modest Growth in Premiums, Higher Worker Contributions at Firms with More Low-Wage Workers. *Health Affairs* 37: 1892–1900.

Irving Levin Associates. (2017). *Health Care M & A in the 21st Century: 2000–2017.* 3rd ed. https://issuu.com/irvinglevinassociates/docs/hc21_2017.

Kaiser Family Foundation. (2021). *Health Insurance Coverage of the Total Population.* www.kff.org/other/state-indicator/total-population/.

Laughlin, Lynda, Augustus Anderson, Anthony Martinez, and Asiah Gayfield. (2021). *Who Are Our Health Care Workers? 22 Million Employed in the Fight Against COVID-19*. Washington, DC: US Census Bureau. www.census.gov/library/stories/2021/04/who-are-our-health-care-workers.html.

Waters, Rob. (2020). *California's Sutter Health Settlement: What States Can Learn about Protecting Residents from the Effects of Health Care Consolidation*. New York: Milbank Memorial Fund. www.milbank.org/wp-content/uploads/2020/09/Sutter-History-Report_v3.pdf.

2 Antitrust Policy in the United States

The fundamental premise of the antitrust laws is that competitive market forces can be relied upon to guide resource allocation in the most efficient way. In the absence of market failure, which may be due to market power, externalities, asymmetric information, or public goods, competitive markets maximize social welfare. US antitrust policy aims to protect and promote competition through the public and private enforcement of the antitrust statutes as interpreted by the judiciary. In this chapter, we provide a brief overview of US antitrust policy.

In the next section, we examine the economic foundation for having public policy that encourages competition. Section 2.3 provides a brief sketch of the historical forces that resulted in our federal antitrust statutes. Section 2.4 addresses the Sherman Act, its prohibitions, and the sanctions for violations. In Section 2.5, we examine the additional prohibitions contained in the Clayton Act. Private enforcement of the antitrust laws is explained in Section 2.6. As we will see in Section 2.7, class action suits may be filed when large numbers of antitrust victims have been injured by the same antitrust violation. We close this chapter with some concluding remarks in Section 2.8.

2.2 THE ECONOMIC RATIONALE FOR ANTITRUST POLICY

In a competitive market, there are many buyers and many sellers. No one has any discernible control over price, and there are no barriers to entry by others. Competitive markets in the health care sector include some health care labor markets, supplies of hospital linens and paper products, and plasticware. By contrast, a monopoly is the single supplier of the good or service in question and can therefore set the price by controlling the quantity it produces. Firms in monopolistic markets include the sole provider of spinal surgery in a local market and a pharmaceutical firm with a patented drug. The economic effects of monopoly are familiar: higher prices and reduced output.

If the firm is a monopsony, a single buyer, that firm can control the price it pays for a good or service by controlling the quantity it purchases. If an isolated town has only one key employer of nurses, such as a hospital, that employer constitutes a monopsony. While there may be a large number of nurses seeking employment, there is only one employer. The economic effects of monopsony are less familiar: reduced prices paid and reduced purchases. Although it may seem somewhat counterintuitive, the impact on consumers turns out to be the same as in monopoly: higher prices and lower quantity. In either case – monopoly or monopsony – consumers are worse off than they would be in a competitive environment.

In both cases, scarce resources are misallocated, which leads to reductions in both consumer welfare and social (or total) welfare. Put differently, the misallocation of resources reduces the total size of the pie. In addition, there is a reallocation of wealth from consumers to the monopolist and from input suppliers to the monopsonist.

What generates political support for a vigorous antitrust policy are the prices that affect the distribution of wealth. For economists, however, the concern is with the allocative inefficiency of the output restrictions rather than the effect on wealth distribution. Here, we explore the impact of monopoly and monopsony on both distributive and allocative efficiency.

Monopoly and Its Welfare Consequences

Consider a case of monopolization. Profit maximization will lead the firm to operate where marginal revenue (MR) equals marginal cost (MC). In other words, the monopolist will produce the quantity where the added revenue of selling one more unit is just equal to the added

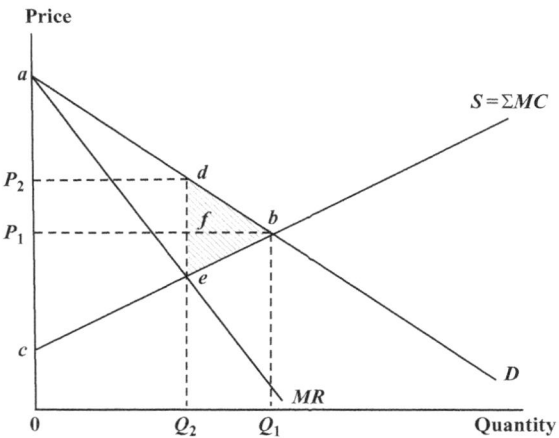

FIGURE 2.1 Competition, monopoly, and social welfare

cost of selling that unit. The economic results are captured in Figure 2.1, where D represents demand, MR is the associated marginal revenue, and S denotes supply, which is the sum of all the individual firm marginal cost curves (ΣMC). The competitive solution, which can be found at the intersection of supply and demand, provides a benchmark for evaluating the adverse economic consequences of monopoly. The competitive price is P_1 and the quantity is Q_1.

In this partial equilibrium setting,[1] our measure of consumer welfare is consumer surplus and our measure of social welfare is the sum of consumer surplus and producer surplus. Consumer surplus is the difference between the consumer's willingness to pay and the price that he or she actually pays. In Figure 2.1, this is the area under the demand curve and above P_1 (i.e., the triangular area abP_1). Producer surplus is the difference between a producer's reservation price and the price actually received. In Figure 2.1, producer surplus is the area above the supply curve and below P_1 (i.e., the triangular area P_1bc). The sum of consumer surplus and producer surplus is a

---

[1] By *partial equilibrium*, we mean that the analysis is confined to this particular market. All other markets are ignored.

measure of social welfare. Given the demand and supply conditions in this market, social welfare is maximized at the competitive equilibrium of P_1 and Q_1. No other price and output will generate a larger social welfare. This is the economic rationale for public policy that promotes and protects competition.

If this market is monopolized, the monopolist will maximize its profits by reducing output to Q_2 (where MR equals MC) and raising price to P_2. Profit maximization by the monopolist reduces consumer surplus from area abP_1 to area adP_2. Some of the lost consumer surplus, area P_2dfP_1, is converted into producer surplus (or profit), whereas the rest is simply lost.[2] In terms of social welfare, the loss due to monopoly is equal to area dbe. This area is the sum of the forgone consumer surplus and producer surplus from not producing at Q_1.

Figure 2.1 shows how monopoly alters the distribution of the surplus by converting some consumer surplus into profit. Not surprisingly, consumers find this objectionable. But monopoly also reduces the total surplus because of the output restriction. In Figure 2.1, we can see that price exceeds marginal cost at a quantity of Q_2. Too little output is being produced because the value to consumers of an additional unit of output exceeds the cost to society of producing that added output. The welfare loss of monopoly is measured by this allocative inefficiency. For economists, this is the economic rationale for antitrust policy.

Monopsony and Its Welfare Consequences

Monopsony leads to welfare effects that are analogous to those of monopoly. Figure 2.2 illustrates these effects.[3] Under competitive conditions, demand (D) and supply (S) determine a price of w_1 and a

---

[2] The loss to consumers is represented by higher costs for those consumers who bought products at the monopolistic price and by consumers who were priced out of the market. The latter consumers were foreclosed because they could not afford the monopoly price.

[3] Blair and Harrison (2010).

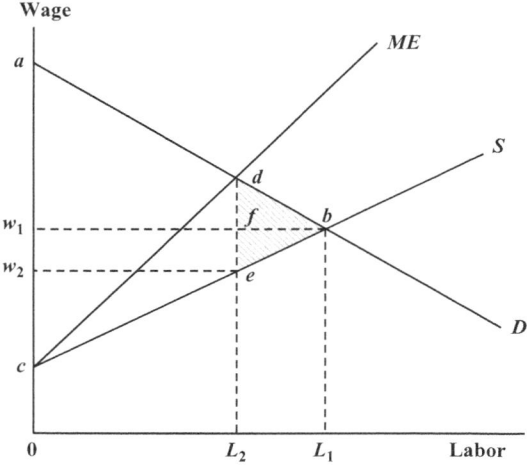

FIGURE 2.2 Competition, monopsony, and social welfare

quantity of L_1, respectively. Buyer surplus[4] is equal to area abw_1, and producer surplus equals area w_1bc. The sum of the two areas, area abc, is social welfare.

Now suppose there is a single buyer, that is, a monopsonist. The monopsonist can take advantage of the positively sloped supply curve by restricting its purchases and thereby depressing the price that it pays for inputs. To maximize its profits, the monopsonist will purchase at the point where the marginal expenditure (ME) equals demand.[5] At this reduced quantity (L_2), the price on the supply curve

---

[4] We are using the term *buyer surplus* because in most monopsony settings, the buyers are firms rather than consumers. The concept, however, is the same: the difference between the buyer's reservation price and the price actually paid.

[5] The profit function for a firm with monopsony power in the market for labor can be written as

$$\pi = PQ(L, x_1, x_2, \ldots, x_n) - w(L)L - \sum_{i=1}^{n} w_i x_i,$$

where P is output price, $Q(L, x_1, x_2, \ldots, x_n)$ is the production function, L is the quantity of labor with a corresponding wage of $w(L)$, and x_i and w_i represent the quantity and price of the other inputs. The first-order condition for profit maximization of interest is is w_2. The result is a reduction in producer surplus from w_1bc to w_2ec. Part of this reduction, area w_1few_2, is converted into buyer surplus and part of it is lost. The net effect on social welfare is a loss equal to triangular area dbe.[6] The figure shows that the welfare results of monopsony are analogous to those of monopoly. A monopsonist reduces social welfare as well as producer welfare. In addition, the monopsonistic restriction on purchases translates into a reduction in the output that the monopsonist produces.[7] With reduced output, the price to the consumer rises.[8] Consequently, both monopoly and monopsony will lead to consumer dissatisfaction and political pressure for change.

2.3   POLITICAL FOUNDATION OF ANTITRUST POLICY

Federal antitrust policy in the United States dates back to 1890 with the passage of the Sherman Act. It is not possible to isolate a single factor that spawned this legislation. Instead, there was a combination of economic and political factors that created the conditions necessary for Congress to pass such important legislation. In his influential book, Hans Thorelli identified four factors that created the necessary political will to challenge monopoly.[9]

$$\frac{\partial \pi}{\partial L} = P\frac{\partial Q}{\partial L} - w - L\frac{dw}{dL} = 0.$$

The value of the marginal product, $P\frac{\partial Q}{\partial L}$, is the demand for L, and $w+L(dw/dL)$ is the marginal expenditure. Since dw/dL is positive, $ME > w$.

[6] Although it may be somewhat counterintuitive, the lower price paid by the monopsonist does not result in lower output prices (Blair and Durrance 2008).

[7] Supreme Court rulings, such as *Mandeville Island Farms*, clearly illustrate that the Court has long understood this parallel. In *Mandeville Island Farms*, sugar beet farmers complained that the refiners colluded in an effort to depress the prices that they paid for the sugar beets. The Court recognized that the sellers were the victims of a collusive monopsony. *Mandeville Island Farms* v. *American Crystal Sugar Co.*, 334 US 219 (1948).

[8] For a more comprehensive exposition of why monopsony leads to higher prices for consumers, see Angerhofer and Blair (2020).

[9] Thorelli (1955).

First, in the years following the Civil War, the agricultural community was financially struggling because the prices of agricultural products were low, the costs of operating farms were high, and farm profits were negligible. The absence of competition among the railroads and local monopolies of essential inputs such as farm machinery and seed increased costs and diminished profits. Ultimately, the farmers' dissatisfaction resulted in the formation of politically powerful interest groups that demanded change.

Second, price-fixing agreements of one sort or another existed in a wide array of industries, including beer, candles, coal, cottonseed oil, ice, lumber, oatmeal, packed meats, sugar, tile, and whiskey. This cartel activity resulted in higher prices for consumers, to their obvious detriment.

Third, as the problems for both farmers and consumers persisted, a more general public sentiment averse to "big business" was developing. This sentiment stemmed from reports of financial scandals that were laid at the feet of big business. In addition, there were revelations of a variety of improprieties, such as industrial espionage, bribery of judges and politicians, and the use of predatory business practices.

Finally, there was widespread criticism of the business community. In the final years before passage of the Sherman Act, public objections to cartels and monopolies continued to grow. At the time, there appeared to be a great deal of truth in the charges that monopolies (1) corrupted public employees and legislators, thereby threatening political democracy; (2) enjoyed a degree of insulation afforded by protective tariffs; (3) hurt consumers by charging higher prices; (4) engaged in questionable financial practices; and (5) caused serious dislocations by suddenly closing plants. The American public felt abused by the monopolies and wanted a law that would prohibit their worst abuses and curtail their power.

These five factors combined to pressure Congress to keep the power of the monopolies and cartels in check. The result was the

Sherman Act of 1890. This Act remains the cornerstone of US anti-trust policy today and affects nearly all industries.

The Sherman Act has two substantive provisions that address the monopoly problem. Section 1 prohibits agreements among ostensible competitors to refrain from competing and thereby act like a monopoly:

> Section 1. Every contract, combination in the form of trust or otherwise, or conspiracy, in restraint of trade or commerce among the several States, or with foreign nations, is hereby declared to be illegal. Every person who shall make any such contract or engage in any such combination or conspiracy shall be deemed guilty of a felony.[10]

Because all contracts restrain trade to some extent, Section 1 could not be read literally. The general language of Section 1 required judicial interpretation. Through decades of litigation, the courts have put flesh on the bare-bones language of Section 1. In so doing, the courts have distinguished between reasonable and unreasonable restraints of trade. Restraints that prove to be unreasonable are deemed to be unlawful, whereas those found to be reasonable are deemed lawful. Whether a business practice is reasonable depends on its impact on consumer welfare or social welfare. Restraints that promote competition and thereby enhance consumer welfare or social welfare are reasonable and, therefore, lawful. Restraints that impair competition and thereby reduce consumer welfare and social welfare are unreasonable and, therefore, are unlawful. The courts have found the following activities to be unlawful because they restrain competition: price-fixing agreements, bid rigging, market allocation schemes, agreements on credit terms, and information exchanges on prices.[11]

---

[10] 15 USC §1.

[11] If two divisions of a firm agree on prices, they cannot be sued under Section 1 of the Sherman Act. As a legal matter, they are incapable of conspiring. But the organization must be a single entity, as the Franciscan Health System found out. See Wu and O'Connor (2019) for more details.

In Part II and Part IV, we discuss various Section 1 violations that include price fixing by generic drug manufacturers and wage fixing in the nurse labor market.

Section 2 of the Sherman Act addresses single-firm conduct that results in monopoly or is likely to lead to monopoly. The language of Section 2 does not outlaw the structural condition of monopoly. Instead, it condemns the act of becoming a monopoly or trying to do so:

> Section 2. Every person who shall monopolize, or attempt to monopolize, or combine or conspire with any other person or persons, to monopolize any part of the trade or commerce among the several States, or with foreign nations, shall be deemed guilty of a felony.[12]

This general language also required judicial interpretation to separate the monopolies that deserve prosecution from those that do not. Once again, the result is based on the impact of the conduct on consumer welfare or social welfare. For example, the firm that monopolizes by building a better mousetrap than its competitors should escape antitrust scrutiny, whereas a firm that disparages or sabotages its rivals should not.[13] In Chapter 3, we discuss the legal monopolies that pharmaceutical firms are granted through patents. But when pharmaceutical firms attempt to extend their patent rights through underhanded tactics, such as exclusionary product hopping, those actions may be considered violations of Section 2 of the Sherman Act. We discuss this possibility in Chapter 4.

The penalties for violating either Section 1 or Section 2 of the Sherman Act are the same. For corporations, these sections provide maximum fines of $100 million. In some instances, however, even

---

[12] 15 USC §2.

[13] For example, Bracco Diagnostics Inc., which produces barium sulfate suspension products, allegedly maintained its monopoly power by abusing the Food and Drug Administration (FDA) approval process in order to force its rival, Genus Medical Technologies LLC, to suspend production of barium sulfate. See Leonard (2019a) for more details.

this substantial penalty may not be enough. After all, the rewards for monopolization – either by agreement or ownership – may be far in excess of the maximum fine. Congress recognized this problem and passed the Criminal Fine Improvements Act in 1987.[14] This Act permits the court to impose a fine equal to twice the pecuniary gain that the corporation obtained from the violation or twice the pecuniary loss suffered by the victims.

For individuals who violate the antitrust laws, the sanctions include provisions for imprisonment as well as fines. An individual may be imprisoned for up to 10 years and fined as much as $1 million for violating the Sherman Act. And, again, at the court's discretion, the fine may equal twice the pecuniary gain that the individual derived from the offense or twice the injury experienced by the victims. Once rare, prison sentences are becoming more common. So far, Frank Peake has been sentenced to the single longest prison term, five years, in 2013, for his role in a price-fixing conspiracy of ocean freight between the US mainland and Puerto Rico. More common sentences are around 24 months.[15]

2.4 ANTITRUST TREATMENT OF MONOPOLY AND CARTELS

Although both monopolies and cartels reduce social welfare, antitrust enforcement of them is altogether different.[16] This difference flows from the recognition that monopoly may result from competition in the market, whereas cartels invariably try to avoid competition.

Monopoly

In spite of the welfare consequences of monopoly, the structural condition of monopoly is not unlawful unless it is accompanied by

---

[14] Criminal Fine Improvements Act, H.R. 3483, 100th Congress (1987).

[15] Recently, the CEO of Bumblebee, Christopher Lischewski, was sentenced to 40 months in prison for his role in a price-fixing scheme among major tuna-canning companies (Department of Justice Antitrust Division 2020).

[16] We discuss issues of monopoly in Part I and seller cartel issues in Part II of this book.

exclusionary conduct. Section 2 of the Sherman Act condemns "[a]ny person who shall monopolize, attempt to monopolize, or conspire with others to monopolize."[17] This language suggests that the law is concerned with conduct rather than mere structure – and that is how the Supreme Court has interpreted the law.[18] The *Grinnell* test has emerged as a summary of what it takes to monopolize unlawfully:

> The offense of monopoly under §2 of the Sherman Act has two elements: (1) the possession of monopoly power in the relevant market, and (2) the willful acquisition or maintenance of that power as distinguished from growth or development as a consequence of a superior product, business acumen, or historic accident.[19]

The structural condition of monopoly is a necessary but not sufficient condition for illegality. This makes economic sense in spite of the static welfare loss described above. When monopoly is attributable to a superior product, consumers value this product at a monopoly price more than they value alternative products at competitive prices. It would make no sense to punish a firm for developing such a desirable product. Such a public policy would create perverse incentives that would reduce innovation and ultimately reduce social welfare.[20] When a monopoly is due to business acumen, this leads to superior economic efficiency in the form of lower costs, which conserves society's scarce resources. Both of these foundations for market dominance deserve encouragement, not condemnation.[21] But when the monopoly is due to exclusionary or predatory conduct, antitrust sanctions are appropriate because dominance does not result from

---

[17] 15 USC §2.

[18] In *United States* v. *United States Steel Corporation*, the Supreme Court observed that "the law does not make mere size an offense, or the existence of unexerted power an offense. It ... requires overt acts." *United States* v. *United States Steel Corporation*, 251 US 417 (1920) at 451.

[19] *United States* v. *Grinnell Corps.*, 384 US 563, 570–71 (1966).

[20] In Chapter 3, we explore the trade-off between monopoly prices and innovation in the market for pharmaceutical drugs.

[21] It is also hard to condemn a firm for "historic accident" or just dumb luck.

competitive superiority.[22] Instead, dominance results from anticompetitive conduct. It is one thing to outperform your rivals and quite another to prevent them from competing.

The standards for unlawful monopsony are analogous to those for unlawful monopoly. First, a plaintiff must prove the existence of monopsony power in the relevant market. Second, the plaintiff must prove the willful acquisition or maintenance of that power. In other words, the monopsonist must have engaged in predatory or exclusionary practices that resulted in or maintained the structural condition of monopsony.

Cartels

There is a wide array of collusive conduct that is condemned under Section 1 of the Sherman Act, which forbids contracts, combinations, and conspiracies that unreasonably restrain trade.[23] The quintessential horizontal restraint is price fixing among ostensible competitors.[24] The sole purpose of this activity is to emulate the conduct of a multiplant monopoly.[25] In this case, however, the monopoly outcome is not due to a superior product, business acumen, or even just luck. It is due to a conscious decision to collude rather than compete. As a result, price fixing receives the harsh antitrust treatment that it deserves. Similar to monopolies, cartels cause both consumer welfare and social welfare to decline.[26] This is why price fixing is per se

---

[22] Easterbrook (1986) warned that aggressive, competitive conduct and aggressive, exclusionary conduct often look very similar. Consequently, care must be taken to avoid stifling competition that would promote both consumer welfare and social welfare.

[23] 15 USC §1. Since all contracts restrain trade to some extent, the antitrust laws condemn only unreasonable restraints, which can be interpreted as restraints that permit collusive monopoly (or monopsony) behavior.

[24] In Chapter 7, we examine collusion among manufacturers of generic drugs that resulted in increased prices and thereby redistributed surplus from consumers to the cartel.

[25] This analogy is developed analytically in Blair and Kaserman (2009).

[26] The cartel outcome is often even worse than that of monopoly because average costs will tend to be higher since there are too many production sites, and, therefore, each site will be operating at an inefficient rate.

unlawful.[27] Challenging conduct that is per se unlawful does not require proof of anticompetitive effects, just proof that the conduct occurred.

There is a wide array of business practices that suffer a similar fate for similar reasons. Any "naked" restraint that is economically equivalent to monopoly pricing is usually unlawful under the per se label. These practices include bid rigging, market division,[28] minimum fee schedules, agreements not to compete on price, agreements on credit terms, exclusionary boycotts,[29] and agreements to control quantity.[30] As the Supreme Court ruled in *Socony-Vacuum*, "any effort to raise, depress, fix, peg, or stabilize price is illegal *per se*."[31]

2.5 THE CLAYTON ACT

The vague language of the Sherman Act's prohibitions caused Congress to pass the Clayton Act in 1914. Section 2 of the Clayton Act, as amended by the Robinson-Patman Act, prohibits price

---

[27] Naked price-fixing agreements are unlawful per se; see *United States* v. *Socony-Vacuum Oil Co., Inc.*, 310 US 150 (1940). There are, however, some agreements that technically involve agreements on price that may pass muster under a rule of reason analysis. Such agreements are not characterized as per se unlawful.

[28] Florida Cancer Specialists (FCS) and a rival oncology group divided the market for cancer treatment in southeast Florida. FCS limited its treatments to chemotherapy, and its rival limited itself to radiation therapy. In exchange for deferred prosecution, FCS paid a fine of $100 million (Bolado 2020).

[29] IQ Dental Supply, Inc., sued Henry Schein, Inc., Patterson Companies, Inc., and Benco Dental Supply Company, Inc., alleging a group boycott. The three defendants controlled some 80 percent of the market for dental supplies. IQ Dental alleged that the defendants colluded to boycott an online distribution portal and all of its suppliers in order to maintain their market power. See Leonard (2019b) for more details.

[30] Another example of monopolizing conduct arose in *BCBSM, Inc.* v. *Vyera Pharmaceuticals, LLC*, No. 1:21-cv-01884 (S.D.N.Y.). To preserve its monopoly in the market for Daraprim, an antiparasitic drug, Vyera Pharmaceuticals blocked generic competition by restricting the resale of their drug, which precluded rival firms from carrying out bioequivalence testing. They used exclusive supply agreements that foreclosed rivals from accessing the active ingredient and did not provide the data generic manufacturers would need to create a generic. Because of these restrictions, the price of Daraprim rose from $17.50 to $750. This conduct is exclusionary rather than competitive.

[31] *United States* v. *Socony-Vacuum Oil Co., Inc.*, 310 US 150 (1940).

discrimination when it may substantially reduce competition or tend to create a monopoly. A seller cannot disguise price discrimination by providing free goods or services, paying brokerage fees, or providing promotional materials or services on an unequal basis. The Robinson-Patman Act also forbids monopsonistic demands for discriminatory price concessions.

Section 3 of the Clayton Act forbids conditional sales if they substantially reduce competition or tend to create a monopoly. This prohibition covers an assortment of vertical agreements, including resale price maintenance, tying, requirements contracts, full-line forcing, exclusive dealing, and exclusive territories.[32] These arrangements often appear to be anticompetitive, but in many instances, they are competitively neutral or even procompetitive.

Section 7 of the Clayton Act prohibits any type of merger that is apt to have the prohibited effect of substantially lessening competition or to create a monopoly. We discuss mergers in detail in Part V of this book, where we review mergers between health insurers, hospitals, and physician practices, as well as conglomerate mergers between hospitals and physician practices.

2.6   PRIVATE ANTITRUST SUITS

Violations of the antitrust laws cause public harm, which is the underlying rationale for US antitrust policy. But these violations also cause private harm to their victims. In order to provide some remedy for these victims, Congress included a right of private action in the antitrust laws. Under Section 4 of the Clayton Act, some – but not all – firms and individuals who have been injured by antitrust violations may have standing to sue for the injuries they have suffered. For the antitrust victims who have standing to sue, Section 4 of the

---

[32] Not all exclusive dealing contracts are unlawful. Mylan offered large rebates to those who agreed to refrain from offering Sanofi's epinephrine auto-injector, which is a substitute for Mylan's EpiPen. The court found no coercion in Mylan's offer, and, therefore, the offer was not illegal (Leonard 2021).

Clayton Act provides a powerful financial incentive for private enforcement of the antitrust laws:

> [A]ny person who shall be injured in his business or property by reason of anything forbidden in the antitrust laws may sue therefor ... without respect to the amount in controversy, and shall recover threefold the damages by him sustained, and the cost of suit, including a reasonable attorney's fee.[33]

At first glance, this provision for private actions appears to be quite clear, but appearances are sometimes deceiving. As with all laws, the courts have to interpret the antitrust statutes and thereby give meaning to what seems to be plain English. More specifically, the courts have had to clarify the types of injuries that are cognizable under Section 4 and put limits on precisely who may sue for private damages.

Antitrust Standing

The term *antitrust standing* refers to the status of being a (legally) proper party to pursue a private antitrust suit.[34] If someone lacks antitrust standing, he or she does not have the right to sue for treble damages. It is therefore crucial to determine the dimensions of antitrust standing.

The language of Section 4 of the Clayton Act seems fairly clear. It appears to confer a property right on *any* person who has been injured due to an antitrust violation. But this apparently clear language has been limited by various judicial rulings. We will examine several criteria for standing that have emerged from these rulings. Specifically, we will consider who is a *person*, what is a *business or property*, what is *antitrust injury*, and the requirement of *direct injury*.

---

[33] 15 USC §15.
[34] The single best survey of the law and economics of standing is Areeda et al. (2021).

The definition of a *person* for purposes of antitrust standing is more expansive than one might suppose. For the cases that we will consider, it is sufficient to observe that the statutory language, *person*, refers to human beings. In addition, it includes corporations, partnerships, and other businesses. Section 4 permits a person to be compensated when an antitrust violation has caused injury to his or her *business or property*. For the most part, an injury to a person's financial interests is compensable. This injury includes the lost profits of a firm as well as the financial interests of a consumer who has been overcharged or a supplier who has been underpaid pursuant to an antitrust violation.

The Supreme Court introduced the concept of *antitrust injury* in its *Brunswick* decision.[35] This concept is useful in identifying compensable injuries. It is an element of standing since it limits private suits to those who have suffered an injury that flows from the anticompetitive consequences of an antitrust violation.

In *Brunswick*, the Court provided some further guidance on what constitutes antitrust injury:

> Plaintiffs must prove *antitrust* injury, which is to say injury of the type the antitrust laws were intended to prevent and that flows from that which makes defendants' acts unlawful. The injury should reflect the anticompetitive effect either of the violation or of anticompetitive acts made possible by the violation.[36]

The antitrust injury doctrine appears to be straightforward to apply in practice. First, one must identify the anticompetitive effects that flow from a particular violation. Then one must infer the logical economic consequences of those anticompetitive effects. If a plaintiff has been injured in his or her business or property due to the anticompetitive effects of an antitrust violation, then he or she would have

---

[35] *Brunswick Corp.* v. *Pueblo Bowl-O-Mat, Inc.*, 429 US 477 (1977). For an economic analysis of antitrust injury, see Page (1980). In addition, see Blair and Harrison (1989) and Blair and Page (1996).

[36] *Brunswick Corp.* v. *Pueblo Bowl-O-Mat, Inc.*, 429 US 477 (1977).

suffered antitrust injury under the *Brunswick* rule. Any injury that is not a consequence of the anticompetitive effects of an antitrust violation does not constitute antitrust injury. Such an injury, therefore, would not be compensable under the remedial provisions of Section 4 of the Clayton Act.

The Supreme Court introduced the requirement that a plaintiff be injured directly in order to have standing to sue in its *Hanover Shoe* and *Illinois Brick* decisions.[37] The Court's goal was to simplify the process for plaintiffs to prove damages when the guilty parties do not sell directly to the plaintiff.

In *Hanover Shoe*, a producer of shoes who leased shoe machinery from United Shoe claimed that United's lease policy was an instrument of illegal monopolization of the shoe machinery industry. Hanover argued that it was entitled to receive the difference between what it paid in rentals and what it would have paid if United had sold its machines. In response, United argued that Hanover suffered no cognizable injury because the illegal overcharge was passed on to Hanover's customers in the form of higher shoe prices. The Supreme Court rejected United's argument and held that Hanover was entitled to the full overcharge. The Court expressed concern that if the pass-on defense were permitted, it would be used by defendants to substantially raise the cost of bringing a case because "[t]reble-damage actions would often require additional long and complicated proceedings involving massive evidence and complicated theories."[38]

The *Illinois Brick* decision made the rule regarding pass-on symmetric. Whereas *Hanover Shoe* precluded the use of pass-on by a defendant, *Illinois Brick* precluded the use of pass-on by a plaintiff. The defendants in this case manufactured concrete block, which they sold primarily to masonry contractors in the Chicago area. These contractors submitted bids to general contractors for the masonry

---

[37] *Hanover Shoe* v. *United Shoe Machinery Corp.*, 392 US 481 (1968) and *Illinois Brick Co.* v. *Illinois*, 431 US 720 (1977).

[38] *Hanover Shoe* v. *United Shoe Machinery Corp.*, 392 US 481 (1968) at 494.

portion of construction projects. In turn, the general contractors submitted bids to the State of Illinois and some 700 governmental entities
that were indirect purchasers of concrete block. The issue before the
Supreme Court was whether these indirect purchasers could sue the
concrete block manufacturers for treble damages. The plaintiffs
alleged that some of the overcharges had been passed on to them.
The defendants pointed out, however, that giving the plaintiffs standing to sue would result in duplicative awards unless *Hanover Shoe*
were overruled.

The Supreme Court refused to overrule its *Hanover Shoe* decision and went on to point out that

> [p]ermitting the use of pass-on theories under §4 essentially would
> transform treble-damage actions into massive efforts to apportion
> the recovery among all potential plaintiffs that could have absorbed
> part of the overcharge – from direct purchasers to middlemen to
> ultimate consumers. However appealing this attempt to allocate
> the overcharge might seem in theory, it would add whole new
> dimensions of complexity to treble-damage suits and might
> seriously undermine their effectiveness.[39]

The Supreme Court's rule regarding a pass-on argument is symmetric. In price-fixing cases, only direct purchasers have standing to
sue.[40] If the price-fixing conspiracy involved buyers, the underpaid
suppliers would be the direct victims and therefore have standing to
sue for damages.

2.7   CLASS ACTION SUITS

In many instances involving health care markets, a single (alleged)
antitrust violation will have many victims with claims that are too
small to warrant individual suits. This may result in class action
litigation. Under some conditions, class treatment may be an

---

[39] *Illinois Brick Co.* v. *Illinois*, 431 US 720 (1977).
[40] For an evaluation, see Blair and Harrison (1999).

appropriate way to preserve the compensatory and deterrent roles of Section 4 of the Clayton Act. By aggregating possibly hundreds of small claims into a single litigation, those antitrust victims can be compensated for their losses.[41] In addition, the threat of a class action suit should serve as a deterrent that will reduce the frequency of antitrust violations. Finally, through class actions, substantial judicial economies may be realized since the court need not try the issue over and over. For these economies to materialize, however, it is necessary that issues affecting each member of the class are quite similar. If they are not, then the court would have to conduct mini-trials during the course of the litigation, and much of the value of class treatment would be lost.

Before certifying a proposed class, the court must conduct a multipart inquiry. The most common antitrust classes are certified under Rule 23(b)(3), which provides for class certification under a predominance standard.[42] Generally, Rule 23(b)(3) has two requirements. First, "questions of law or fact common to the members of the class predominate over any questions affecting only individual members." Second, a class action must be "superior to other available methods for the fair and efficient adjudication of the controversy." Satisfying Rule 23(b)(3) may be problematic. Proof of a violation is not sufficient to establish civil liability under Section 4 of the Clayton Act. Moreover, Rule 23(b)(3) requires that the proposed class representative demonstrates that common questions predominate over individual questions. For the most part, this involves liability issues rather than damage issues. But liability – even in a per se case – extends beyond proof of a violation and includes impact. That is, it is necessary to prove that all class members suffered injury to their business or property using common proof. To satisfy the predominance requirement,

---

[41] Often class actions are sponsored by the plaintiff attorneys who try the case. Their fees, which they take out of the damages administered, can be quite substantial. For example, when *UFCW & Employers Benefit Trust* v. *Sutter Health*, No. CSG 14-538451 (S.C. Cal. 2014) settled for $575 million, the attorneys asked for 32 percent, or $184 million.

[42] ABA Section of Antitrust Law (2017) provides a compact survey with ample citations. For a more extensive examination, see Blair and Durrance (2015).

therefore, the proposed class representative must prove that the antitrust violation and the fact of injury can be established "on a systematic, class-wide basis." That is, proof for one is proof for all. Otherwise, individual issues will arise. If the court is faced with the prospect of individualized questions of liability, it would have to conduct multiple mini-trials on liability. This would make a class action inappropriate. There is no specific test for determining whether common issues predominate. As a general matter, the best that can be said is that the need for individualized examination of each class member vanishes if there is generalized evidence that either proves or disproves an essential element of the claim on a class-wide basis.

2.8   CONCLUDING REMARKS

The antitrust laws are aimed at promoting market competition and eliminating or reducing business conduct and market structures that yield noncompetitive outcomes. In subsequent chapters, we will see that antitrust enforcement is needed in many health care markets. The lure of higher profit often leads to antitrust violations that cost society billions of dollars and a good deal of human misery.

REFERENCES

ABA Section of Antitrust Law. (2017). *Antitrust Law Developments.* 8th ed. Chicago: ABA Publishing.

Angerhofer, Tirza J., and Roger D. Blair. (2020). *Collusion in the Labor Market: Intended and Unintended Consequences.* Competition Policy International: Antitrust Chronicle, May II. www.competitionpolicyinternational.com/collusion-in-the-labor-market-intended-and-unintended-consequences/.

Areeda, Phillip E., Herbert Hovenkamp, Roger D. Blair, and Christine Piette Durrance. (2021). *Antitrust Law.* 5th ed. Vol. IIA. New York: Aspen Law & Business.

Blair, Roger D., and Christine Piette Durrance. (2008). The Economics of Monopsony. In W. Dale Collins, ed., *Issues in Competition Law and Policy.* Chicago: ABA Publishing, 393–407.

Blair, Roger D., and Christine Piette Durrance. (2015). The Economics of Class Actions. In Roger D. Blair and D. Daniel Sokol, eds., *The Oxford Handbook of*

International Antitrust Economics. New York: Oxford University Press, 187–204.

Blair, Roger D., and Jeffrey L. Harrison. (1989). Rethinking Antitrust Injury. *Vanderbilt Law Review* 42: 1539–1573.

Blair, Roger D., and Jeffrey L. Harrison. (1999). Reexamining the Role of Illinois Brick in Modern Antitrust Standing Analysis. *George Washington Law Review* 68: 1–43.

Blair, Roger D., and Jeffrey L. Harrison. (2010). *Monopsony in Law and Economics*. New York: Cambridge University Press.

Blair, Roger D., and David L. Kaserman. (2009). *Antitrust Economics*. 2nd ed. New York: Oxford University Press.

Blair, Roger D., and William H. Page. (1996). The Role of Economics in Defining Antitrust Injury. *Managerial and Decision Economics* 17: 127–142.

Bolado, Carolina. (2020). Fla. Cancer Group Nabs Partial Win in Adventist Antitrust Suit. *Law360*. Bloomberg Law. www.law360.com/articles/1316731/fla-cancer-group-nabs-partial-win-in-adventist-antitrust-suit.

Department of Justice Antitrust Division. (2020). Former Bumble Bee CEO Sentenced to Prison for Fixing Prices of Canned Tuna. Department of Justice. www.justice.gov/opa/pr/former-bumble-bee-ceo-sentenced-prison-fixing-prices-canned-tuna.

Easterbrook, Frank H. (1986). On Identifying Exclusionary Conduct. *Notre Dame Law Review* 61: 972–980.

Leonard, Mike. (2019a). Bracco Unit Monopolizes Medical Barium, Suit Says (Corrected). Bloomberg Law. https://news.bloomberglaw.com/antitrust/bracco-unit-monopolizes-barium-for-medical-imaging-suit-says.

Leonard, Mike. (2019b). Henry Schein, Patterson Face Revived Dental Supply Boycott Suit. Bloomberg Law. https://news.bloomberglaw.com/antitrust/henry-schein-patterson-face-revived-dental-supply-boycott-suit.

Leonard, Mike. (2021). Mylan Defeats EpiPen Antitrust Lawsuit Brought by Rival Sanofi. Bloomberg Law. https://news.bloomberglaw.com/antitrust/mylan-defeats-epipen-antitrust-lawsuit-brought-by-rival-sanofi.

Page, William H. (1980). Antitrust Damages and Economic Efficiency: An Approach to Antitrust Injury. *University of Chicago Law Review* 47: 467–504.

Thorelli, Hans B. (1955). *The Federal Antitrust Policy*. Baltimore: Johns Hopkins University Press.

Wu, Stephen, and Katherine O'Connor. (2019). Federal Court Opinion Reminds Health Care Providers to Assess the Antitrust Risks of Competitor Affiliations. Jdsupra. www.jdsupra.com/legalnews/federal-court-opinion-reminds-health-31726/.

PART I **Monopoly**

In Chapter 2, we introduced the theory of monopoly. A monopolist is a firm that is the sole provider of a good or service with few or no close substitutes. In order to maximize profits, a monopolist will raise price and sell fewer goods and services than would be the case in a competitive market, thereby harming consumers and creating social welfare loss. In Part I, we will examine monopoly in health care markets and discuss ways to mitigate its harmful effects on society.

When a firm accounts for 70–75 percent of the output in a market, the Antitrust Division of the US Department of Justice considers it a monopolist. Consumers would benefit from fewer monopolies, but unfortunately antitrust remedies do not always exist. Patents, for example, may create legal short-term monopolies. A patent grants an innovator the exclusive right to sell an innovation for 20 years from when the patent application is filed. When no close substitutes exist, the patentee will price at the monopoly level, leading to social welfare loss. But patents incentivize beneficial innovation by ensuring that innovators retain the benefits of their innovation for a limited period of time. Without patent policy, innovators could see their profits swiftly disappear as free riders copy and sell their invention without expending the same investment costs.

In Chapter 3, we discuss the procompetitive rationale for patents in the context of pharmaceutical drugs. Pharmaceutical firms often pay billions of dollars to develop life-saving drugs. Worse, a firm must invest this money before its product can even be brought to the market, leading to substantial risk. By protecting a firm's right to exclusively sell its products with a patent, public policy aims to incentivize the development of useful medications. But firms often charge extremely high prices for the drugs that they have developed when they receive a patent. In Chapter 3, we analyze the trade-off between incentivizing research and development while ensuring equitable patient access to health-improving drugs.

Monopolies are illegal, however, when they arise from a firm's efforts to limit competition in the marketplace by engaging in competitively unreasonable conduct. For example, a monopolist may violate the antitrust laws by engaging in predatory or unreasonable exclusionary practices. In order to maintain their monopolies for pharmaceutical drugs, some pioneer firms have adopted the strategy of product hopping, where a pharmaceutical firm extends its patent (and period of exclusivity) by slightly modifying a drug that is under patent protection and encouraging doctors to switch their patients to that modified drug. While the modifications to the drug are often rather minor, extended patent protection generally excludes generic firms from entering, competing, and driving prices down. To the extent that the benefits of the modification are less than the cost of reduced competition, consumers are harmed. We discuss product hopping and various remedies in Chapter 4.

In Chapter 5, we examine bundled discounts. A firm with multiple products may provide discounts to its customers based on their purchase of multiple products. In some cases, this bundled discount may exclude similarly efficient firms that produce only one product. We discuss some relevant litigation and various antitrust remedies.

In pursuit of profit maximization, monopolists invariably harm consumers and reduce social welfare. When monopolies arise due to natural or legal means, the antitrust Agencies – the Antitrust Division of the US Department of Justice and the Federal Trade Commission – cannot intervene. But Section 2 of the Sherman Act prohibits the formation or maintenance of monopolies that limit competition in the marketplace by excluding rivals and also grants victims the right to sue to recover damages.

3 Patents and Monopoly Pricing of Pharmaceuticals

3.1 INTRODUCTION

In 2019, US health care expenditures amounted to $3.8 trillion. Of this sum, prescription drug expenditures accounted for 9.7 percent, or $369.7 billion, of all health care expenditures.[1] To put this in perspective, these pharmaceutical expenditures amounted to about $1,128 for every man, woman, and child in the United States.[2] As Table 3.1 shows, these expenditures have been steadily increasing over time.

In recent years, there have been many highly visible accounts of extremely high prescription drug prices. For example, after acquiring the multiple sclerosis drug Acthar, Mallinckrodt ARD raised the price from $40 to $40,000 for a vial.[3] These accounts have raised concerns about equity, price gouging, and social conscience, and have led to demands for relief. But the high prices of prescription drugs are often imposed by legal monopolists, which have been created by patents. For our purposes, a central question is whether an antitrust remedy exists. The short answer is probably not, but there have been numerous policy proposals aimed at reining in prescription drug prices.

There is an undeniable tension between antitrust law and intellectual property (patent) law. The former seeks to promote and protect competition by limiting the formation of monopolies and cartels. The latter rewards innovators by conferring legal monopolies on their inventions. In spite of this tension, the ultimate aim of both antitrust

---

[1] Centers for Medicare & Medicaid Services (2020a).

[2] Centers for Medicare & Medicaid Services (2020b).

[3] *United Ass'n of Plumbers & Pipefitters Local 322 of S.N.J.* v. *Mallinckrodt ARD LLC,* No. 20-cv-188 (D.N.J. 2020). Mallinckrodt defended its price increase by claiming that the high value of the treatment was "the obvious reason for that price."

Table 3.1. *US expenditures on prescription drugs, 2003–2019*

Year	Amount (in billions)	Annual percentage change
2003	$176.70	–
2004	$195.60	8.90
2005	$208.60	6.60
2006	$228.10	9.40
2007	$239.30	4.90
2008	$244.30	2.10
2009	$254.30	4.10
2010	$253.40	–0.30
2011	$256.30	1.20
2012	$257.00	0.30
2013	$262.60	2.20
2014	$298.00	13.50
2015	$324.40	8.80
2016	$329.90	1.70
2017	$337.10	2.20
2018	$349.80	3.80
2019	$369.70	5.70

Source: Centers for Medicare & Medicaid Services (2020b).

and patent law is to protect and promote consumer welfare. Protecting competition promotes consumer welfare by reducing deadweight social welfare losses that result from monopolistic restrictions on output and the accompanying allocative inefficiency. Protecting monopolies that result from the production of information that qualifies for patent protection enhances social welfare by encouraging inventors and firms to allocate time, money, and other resources to research and development (R&D).

The economic rationale for patent protection flows from the fact that inventors and companies must make necessary investments before they receive any financial benefits from the discovery of new products or more efficient production processes. Patent law prevents copiers from free riding on the innovation efforts of pioneer firms.

Thus, the antitrust–patent tension involves the sacrifice of some consumer welfare in the present for enhanced consumer welfare in the future. When it comes to pharmaceuticals, many consumers complain bitterly about prescription drug prices, which the pharmaceutical companies justify by pointing to the high costs of researching and developing a new drug.

In Section 3.2, we examine the patent system and the rationale for patent protection. In Section 3.3, we examine the monopoly pricing that prescription drug patents make possible. In Section 3.4, we look at the strategy of patent licensing, whereby patent holders permit other producers to manufacture their patented drugs for a fee. We also discuss the advantages and disadvantages of compulsory licensing. Section 3.5 discusses antitrust remedies. In Section 3.6, we consider pharmaceutical price regulation in other countries and the proposals that the United States is considering to mitigate high prices. Section 3.7 includes some extensions of monopoly pricing, such as medical devices and orphan drugs. We close the chapter with some concluding remarks in Section 3.8.

3.2   THE PATENT SYSTEM

Pharmaceutical firms spend enormous sums on R&D in an effort to invent new (or improved) drugs. In 2019, the US pharmaceutical industry spent over $83 billion on R&D.[4] Whether those investments are profitable depends on several factors, including (1) whether a new molecular entity is successfully discovered, (2) the time and resources needed to win Food and Drug Administration (FDA) approval, (3) competition – albeit imperfect – from other pharmaceuticals, (4) marketing success, and (5) the length of the effective patent protection.

The risks associated with such investments are numerous. First, the R&D effort may not bear fruit. Second, the FDA may withhold approval if the potential side effects of a new drug appear to be

---

[4] Austin and Hayford (2021).

undesirable and significant. Third, a new drug may not supplant existing drugs in the market. Fourth, a new drug's success may be undermined by other drugs introduced by rival pharmaceutical producers. Finally, policymakers have proposed price regulation, which would reduce the profit pharmaceutical firms could earn. For an investment in a pharmaceutical R&D project to make economic sense, it must have a reasonable expectation of being profitable. Put differently, an investor will invest only if expected revenue exceeds expected costs. Complicating the analysis is the fact that the costs and revenues are incurred at different points in time. Thus, we examine the expected net present value (NPV) of the investment over its lifetime.

For a pharmaceutical project, there are two general types of costs that are incurred before any revenues can be realized. First, of course, are the costs incurred in the R&D process. We denote these expected costs as R_t, where t represents the year in which the cost is incurred. Assuming that a new molecular entity has been discovered, the firm will apply for a patent and begin the testing required by the FDA. The expected costs of this application and testing, which usually involve several stages, including pre-trials, clinical trials (Phases 1, 2, and 3), and FDA approval, will be identified as C_t. Both the pre-discovery and post-discovery costs must be incurred before any revenues are realized. Once sales begin, the firm will experience expected profits (or perhaps losses) for the remaining life of the patent. For simplicity, we assume that the profits on the production and distribution will be positive. We also assume that profits (Π_t) do not survive the expiration of the patent. We can write the expected NPV as follows, where Σ denotes the summation operator, i represents the discount rate, and t indicates time:

$$NPV(\Pi) = -\sum_{t=1}^{T_1} \frac{R_t}{(1+i)^t} - \sum_{t=T_1+1}^{T_2} \frac{C_t}{(1+i)^t} + \sum_{t=T_2+1}^{20+T_1} \frac{\Pi_t}{(1+i)^t}.$$

In this expression, T_1 is the number of years needed to invent the new molecular entity and $T_2 - T_1$ is the number of years spent on the patent application and FDA approval process. The remaining patent life is $20 - (T_2 - T_1)$ years since the patent clock begins as soon as the patent application is filed. In our expression, we assume that all costs are incurred and all profits are received at the end of the year. It is important to recognize that all these variables are subject to considerable uncertainty.

Inventors of new products or new production processes must invest their time, money, and other resources before – sometimes *long* before – they realize any return.[5] There are, however, other difficulties for inventors.

For example, investing in the production of information, such as R&D for pharmaceutical drugs, is a highly risky venture. There is a substantial stochastic element in the production process for drugs, and, therefore, the output will be a random variable. Many innovative efforts will produce no output at all. Others will produce some output that could turn out to be of little economic value. For example, the innovation may be scooped by other inventors, who may have filed a patent on the drug first. Some projects will produce positive profits to one degree or another. The decision to invest in such a risky venture is the result of an inventor or a firm weighing the discounted expected costs and expected benefits. If the latter outweighs the former, the people involved should make the investment.

After assessing all the uncertainties, suppose that the NPV is positive. The vast majority of the cost will be borne before any positive returns can be realized. Consequently, there must be some assurance that the flow of future profits will not be undermined by rivals who simply copy the results of the firm's R&D efforts. Preserving the incentive to invest resources in a risky venture demands a means of appropriating the economic value of the new product or production process.[6]

---

[5] This is particularly troublesome for pharmaceuticals since the prolonged FDA approval process must be tacked on to the time that the inventive process requires.

[6] Arrow (1962) explored various incentive problems surrounding investments in the production of information. A central focus of his analysis was appropriability of the information.

This is precisely the goal of the US patent system. Patents protect these future returns and thereby incentivize investment in innovation.

The US system of patent rights shields an inventor from opportunistic competition, or, in other words, simple copying or imitation. But the patent system cannot insulate the invention from all forms of competition, nor should it. If a rival invents a new product that is superior to the original, that rival is entitled to patent protection of his or her own. A rival, however, is not the only danger for inventors. Future operating profits may be undermined by a variety of other factors, including the emergence of unfortunate side effects, changes in consumer preferences or demand for the product, government regulations, or financial conditions. Consequently, the future returns to inventive effort face various degrees of uncertainty that reduce the incentive to innovate. All that our patent system can do (or should do) is limit uncertainty by outlawing patent infringement.

3.3   PATENTS AND MONOPOLY PRICING

If a pharmaceutical firm has a patent on a drug, it may charge any price that it sees fit. Nothing in the patent or antitrust laws constrains the unilateral pricing freedom of the patentee. This freedom often leads to extremely high markups over production costs. The reason for this result is the low elasticity of demand at the point where profits are maximized.[7]

By definition, a monopolist is the sole supplier of a well-specified product for which there are no close substitutes.[8] Being a monopolist, however, does not confer unlimited power over the market. In typical circumstances, a monopolist cannot *coerce*

---

[7] Elasticity refers to the quantity response to a given change in price. If the price increases by 1 percent and elicits a less than 1 percent decrease in quantity, the elasticity would be considered low, or inelastic.

[8] If an invention qualifies for patent protection, the inventor will be the sole source of that specific product, but that does not necessarily mean that there are no close substitutes. For example, Apple has a patent monopoly on the production and sale of its iPhone models. Nonetheless, Samsung's Galaxy smartphones are imperfect (but not necessarily inferior) substitutes.

consumers to pay more for its wares than the amount that they are voluntarily willing to pay. Put differently, the monopolist's ability to raise the price is limited by demand for the monopolized product. The power that a monopolist has derives from the simple fact that it is the sole source of supply. Due to the absence of competition, the monopolist can control the total quantity of its product that is offered for sale and thereby control the price. In maximizing its profit, the monopolist restricts output below the competitive level and raises the price above the competitive level. Thus, the economic concept of monopoly power is the ability to *profitably* charge prices above the competitive level and to maintain those prices for some period of time. The latter requirement necessarily implies that some barriers to entry must be present if the monopoly is to survive for very long. This is where patent rights play a vital role.

Although the patent holder must be the guardian of his or her patent rights, a patent prohibits the obvious and easiest avenue into the market: simply copying the product or the production process. Consequently, an entrant must discover another way of entering. In some cases, this may be relatively easy through reverse engineering, but in others it can be quite difficult.[9] When it is hard to invent around the patent protection, noncompetitive prices can persist as long as the patent protection lasts.

Monopoly Markups and Demand Elasticity

It is straightforward to show that markups, or the difference between price and marginal cost, are driven by the elasticity of demand. The cost of getting the pharmaceutical to market, however, does not affect the markup.[10] For a profit-maximizing monopolist, the optimal

---

[9] In some cases, pharmaceutical companies will refuse to give drug samples to generic companies, which hinders the development of generic substitutes. For example, Celgene refused to sell samples of its drug Revlimid to Mylan Pharmaceuticals (Pear 2018).

[10] The profit-maximizing price of a good is always determined by the demand and marginal cost. Consumers' willingness to pay for a good is not affected by the firm's costs. Additionally, marginal cost does not include fixed or sunk costs. Since the

output is found where marginal cost (MC) is equal to marginal revenue (MR):

$$MC = P + Q\frac{dP}{dQ}.$$

Thus, the markup is given by

$$P - MC = -\frac{P}{\eta},$$

where P represents price, Q represents quantity, and η represents the demand elasticity. As the demand becomes less elastic, that is, η becomes smaller in absolute value,[11] $P - MC$ (the markup) increases.

Very large markups result from profit maximization by a patentee in the presence of decidedly inelastic demand. Specific pharmaceutical products provide excellent examples of substantial markups due to demand inelasticity. Consider Gilead Science's hepatitis C drug, Sovaldi. Compared to rival treatments, it was much more effective and had far fewer disagreeable side effects. The treatment required the patient to take one pill per day for twelve weeks. The price per pill was $1,000, whereas the cost of production may have been about $2 per pill.[12] Thus, the markup per pill was approximately $998 above the marginal cost. This markup would be consistent with profit maximization if the demand were sufficiently inelastic.

We can find the price elasticity of demand for Sovaldi by substituting for P and MC:

$$\frac{(1{,}000 - 2)}{1{,}000} = -\frac{1}{\eta} \Rightarrow \eta = \frac{-1{,}000}{998} = -1.002.$$

initial investment in drug development is a sunk cost, it plays no role in informing the price.

[11] The markup is also related to the Lerner index of monopoly power: $\lambda = \frac{P-MC}{P} = -\frac{1}{\eta}$. See Lerner (1934) for his seminal work.

[12] Gilead did not release marginal cost data for producing a Sovaldi pill. We estimate these data for the purposes of our example (Knox 2013).

Thus, Gilead's dramatic markup, which had garnered a great deal of criticism, is consistent with profit maximization, which occurs when demand is close to being unitary elasticity (i.e., η is equal to 1) at the quantity where marginal revenue equals marginal cost. After substituting for P and MC, we find $\eta = -1.002$. Thus, the patent monopolist operates in the elastic region of the demand, but just barely.

Whenever we observe substantial markups and the corresponding economic profits that result, consumers and policymakers raise questions about the wisdom of patent protection. In the Sovaldi example, the price per pill was 500 times the marginal cost of production.[13] This extreme markup may seem excessive, but the substantial profits Gilead received provided an incentive for other firms to invest in creating a better drug or treatment that would displace Gilead. In fact, this is precisely what happened. Gilead's Sovaldi displaced an inferior treatment that Merck previously sold. In response to Gilead's success, Merck developed elbasvir and grazoprevir, which Merck sold for much less than Gilead's Sovaldi. Thus, market forces are doing their work of spurring innovation of new and improved products.

There are several reasons why the elasticity of demand tends to be low for prescription drugs. First, the consumption of prescription drugs is often not discretionary in the usual sense because they are needed for a patient's good health and to alleviate pain and suffering. Second, the patient ordinarily does not choose the prescription drug. Instead, the physician makes the choice and may be unaware of the relative price of medications to treat a specific condition. Third, there may be few, if any, substitutes for the drug in question. Even in cases where there are substitutes, the patient cannot switch medications without a new prescription from a physician. Fourth, the prevalence of health insurance coverage blunts the incentives of physicians and patients alike to fully investigate their options. When these conditions hold, it is quite possible to observe very high markups over production costs.

[13] The Massachusetts Attorney General strongly urged Gilead to reduce its price and suggested that its pricing may constitute an unfair business practice; see Pollack (2016) for a more extensive discussion.

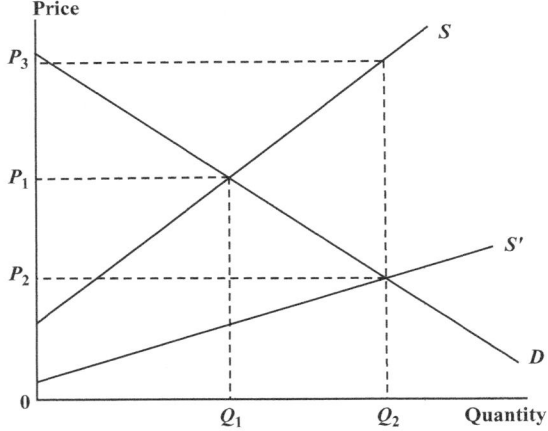

FIGURE 3.1 Distortion of quantity and pharmaceutical prices due to insurance

The Effect of Health Insurance on Drug Prices

If a health insurance policy covers a prescription drug, the policy-holder pays only a portion of the price, say, 10 percent. In that event, consumption would be larger than in the absence of insurance. This result is illustrated in Figure 3.1, where D is demand, S is supply, and S' is the perceived supply due to insurance coverage. In the absence of health insurance, the price and quantity would be P_1 and Q_1, respectively. With insurance, the perceived supply is S'. At each quantity, the height of S' is 10 percent of the height of S. Consumers will then consume Q_2 and pay P_2 out of pocket. The pharmaceutical company, however, will receive P_3 for this quantity.

Consider the following numerical example. In the absence of insurance, demand can be written as

$$P_d = 100 - 0.5Q,$$

and supply can be written as

$$P_s = 10 + Q.$$

The market equilibrium price is determined by the equality of supply and demand:

$$100 - 0.5Q = 10 + Q,$$

which yields $Q = 60$ and $P = \$70$.

With insurance, suppose that the policyholders have a 10 percent copayment. In other words, the consumer pays only 10 percent of the price on the supply curve for any quantity. The effective supply therefore shifts to

$$P_s = 1 + 0.1Q.$$

With insurance, the new price and output are determined by the equality of demand and the altered supply:

$$100 - 0.5Q = 1 + 0.1Q,$$

which yields $Q = 165$ and a policyholder price of $\$17.50$. The price actually received by the suppliers is found by substituting 165 for Q in the original supply function:[14]

$$P = 10 + Q = \$175.$$

Clearly, the presence of insurance drives up prices. Although the policyholders seem to be getting a good deal, the price increases are reflected in the insurance premiums they must pay. Additionally, those without insurance must bear the harm of paying inflated prices.

3.4 PATENT LICENSING

When a patent has been awarded on a pharmaceutical product, no one may produce, sell, or consume that product without the patentee's permission. The patentee may grant or withhold its permission as it sees fit – at least in most cases. The patentee may license its patent to

---

[14] This is an example of the moral hazard examined by Arrow (1962). Insurance distorts choices. The value of the marginal unit to the patient is now well below the social cost.

one or more rival producers for a fee. Under some circumstances, the patentee will be able to extract the full economic benefit through licensing.

Fundamentally, there are two main licensing options that will permit the patentee to extract the monopoly profit. First, the patentee could issue an unlimited use license to a single pharmaceutical producer for a lump sum. Second, the patentee could award licenses to a wide array of rival producers and charge a per unit license fee. In either case, the patentee will be able to extract the profit that is embodied in its patent.

Lump-Sum License Fee

The maximum lump-sum license fee that the patentee can charge depends on the demand for the patented product as well as the costs of production and distribution. In Figure 3.2, demand (D) and the corresponding marginal revenue (MR) are displayed along with the marginal (and average) cost of production and distribution (MC). The profit-maximizing price and output are P_1 and Q_1, respectively. The profit potential is equal to the markup, $(P_1 - MC)Q_1$.

If there are a number of equally efficient pharmaceutical producers bidding for the license, the lump-sum fee will sell at a price equal to $(P_1 - MC)Q_1$. In that event, the winning bidder will earn no more than a competitive return, as the lump-sum license fee equals the monopoly profit. Profit maximization will lead the licensee to produce at Q_1 and sell at P_1, but the surplus over the costs of production and distribution will be just enough to cover the lump-sum license fee.[15]

Per Unit License Fee

If the patentee issues per unit licenses to a large number of rival producers, it can also extract all of the monopoly profit. The optimal

---

[15] There is inherently more risk involved with lump-sum fees since a licensee must invest a substantial amount of cash before earning revenue. There is a risk that demand for the product may fall leading to negative profits. Assuming that potential buyers are risk-averse, a lump-sum fee may be lower than the total cost for per unit fees.

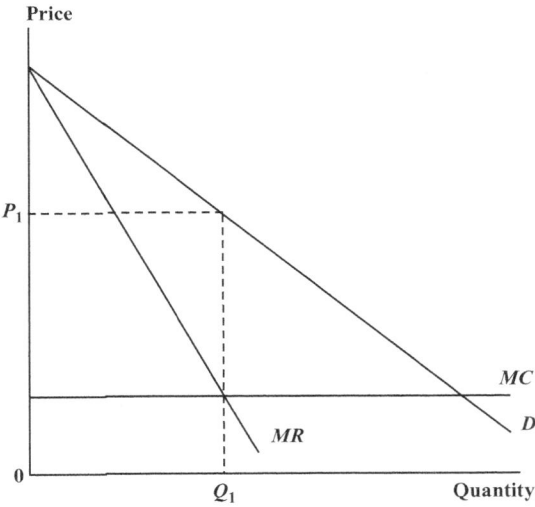

FIGURE 3.2 Licensing options for the patent monopolist

license fee will be the profit-maximizing markup, $P_1 - MC$. Each producer's per unit cost then becomes $MC + (P_1 - MC)$, which is P_1. Since the rivals are competing, the price will be P_1 and the total quantity produced will be Q_1. The total license fee will be equal to $(P_1 - MC)Q_1$, which is again equal to the monopoly profit.

Suppose that the demand for the patented drug is given by $P = 100 - 0.01Q$ and the constant marginal cost of production and distribution is $MC = 20$. The profit-maximizing quantity will then be 4,000 and the corresponding price will be $60. The profit will be $(60 - 20)(4,000) = \$160,000$. If the patentee charged a per unit license fee of $40 to a large number of licensees, the patentee would earn $160,000. A reasonable lump-sum license fee would be $160,000.

Compulsory Licensing

In some circumstances, a patentee may be forced to license its patent. If the license fee is not confiscatory, it is unclear why compulsion would be necessary. Moreover, if the license fee is not confiscatory, compulsion will not reduce pharmaceutical prices.

Under a compulsory license, a patented innovation can be used without the consent of the patent owner but with compensation in the form of a license fee. The Bayh-Dole Act of 1980 stipulated that the US government had the right to license a drug itself or issue compulsory licenses if a pharmaceutical firm was not fulfilling its objectives. Additionally, the Trade-Related Aspects of Intellectual Property Rights (TRIPS), which is an international agreement among the World Trade Organization (WTO) countries, allows countries to issue a compulsory license to produce foreign-patented drugs when there is a national medical emergency. For example, there were calls to force Gilead Sciences to license its pharmaceutical drug, Remdesivir, which had shown promising signs of treating the novel 2019 coronavirus. Since Gilead would not have had the capacity to produce all of the treatments necessary to satisfy global demand, there were questions as to whether the company should be forced to license its patent to ensure a steady global supply.[16]

Using compulsory licensing in a misguided effort to lower prices may backfire since it will reduce incentives to innovate. If a patentee employs the patent in making a product that no one else can produce due to patent protection, that patentee will be able to extract whatever monopoly profit is feasible given the market demand and its cost conditions. Assuming that the patentee maximizes its profit, the monopoly markup represents a reasonable royalty for permission to employ the patent.

If the patentee's royalty is limited to some amount below the profit-maximizing amount, the compulsory licensing will, in effect, confiscate some of the return to the patentee's inventive effort. This possibility will reduce the incentives of others to make similar investments since there is a chance that returns will be depressed.

If a reasonable royalty is paid to the patentee, it is unclear why compulsory licensing is necessary. If the patentee is not capacity

---

[16] Reuters (2020).

constrained,[17] the increased demand for its product should cause the patentee to expand its supply of the needed drug. If it is capacity constrained, the pursuit of profits should lead the patentee to contract voluntarily with a competent pharmaceutical manufacturer for the extra production. If compulsory licensing is not confiscatory, the gains are unclear. Since the license fee would be equal to the markup, the patentee should be indifferent between licensing and not licensing. To the extent that compulsory licensing makes the patentee worse off, this system will weaken the incentives to invest in inventive activity. Would-be inventors may fear confiscation through compulsory licensing and alter their investment decisions in ways that are predictable but difficult to measure. This confiscation will serve to retard progress of research into lifesaving drugs.

3.5   ANTITRUST REMEDIES

Although pharmaceutical companies are involved in many anticompetitive schemes, charging profit-maximizing prices under patent law is not one of them. Indeed, monopoly profits (for a time) are a rightful reward for innovation. Criminalizing such behavior would only lead to a society's devoting suboptimal amounts of resources to innovation. In this sense, there are no appropriate antitrust remedies. Antitrust remedies, however, play an important role in anticompetitive schemes outside of the jurisdiction of patent law, such as strategies to extend monopoly rights beyond what is due and delay generic competition.[18] We discuss these issues and relevant antitrust remedies in Chapters 4, 7, and 8.

Unlike the United States, the European Union (EU) does have laws against excessive pricing.[19] Yet, these laws are rarely invoked

---

[17] A firm is capacity constrained when it does not have the ability to expand production to satisfy an increased demand.

[18] Takeda Pharmaceutical Company allegedly exaggerated the scope of its patent to regulators and was involved in other underhanded tactics to delay generic entry (Leonard 2021).

[19] In 2016, the United Kingdom fined Pfizer Inc. and Flynn Pharma Ltd. for charging "unfairly high prices" for the anti-epilepsy drug Epanutin, whose prices increased by 2,600 percent in 2012 (Bodoni 2021).

and then only in cases deemed to have some sort of market failure. Debate still exists around the issue of what is considered an "excessive" price. In the EU, comparators are used to determine prices, although a "reasonable" rate of return is strictly contested.[20] Antitrust authorities do not have the knowledge or expertise to determine reasonable prices, nor should they since doing so falls outside of their jurisdiction. Instead, we turn to regulatory policy proposals that seek to reduce drug prices.

3.6 GOVERNMENT POLICY PROPOSALS TOWARD PRESCRIPTION DRUG PRICING

There have been a plethora of proposals from Congress that would use public policy to reduce pharmaceutical drug prices. President Joe Biden and his administration have put forward a number of proposals targeting prescription drug pricing, which echo the sentiment of a series of executive orders issued by President Donald Trump during his term.

In this section, we review several broad approaches proposed by congressional bills or mandated by presidential executive orders, including arbitrage, government negotiation, and price regulation, as well as other proposals that have received attention in the United States. People living in other developed countries pay much less, on average, for prescription drugs. Here, we also review the policies of other countries that are aimed at reducing pharmaceutical drug prices and consider whether such policies would work in the US market.[21]

Arbitrage

Due to price controls or hard bargaining by foreign governments, successful drugs sell at much lower prices in foreign markets than in the United States, where prices are usually higher than anywhere else. A 2019 report found that consumers in the United States paid 70–4,833 percent more for their prescription drugs than the average

---

[20] ABA Antitrust Section (2020).   [21] Ways and Means Committee Staff (2019).

of consumers in 11 similar countries.[22] The highest disparity occurred with Dulera, a prescription asthma medication that costs $23.95 per dose in the United States but only $0.49, on average, in other countries. Permitting arbitrage would allow US consumers to buy less expensive drugs from other countries, such as Canada. In Ontario, for example, Canadians pay only 28.4 percent of US prescription drug prices.

Arbitrage undermines efforts to price discriminate. For price discrimination to be a successful business strategy, a firm must be able to identify two or more markets with different demand elasticities, such as the United States and Canada, and prevent arbitrage.[23] The firm's marginal cost of producing drugs is the same in both markets,[24] but the demands are different.[25] Thus, the profit-maximizing price will be different in each market, and consequently the price will be higher in one market. In this example, the United States pays the higher price. Arbitrage allows drugs to flow freely between the two markets. Naturally, drugs will flow from the lower-price market to the higher-price market. Demand for drugs in Canada would increase, whereas demand for drugs in the United States would decrease. Thus, drug prices would increase in Canada but decrease in the United States. Eventually, the prices would be the same.[26] Consequently, US consumers benefit while Canadians are worse off.

The European Union's (EU) experience with arbitrage is a useful example. The EU is a union of 27 European countries with

---

[22] Ways and Means Committee Staff (2019, 3). These countries included the United Kingdom, Japan, Canada (Ontario), Australia, Portugal, France, the Netherlands, Germany, Denmark, Sweden, and Switzerland.

[23] Of course, pharmaceutical drug prices in the United States and Canada are not different just because of different demand functions, but, rather, from tight cost controls in Canada's national health insurance system.

[24] In reality, the marginal costs may be different due to transportation costs and government regulations that require specific modifications.

[25] Prices for prescription drugs are not solely determined by demand. The Canadian government has strict price controls that force pharmaceutical firms to offer lower prices to Canadian citizens.

[26] There may still be differences in prices due to transaction costs.

bureaucratic and regulatory power over the union, although members often act autonomously. Importantly, the EU functions as a free market with no barriers to trade. The policy of "community exhaustion" or "regional exhaustion" allows a good that is on the market in the EU to be resold anywhere within the EU with no restraints. Since each EU country negotiates its own prescription drug prices, drugs are moved from lower-price countries to higher-price countries. Thus, drug prices in Europe, although not the same everywhere, have converged because of arbitrage.[27] Arbitrage, however, reduces access. Because of arbitrage, firms may limit access to their drugs in lower-income countries to ensure that the drugs cannot be resold and undermine their profit margins in higher-income countries. This limit can lead to supply shortages, unaffordable prices, and marketing delays in those countries, thereby limiting lifesaving treatment for patients.[28]

The United States faces some substantial obstacles to an arbitrage proposal. First and foremost is the FDA, which is vulnerable to industry interests.[29] The FDA has warned that imported drugs may not be safe. For example, some of the drugs could be counterfeit and threaten the health and safety of US residents. Other drugs may be mishandled, for example, by being transported at room temperature when they should be refrigerated. The FDA has published a proposal with step-by-step instructions for drug importation by states that would ensure the safety of drugs. Some responsibilities of importers include screening drugs for damage and counterfeiting, checking samples from shipments at an approved FDA laboratory, and gaining FDA approval for each shipment, which would increase the costs of reselling drugs from other countries. The FDA also advocates for a simple "manufacturer to exporter to importer to patient" model, which would ensure the shortest supply chain.[30]

---

[27] Towse et al. (2015).   [28] Towse et al. (2015).   [29] Hayes and Prasad (2018).
[30] Spatz (2020).

Second, the drug manufacturers that would be reluctant to see their US profit margins shrink must also be on board. These manufacturers would have no incentive to sell drugs to Canadian exporters that would resell those drugs to the United States. These pharmaceutical companies may limit shipments to Canadian exporters in order to curtail arbitrage.[31] The drug companies could refuse to sell drugs to pharmacies above what they consider to be a reasonable demand for Canadian citizens.

Finally, Health Canada issued a warning that it would not jeopardize the supply of drugs to its citizens. Since Canada regulates its drug prices, a huge increase in demand for Canadian drugs may lead to shortages, and perhaps higher prices for exported drugs.[32] Instead, Canada recommended that the United States should implement some of its drug price initiatives, which reduced the cost of prescription drugs for Canadians.

In 2020, President Trump issued an executive order permitting the importation of drugs from other countries, specifically Canada. The order specified that this importation would not pose additional risk to public health and would require support from the FDA, drug manufacturers, and Canada.[33] Approval for importing drugs has moved slowly under the Biden administration, but six states have passed laws that would allow them to begin this process.[34] The Affordable and Safe Prescription Drug Importation Act[35] would permit the Department of Health and Human Services to import pharmaceutical drugs from Canada. After two years, imports would be considered from other countries with safety standards comparable to those of the United States.

---

[31] Harris (2003).   [32] Martell (2019).

[33] A number of US citizens who live near the Canadian border routinely buy their drugs across the border. This, however, is not a viable option for US citizens living in more southerly states. A nationwide program would require significant support from Canada.

[34] Galewitz (2021).

[35] Affordable and Safe Prescription Drug Importation Act, S.R. 920, 117th Congress (2021).

Drug importation has been a popular proposal among policy-makers, but due to the obstacles described in this section, arbitrage may not be as effective as policy analysts indicate.

Price Negotiations

In the current US system, many insurance companies and pharmacies (through pharmacy benefit managers [PBMs]) negotiate prices with drug manufacturers. In this market structure, a monopolist sells to a large group of buyers, which grants the monopolist significant bargaining power in negotiating prices with each buyer. The drug manufacturer can afford to walk away from a deal it dislikes because it knows it will not lose a large portion of the US market in doing so. Thus, buyers must accept higher prices to have access to the drug.

The US government or US health care agencies could instead negotiate directly with pharmaceutical companies for a specific quantity of drugs at a specific price. Medicare in the United States, for example, would have substantial bargaining power to negotiate better drug prices due to the large number of customers that it represents.[36] In 2019, Medicare provided health care to approximately 53 million individuals over the age of 65 and 9 million disabled individuals under age 65.[37] Prescription drug benefits are provided through Medicare Part D and were added to Medicare through the Medicare Modernization Act of 2003. In 2019, Medicare spending made up 14 percent of federal mandatory spending (almost $800 billion). Medicare Part D, which provides prescription drug benefits to 45 million Americans, accounted for over $100 billion in pharmaceutical drug spending (approximately 30 percent of all drug spending).[38]

In its noninterference clause, however, the Medicare Modernization Act of 2003 prohibited Medicare from interfering with negotiations between drug manufacturers and pharmacies or

---

[36] We discuss the economics of buyer power in Part IV.
[37] Kaiser Family Foundation (2019) and Cubanski, Neuman, and Freed (2019).
[38] Freed, Cubanski, and Neuman (2019).

insurance companies in order to promote competition.[39] This prevents a bilateral monopoly solution that would maximize social welfare.[40] Currently, a number of policy proposals in the United States, such as the Lower Cost Drugs Now Act[41] and the Medicare Drug Price Negotiation Act,[42] seek to remove the noninterference clause from the 2003 law and permit the Secretary of Health and Human Services to negotiate drug pricing for Medicare.[43] The Lower Cost Drugs Now Act also has a provision that would penalize drug manufacturers whose prices rise faster than inflation. Additionally, in the 2022 budget, President Biden called for Congress to address Medicare's ability to negotiate prescription drug prices.[44]

Both Germany and Australia have implemented successful price negotiation strategies. Germany uses a system of internal reference prices and consolidated negotiation to keep drug prices affordable. The Federal Association of Sickness Funds determines suitable reference prices for drugs within a certain class of therapeutically comparable drugs. The National Association of Statutory Health Insurance Funds, meanwhile, negotiates directly with manufacturers of drugs that prove to have a significant clinical benefit over existing drugs.[45] If initial negotiations fail, prices are determined through arbitration with the manufacturer, insurers, and a third party. Eventually, manufacturers can pull their product from the market if they are dissatisfied with the price. Drug manufacturers want high

---

[39] Medicare Prescription Drug, Improvement, and Modernization Act of 2003, H.R. 1, 108th Congress (2003).

[40] We discuss the bilateral monopoly solution in detail in Chapter 12.

[41] Elijah E. Cummings Lower Drug Costs Now Act, H.R. 3, 116th Congress (2019). This bill passed the House in December 2019.

[42] Medicare Drug Price Negotiation Act, S. 908/H.R. 2139, 117th Congress (2021). A similar bill was introduced in 2019: Medicare Negotiation and Competitive Licensing Act of 2019, H.R. 1046, 116th Congress (2019).

[43] Two other bills also permit the Secretary of HHS to negotiate prices for Medicare: Empowering Medicare Seniors to Negotiate Drug Prices Act, S. 62/H.R. 2071, 116th Congress (2019), and Consumer Health Options and Insurance Competition Enhancement (CHOICE) Act and Medicare-X Choice Act, S. 386, 117th Congress (2021).

[44] White House (2021).   [45] Morgan (2016).

prices and Germany wants low prices, but both negotiators have cards to play. Drug manufacturers can refuse to sell their drug in the German market if they do not want to take the price offered; however, they would have to forego sales in the large German market. In most cases, a price is ultimately agreed upon.

Australia similarly negotiates drug prices through their Pharmaceutical Benefit Scheme (PBS), which subsidizes pharmaceutical drug costs. The Pharmaceutical Benefits Advisory Committee determines which drugs should be reimbursable through the program and negotiates prices. The prices of non-PBS drugs are not regulated, and manufacturers set their own prices.[46] Patients, however, would need to pay the unsubsidized price.

Among other things, the US Lower Cost Drugs Now Act would amend the noninterference clause and allow price negotiation of at least 25 and up to 250 drugs in Medicare Part D. Reasonable prices would be considered on the basis of research and development costs, market data, marginal cost of production and distribution, existence of therapeutic equivalents, and international prices. Those drugs with the highest Medicare spending would be first in line. If the drug companies refused to negotiate, they could face strict penalties and large fines. The proposal is estimated to generate $345 billion in savings between 2023 and 2029.[47] The Medicare Drug Price Negotiation Act, Empowering Medicare Seniors to Negotiate Drug Prices Act, CHOICE Act, and Medicare-X Choice Act would also permit drug price negotiation by the Department of Health and Human Services.[48]

---

[46] Morgan (2016, 2–3).   [47] Cubanski, Neuman, True, et al. (2019).

[48] Commonwealth Fund (2021). The Medicare Negotiation and Competitive Licensing Act of 2019 would annul the noninterference clause and set no drug minimum or maximum price for negotiations of Part D drugs. The Secretary of Health and Human Services would determine a reasonable price based on effectiveness, consumer financial burden, therapeutic alternatives, research and development costs, and global revenue. This Act differs from the previous proposal in the way that it treats failed negotiations. Rather than imposing fines, the government would issue a license to another manufacturer (i.e., compulsory licensing) to produce a similar drug for Medicare (Cubanski Neuman, True, et al. 2019).

In these proposals, however, the bargaining power shifts to the government, which could depress pharmaceutical drug prices below the optimal, competitive level. Drug manufacturers could threaten to withdraw their drugs from the market. Between 2011 and the beginning of 2019, for example, Germany was able to successfully negotiate or arbitrate the price of 212 drugs, but 28 drugs were withdrawn from their market, 15 of which were withdrawn due to price disagreements.[49] Fining the firms that refuse to negotiate would limit the effectiveness of this bargaining threat. But these fines could further depress returns on investment, which would lead to a reduction in the number of innovative drugs.

Price Regulation

The most direct method of reducing prices is to mandate lower prices through direct government action, such as setting a maximum price for a drug. A common practice is international reference pricing (IRP),[50] where the maximum price is determined by the average price of the drug in a set of comparative countries.

In 2020, New Jersey Senator Cory Booker introduced the Prescription Drug Affordability and Access Act, which would create an independent federal agency tasked with determining appropriate drug prices and policing them.[51] The agency's pricing formula would take into account the cost of research and development for the drug, the manufacturing cost, comparable drug prices in other countries, and federal investments and grants that contributed to the development of the drug. If the manufacturer sells the drug at higher prices, the agency could grant licenses to other companies to produce the drug. This policy is quite similar to one used in Canada, the Patented Medicine Prices Review Board (PMPRB), which sets the maximum price of the drug at the median drug price of seven other countries (France, Germany, Italy,

---

[49] Greiner, Witte, and Gensorowsky (2019).

[50] This is also called external reference pricing.

[51] Prescription Drug Affordability and Access Act, S. 3166, 116th Congress (2020).

Sweden, Switzerland, the United Kingdom, and the United States)[52] or at a maximum price determined by the prices of comparable drugs in Canada.[53] If the average drug price was higher than the maximum, the drug manufacturer would need to pay fines to the government.[54]

In the United States, President Trump issued an order targeting the cost of insulin to patients with diabetes. Specifically, the 2020 order required the Secretary of Health and Human Services to ensure that Federally Qualified Health Centers (FQHCs) would make low-cost insulin available to low-income individuals or individuals with high cost sharing (i.e., high out-of-pocket costs relative to what insurance covers). For the time being, this order has been put on hold by the Biden administration.[55] In the same year, President Trump also signed an executive order for IRP or "most favored nation" pricing. Under this order, Medicare would not pay more than the lowest price paid among Organisation for Economic Co-operation and Development (OECD) countries, adjusting for differences in country gross domestic product (GDP). This executive order was stalled by a temporary court injunction and has been withdrawn by the Biden administration.[56]

Direct price regulation, however, often leads to suboptimal solutions. Pricing decisions are shifted from companies that know the average cost of their product to the government, which would be less equipped with the knowledge to set the socially optimal price. In the past, the United States has engaged in price regulation in several industries, including railroads, airlines, cable television, trucking, telephones, and electricity. This experience with price regulation has not gone well and has largely been abandoned.[57]

---

[52] Canada may remove the United States from their list due to exorbitant prices (Booker 2019).

[53] Morgan (2016).

[54] In many countries, drug price increases are capped at the inflation rate. The Elijah E. Cummings Lower Drug Costs Now Act proposes a similar policy. Elijah E. Cummings Lower Drug Costs Now Act, H.R. 3, 116th Congress (2019).

[55] Rood (2021).   [56] Cohen (2021); Church and Richardson (2021).

[57] For the complexities surrounding price regulation, see Viscusi, Harrington, and Sappington (2018).

But the United States continues to entertain price regulation proposals in prescription drug markets. For example, the Prescription Drug Price Relief Act would use international reference pricing based on the median price in Canada, France, Germany, Japan, and the United Kingdom. If drug companies failed to abide by these prices in the United States, the Department of Health and Human Services would be permitted to void patent agreements and allow generic firms to manufacture the drug.[58]

The Lower Cost Drugs Now Act would also cap prices through international reference pricing using an index of drug prices from Australia, Canada, France, Germany, Japan, and the United Kingdom. Of the six, only the United Kingdom does not have an IRP system.[59] Fortunately, these countries do not solely rely on international prices to determine their own prices; thus, the policy does not require constant adjustments. The IRP policy in these countries has been quite successful and may have contributed to an 11.5 percent mean reduction in the price of some drugs, according to a 2012 review study.[60]

IRP connects different drug markets around the world. Thus, drug manufacturers must consider how a negotiated price in one country will affect the prices they can charge in other countries. Although imposing no welfare loss on the country that imposes the policy, this may cause externalities for countries that are included in the reference list. For example, it may make more sense for a drug company to forego sales in, say, Germany, which is included in pricing decisions in at least 13 countries, than to allow a cheaper price in Germany to reduce prices across multiple other countries. Additionally, the introduction of drugs may be delayed in lower-income countries that are included in reference lists. One study estimated that the elimination of IRP policies would bring drugs to market 14 months earlier in Eastern Europe.[61] If the United States were to adopt an IRP policy, drug companies may demand higher drug

[58] Prescription Drug Price Relief Act, S. 909/H.R. 2148, 117th Congress (2021).
[59] Capretta (2019).   [60] Lee et al. (2012).   [61] Maini and Pammolli (2017).

prices or increase delays in the countries that would determine the US drug prices.

Other Proposals

There have been a variety of other proposals designed to reduce prescription drug pricing through other mechanisms. Specifically, there are several bills that would increase the price transparency of prescription drugs. The FAIR Drug Pricing Act[62] would require pharmaceutical drug manufacturers to report and justify increases in prescription drug prices for specific drugs, namely, drugs that cost more than $100 and where a price increase amounts to 10 percent over one year or 25 percent over three years. Although this proposal does not impose consequences on drug manufacturers for price increases, it would provide public information and increase drug pricing transparency. Other proposals would limit the power of pharmacy benefit managers (PBMs), who act as intermediaries between drug manufacturers and health insurers (we discuss PBMs in more detail in Chapter 9). For example, the Lower Costs, More Cures Act contains a provision that would limit PBM spread pricing, or the difference between the payment the PBM receives and the pharmacy reimbursement it pays. The Lower Cost Drugs Now Act, Prescription Drug Pricing Reduction Act,[63] and Lower Costs, More Cures Act also include proposals to reduce drug prices through greater information and pricing transparency.

In 2018, former President Trump signed the Patient Right to Know Drug Prices Act into law. While 28 states had previous policies in place, this law formally eliminates gag clauses, or contractual requirements between insurers and pharmacies prohibiting pharmacists from informing consumers about the least expensive way to purchase a prescription drug – with insurance or out of pocket.[64]

---

[62] Fair Accountability and Innovative Research (FAIR) Drug Pricing Act, S. 898, 177th Congress (2021).

[63] Prescription Drug Pricing Reduction Act of 2020, S. 2543, 116th Congress (2019).

[64] Patient Right to Know Drug Prices Act, S.B. 2554, 115th Congress (2018).

Finally, some proposals seek to increase the rate of generic entry into prescription drug markets, which would increase competition and thereby reduce prices. Both the Lower Costs, More Cures Act and the Protecting Consumer Access to Generic Drugs Act[65] would prohibit pay-for-delay agreements, where a drug manufacturer compensates a generic producer to delay entry (we discuss this issue in Chapter 8). Failure to comply could result in civil action and possible penalties against the manufacturer by the Federal Trade Commission.

The Price–Access Trade-Off

Higher drug prices pay for innovation. As mentioned in Section 3.2, pharmaceutical firms decide to innovate based on the net future revenues they can expect. Price regulation decreases the expected future revenues and will disincentivize research and development of new drugs. A study estimated that lower pharmaceutical prices in the EU compared to the United States from 1986 to 2004 cost the EU 46 fewer new medications and reduced research and development spending growth. Whereas US research and development spending grew by 8.8 percent, EU spending growth was only 5.4 percent.[66]

In contrast to other countries, new drugs come to the US market almost immediately since the United States is one of the most lucrative markets for drug manufacturers. Drug companies may delay entry of their drugs in other countries due to arbitrage and international reference pricing. Additionally, negotiations can be lengthy and further delay entry. For example, about 96 percent of cancer drugs launched between 2011 and 2018 were available in the United States in 2019, compared to only 71 percent in the United Kingdom and only 59 percent in Japan. Additionally, the United States receives drugs on average within two months from a drug's launch, whereas the United Kingdom receives drugs after 12 months and Japan after 21 months.[67]

---

[65] Protecting Consumer Access to Generic Drugs Act, H.R. 153, 117th Congress (2021).
[66] Golec and Vernon (2006).   [67] PhRMA (2020).

However, citizens in the latter countries often pay much lower prices for prescription drugs. Thus, the decision to regulate prices is one of balancing the trade-off between affordable care for many consumers versus increased innovation and access to novel drugs for a few consumers. The goals of price regulation have merit: lower costs for consumers, private insurance, and government-sponsored insurance (e.g., Medicare and Medicaid). But as Milton Friedman noted, "there is no such thing as a free lunch." Price regulation will necessarily decrease the potential gains from innovation. Such a change could result in some unintended consequences for innovation and drug development. Unfortunately, it is difficult to predict where and how large those unintended consequences would be.

3.7 EXTENSIONS: MEDICAL DEVICES AND ORPHAN DRUGS

The economic analysis presented in this chapter is not confined to pharmaceutical drugs. Medical devices are often covered by one or more patents that permit substantial markups. In addition, the FDA bestows monopoly power on pharmaceutical firms for so-called orphan drugs. We examine these briefly in turn.

Medical Devices

A wide assortment of medical devices is employed in diagnosing illnesses and treating patients. In some cases, there is enough competition to keep prices in check. In others, however, there may be little to no competition, and prices will be at or near monopoly levels. Artificial knees and hips provide a good example. There are five major manufacturers of these artificial joints, so one would expect some amount of competition.[68] All of the devices provide the same function, but each does so in somewhat different ways. The surgical procedure varies by

---

[68] There are five major producers of artificial joints, with a number of smaller firms. These major producers include Zimmer, DePuy, Stryker, Smith & Nephew, and Biomet (Rosenthal 2013).

brand to some extent, so orthopedic surgeons tend to train with one brand and stick with it. As a result, competition takes place at the point when the surgeon selects the brand that he or she intends to use for joint replacement recipients. The manufacturers compete for the surgeon's favor by offering a variety of inducements: technical support, assistance in operating rooms, and financial incentives of one sort or another. While many marketing efforts are legitimate, financial incentives may be seen as unlawful kickbacks. If so, they are treated unfavorably. For example, in 2007, Zimmer, DePuy, Smith & Nephew, and Biomet were fined millions of dollars for paying surgeons "consulting fees" to use their artificial joint products.[69]

Once the surgeons have selected a brand, the market is divided among the various artificial joint producers based on the surgeons' preferences. Consequently, each manufacturer has a monopoly and can price accordingly, with patient ignorance and insurance serving to inflate the cost of the devices. Patients of artificial joint surgery select their surgeon and in doing so select a brand, but most patients will be totally unaware of the brand the surgeon is selecting. In this situation, the surgeon acts like a doctor who is prescribing medication. Additionally, insurance policies generally pay a substantial fraction of the cost of the surgery, which further erodes the patient's sensitivity to the list price of the device.

The artificial joint is an input in the surgical procedure; therefore, the demand for the artificial joint is derived from the demand for the operation. Given this derived demand, the manufacturer can charge a monopoly price free from the worry of competing devices. The demand for the artificial joint is apt to be very inelastic, which permits substantial markups. The Lerner Index of monopoly power is $\lambda = \frac{-1}{\eta}$, that is, the negative inverse of the elasticity of demand. If the elasticity of demand is 1.05 at the profit-maximizing price, the price will be 20 times the competitive price. The patients suffer the higher

---

[69] Stryker, another major manufacturer of artificial joints, cooperated with the investigation and was not fined. See Tanne (2007) for more information.

costs while the surgeons profit from the manufacturer inducements with no real incentive for change.

In some instances, a hospital buys an expensive piece of equipment that requires continuing purchases of supplies. The market for these supplies is referred to as an "aftermarket" since it follows the initial equipment purchase. This situation creates some interesting pricing decisions. To see this, we will examine the case of the CARTO 3, a heart arrhythmia machine that has a price tag of $400,000–$500,000.[70]

Biosense, which manufactures the CARTO 3, also sells the complementary catheters for $1,000–$2,000. The manufacturer has an interesting pricing problem. The hospital knows that once it purchases the CARTO 3, it will be locked into buying catheters from Biosense; therefore, the hospital will expect to pay monopoly prices for the catheters. This recognition influences the purchase decision. Biosense must necessarily lower the price of the CARTO 3 below the level that it could charge if it could credibly commit to charging a competitive price for the catheters. Having gotten a "bargain" price on the original machine, hospitals have an incentive to reduce the price they pay for the catheters.[71] There is an incentive for the hospital to buy refurbished, or reprocessed, catheters instead of brand-new catheters. In order to protect its profits, Biosense induced the hospitals to buy new catheters by refusing to offer clinical support to hospitals that used refurbished catheters.[72] This behavior resulted in a class action suit against Biosense.[73]

Orphan Drugs

Any disease that affects fewer than 200,000 people in the United States is considered to be rare. Since the market is relatively small,

---

[70] Leonard (2020).

[71] For a discussion of this market structure in the printer market, see Kobayashi (2008).

[72] For more information about the complexities of durable good markets, see Blair and Herndon (1996).

[73] *Innovative Health LLC* v. *Biosense Webster Inc.*, No. 19-cv-1984 (C. D. Cal. 2020).

the pharmaceutical industry may neglect to research and develop treatments, or even produce the lifesaving drugs that have already been developed as treatments. Pharmaceutical drugs that treat these relatively rare conditions are therefore known as orphan drugs. With the threat of competition and a lack of economies of scale, it can be risky and possibly unprofitable for a pharmaceutical firm to research and produce these drugs. This disincentive presents a problem for those people who require such medications, so Congress passed the Orphan Drug Act in 1983. The Act incentivizes pharmaceutical firms to research treatments with orphan drugs by allowing the FDA to grant seven-year monopolies for orphan drugs that can extend past a drug's patent. Additionally, there are tax incentives; firms that research orphan drugs get a 50 percent tax credit on the clinical research for that drug. Allowing firms to earn profits above the normal economic return would incentivize production and ensure a steady supply of the orphan drug. To some extent, this legislation was a success. Since 1983, the FDA has approved about 900 orphan drug applications.[74]

However, this legislation has also led to abuse of the system. For example, many orphan drugs are quite commonly prescribed. Due to the many incentives that the orphan label grants, many pharmaceutical firms apply for orphan drug status by claiming that their drug is used to treat a rare disease. After approval, the drug is prescribed for many off-label uses.[75] For example, Rituxan (rituximab) received orphan drug status for treating follicular non-Hodgkin's lymphoma. Yet, it is one of the top 10–selling drugs used for treatment of rheumatoid arthritis in the United States, with 2018 sales of $6.75 billion.[76]

Additionally, prices of orphan drugs are much higher than the prices of non-orphan drugs due to their monopoly status. In 2018, the

---

[74] US Food and Drug Administration (n.d.).

[75] Doctors have the authority to prescribe any drug to their patients for off-label use. The government assumes that doctors have the expertise to know what is best for their individual patients. This rule is often abused by pharmaceutical firms, which often market the off-label uses of their drug to physicians.

[76] Philippidis (2019).

median annual price for the top 100 orphan drugs was $109,723, whereas the median annual price for the top 100 non-orphan drugs was $15,702.[77] For example, once Marathon Pharmaceuticals received orphan drug status for its drug Emflaza (deflazacort), which is used to treat muscular dystrophy, the price jumped from $1,000 a year to $89,000 a year.[78] Even though continued production of the drug is assured, the high prices may preclude patients from getting the drugs that they need.

The FDA could impose two simple rules that would curb the worst of these abuses. First, the FDA could crack down on supposed orphan drugs before a certification is granted by (1) requiring disclosure of all potential uses of the drugs and (2) forcing companies to admit whether a rare disease is a subset of a more common disease. Second, the FDA could remove monopoly status for any orphan drug that was used to treat more than 200,000 patients, including off-label uses. These rules would limit the ability of pharmaceutical firms to gain orphan drug status for drugs that are not truly orphans.

3.8 CONCLUDING REMARKS

Health care costs generally and pharmaceutical drugs specifically have been increasing at staggering rates. In this chapter, we saw that pharmaceutical prices are substantially higher than the production costs due to the legal exercise of monopoly power. In Chapters 4 and 5, we will examine elevated prices that are more amenable to antitrust enforcement.

Our system of intellectual property law creates legal monopolies, but not necessarily economic monopolies. When the demand for the product or process is considerable, intellectual property rights are substantial; the economic monopoly results in supra-competitive prices and supra-competitive profits for the intellectual property rights owners. These noncompetitive outcomes have adverse consequences for social welfare in a static sense. At the same time, the lure

---

[77] Pomeranz (2019).   [78] Schenker (2017).

of economic profits provides inventors and firms with an incentive to invest in the innovation efforts that provide products, processes, and other creations that would not otherwise exist.

In the absence of overt collusion or unlawful attempts to monopolize health care markets, no clear antitrust remedy exists. In some cases, the United States might consider revising its patent system. Such changes are risky, however, because they may reduce innovative incentives and product availability. Regulation, which is the norm in many – if not all – developed countries, is a trade-off between innovation and access. Thus, the problem of soaring health care costs is very real, but an ideal solution is unlikely to be found in US antitrust enforcement or by implementing simple modifications to the existing intellectual property regime.

REFERENCES

ABA Antitrust Section. (2020). *Rising Drug Prices: Is Antitrust the Cure?* Committee Program Audio. June 22. www.americanbar.org/groups/antitrust_law/committees/committee_program_audio/june2020/062220-rising/.

Arrow, Kenneth J. (1962). Economic Welfare and the Allocation of Resources for Invention. In National Bureau of Economic Research, ed., *The Rate and Direction of Inventive Activity: Economic and Social Factors.* Princeton, NJ: Princeton University Press, 609–626.

Austin, David, and Tamara Hayford. (2021). *Research and Development in the Pharmaceutical Industry.* Congressional Budget Office. www.cbo.gov/system/files/2021-04/57025-Rx-RnD.pdf.

Blair, Roger D., and Jill Boylston Herndon. (1996). Restraints of Trade by Durable Good Producers. *Review of Industrial Organization* 11: 339–353.

Bodoni, Stephanie. (2021). *Pfizer, Flynn Pharma Face UK Antitrust Charges Over Price Jump.* Bloomberg Law. www.bloomberg.com/news/articles/2021-08-05/pfizer-flynn-accused-of-abusing-position-in-drug-pricing-probe.

Booker, Cory. (2019). *Booker Unveils Groundbreaking Bill Establishing National Drug Pricing Agency to Lower Costs, Increase Access.* Cory Booker Press Release. www.booker.senate.gov/news/press/booker-unveils-groundbreaking-bill-establishing-national-drug-pricing-agency-to-lower-costs-increase-access.

Capretta, James C. (2019). *A Closer Look at International Reference Pricing for Prescription Drugs.* Real Clear Policy. www.realclearpolicy.com/articles/2019/

03/29/a_closer_look_at_international_reference_pricing_for_prescription_drugs_ 111142.html.

Centers for Medicare & Medicaid Services. (2020a). *NHE Fact Sheet*. www.cms.gov/ Research-Statistics-Data-and-Systems/Statistics-Trends-and-Reports/National HealthExpendData/NHE-Fact-Sheet.

Centers for Medicare & Medicaid Services. (2020b). *NHE Tables, Table 2: National Health Expenditures; Aggregate, Annual Percent Change, Percent Distribution and per Capita Amounts, by Type of Expenditure*. www.cms.gov/files/zip/nhe-tables.zip.

Church, Richard P., and Leah D. Richardson. (2021). CMS Proposes to Rescind Most Favored Nation Drug Pricing Rule. *National Law Review* XI. No. 222. www.natlawreview.com/article/cms-proposes-to-rescind-most-favored-nation-drug-pricing-rule.

Cohen, Joshua. (2021). Court Injunction Temporarily Upends Most Favored Nation Policy to Lower Prices of Medicare Part B Drugs. *Forbes*. www.forbes.com/sites/ joshuacohen/2021/01/02/court-injunction-temporarily-upends-most-favored-nation-policy-to-lower-prices-of-medicare-part-b-drugs/amp/.

Commonwealth Fund. (2021). *Key Provisions of Drug Pricing Proposals*. Commonwealth Fund. www.commonwealthfund.org/publications/2021/apr/ key-provisions-drug-pricing-proposals.

Cubanski, Juliette, Tricia Neuman, and Meredith Freed. (2019). *The Facts on Medicare Spending and Financing*. Kaiser Family Foundation. www.kff.org/ medicare/issue-brief/the-facts-on-medicare-spending-and-financing/.

Cubanski, Juliette, Tricia Neuman, Sarah True, and Meredith Freed. (2019). *What's the Latest on Medicare Drug Price Negotiations?* Kaiser Family Foundation. www.kff .org/medicare/issue-brief/whats-the-latest-on-medicare-drug-price-negotiations/.

Freed, Meredith, Juliette Cubanski, and Tricia Neuman. (2019). *A Look at Recent Proposals to Control Drug Spending by Medicare and Its Beneficiaries*. Kaiser Family Foundation. www.kff.org/medicare/issue-brief/a-look-at-recent-pro posals-to-control-drug-spending-by-medicare-and-its-beneficiaries/.

Galewitz, Phil. (2021). *Biden Administration Signals It's in No Rush to Allow Canadian Drug Imports*. KHN. https://khn.org/news/article/biden-administra tion-signals-its-in-no-rush-to-allow-canadian-drug-imports/.

Golec, Joseph H., and John A. Vernon. (2006). European Pharmaceutical Price Regulation, Firm Profitability and R&D Spending. NBER Working Paper 12676. www.nber.org/papers/w12676.pdf.

Greiner, Wolfgang, Julian Witte, and Daniel Gensorowsky. (2019). *Beiträge zur Gesundheitsökonomie und Versorgungsforschung (Band 29)*. AMNOG Report 2019. www.dak.de/dak/download/amnog-report-2019-pdf-2099700.pdf.

Harris, Gardiner. (2003). Canada Fills US Prescriptions under the Counter. *New York Times*. www.nytimes.com/2003/06/04/business/canada-fills-us-prescrip tions-under-the-counter.html.

Hayes, Michael J., and Vinay Prasad. (2018). Financial Conflicts of Interest at FDA Drug Advisory Committee Meetings. *The Hastings Center Report* 48: 10–13.

Kaiser Family Foundation. (2019). *An Overview of Medicare*. Kaiser Family Foundation. www.kff.org/medicare/issue-brief/an-overview-of-medicare/.

Knox, Richard. (2013). *$1,000 Pill for Hepatitis C Spurs Debate over Drug Prices*, NPR. www.npr.org/transcripts/256885858.

Kobayashi, Bruce. (2008). Spilled Ink or Economic Progress? The Supreme Court's Decision in Illinois Tool Works v. Independent Ink. *Antitrust Bulletin* 53: 5–33.

Lee, Joy Li-Yueh, Michael A. Fischer, William H. Shrank, et al. (2012). A Systematic Review of Reference Pricing: Implications for US Prescription Drug Spending. *American Journal of Managed Care* 18: 429–437.

Leonard, Mike. (2020). *J&J Unit Assails Antitrust Analysis in Cardiac Catheter Case*. Bloomberg Law. https://news.bloomberglaw.com/tech-and-telecom-law/ j-j-unit-assails-antitrust-analysis-in-cardiac-catheter-case.

Leonard, Mike. (2021). *Takeda Loses Antitrust Appeal over Diabetes Drug Patent Listing*. Bloomberg Law. https://news.bloombergtax.com/ip-law/takeda-loses-antitrust-appeal-over-diabetes-drug-patent-listing.

Lerner, Abba. (1934) The Concept of Monopoly and the Measurement of Monopoly Power. *Review of Economic Studies* 1: 157–175.

Maini, Luca, and Fabio Pammolli. (2017). Reference Pricing as a Deterrent to Entry: Evidence from the European Pharmaceutical Market. Working paper. https:// scholar.harvard.edu/files/lucamaini/files/reference_pricing_as_a_deterrent_to_ entry.pdf.

Martell, Allison. (2019). *Exclusive: Canada Warns US against Drug Import Plans, Citing Shortage Concerns*. Reuters. www.reuters.com/article/us-canada-pharmaceuticals-exports-exclus/exclusive-canada-warns-us-against-drug-import-plans-citing-shortage-concerns-idUSKCN1UD2LN.

Morgan, Steven. (2016). *Pharmaceutical Pricing Policies in 10 Countries*, Working Papers for the 2016 Meeting of the Vancouver Group. www .commonwealthfund.org/sites/default/files/2018-09/Steven%20Morgan% 2C %20PhD_Ten%20Country%20Pharma%20Policy%20Summaries_2016%20 Vancouver%20Group%20Meeting.pdf.

Pear, Robert. (2018). Drug Company "Shenanigans" to Block Generics Come under Federal Scrutiny. *New York Times*. www.nytimes.com/2018/04/14/us/politics/ drug-companies-gener.html.

Philippidis, Alex. (2019). *Top 15 Best-Selling Drugs of 2018*. Genengnews. www .genengnews.com/a-lists/top-15-best-selling-drugs-of-2018/.

PhRMA. (2020). *The United States vs. Other Countries: Availability of Cancer Medicines Varies*. www.phrma.org/resource-center/Topics/Medicare/The-United-States-vs-Other-Countries-Availability-of-Cancer-Medicines-Varies.

Pollack, Andrew. (2016). Gilead Faces Fights over Hepatitis C and H.I.V. Drugs. *New York Times*. www.nytimes.com/2016/01/28/business/gilead-faces-fights-over-hepatitis-c-and-hiv-drugshtml.

Pomeranz, Karen. (2019). *EvaluatePharma Orphan Drug Report 2019*. Evaluate. https://info.evaluate.com/rs/607-YGS-364/images/EvaluatePharma%20Orphan %20Drug%20Report%202019.pdf.

Reuters. (2020). *Who Can Make Gilead's Coronavirus Drug, Licence Free?* Reuters. www.reuters.com/article/us-health-coronavirus-gilead-sciences-ex/who-can-make-gileads-coronavirus-drug-licence-free-idUSKBN22I1GP.

Rood, Lee. (2021). Fact Check: Biden Administration Delays Implementation of Trump Rule on Insulin, EpiPens. *USA Today*. www.usatoday.com/story/news/ factcheck/2021/01/30/fact-check-biden-freezes-rule-health-center-insulin-epi pen-prices/4254921001/.

Rosenthal, Elizabeth. (2013). In Need of a New Hip, but Priced out of the US Market. *New York Times*. www.nytimes.com/2013/08/04/health/for-medical-tourists-simple-math.html.

Schenker, Lisa. (2017). FDA Approves Northbrook Company's $89,000 Muscular Dystrophy Drug. *Chicago Tribune*. www.chicagotribune.com/business/ct-mus cular-dystrophy-drug-fda-approval-0210-biz-20170209-story.html.

Spatz, Ian D. (2020). *FDA Calls States' Bluffs on Drug Importation*. Statnews. www .statnews.com/2020/02/18/fda-calls-states-bluffs-on-drug-importation/.

Tanne, Janice Hopkins. (2007). US Makers of Joint Replacements Are Fined for Paying Surgeons to Use Their Devices. *British Medical Journal* 335: 1065.

Towse, Adrian, Michele Pistollato, Jorge Mestre-Ferrandiz, et al. (2015). European Union Pharmaceutical Markets: A Case for Differential Pricing? *International Journal of the Economics of Business* 22: 263–275.

US Food and Drug Administration. (2019). *The United States vs. Other Countries: Availability of Cancer Medicines Varies*. PhRMA. www.phrma.org/-/media/ Project/PhRMA/PhRMA-Org/PhRMA-Org/PDF/G-I/IPI-Model—Comparison-of-Cancer-Medicine-Availability—012819.pdf.

US Food and Drug Administration. (n.d.). Search Orphan Drug Designations and Approvals. www.accessdata.fda.gov/scripts/opdlisting/oopd/index.cfm.

Viscusi, W. Kip, Joseph E. Harrington, and David E. M. Sappington. (2018). *Economics of Regulation and Antitrust*. 5th ed. Boston: MIT Press.

Ways and Means Committee Staff. (2019). A Painful Pill to Swallow: US vs. International Prescription Drug Prices. https://waysandmeans.house.gov/sites/democrats.waysandmeans.house.gov/files/documents/U.S.%20vs.%20International%20Prescription%20Drug%20Prices_0.pdf.

White House. (2021). Budget of the United States Government: Fiscal Year 2022. www.whitehouse.gov/wp-content/uploads/2021/05/budget_fy22.pdf.

4   Patents and Exclusionary Product Hopping

4.1   INTRODUCTION

Ever on the lookout for a way to extend a patent monopoly and thereby earn monopoly profits, some prescription drug manufacturers have hit on a strategy known as *product hopping*. The initial patent on a prescription drug covers the active ingredient that is delivered in a specific form and dosage with a specific absorption rate. A simple modification to the prescribed drug can lead to a new patent and a continued stream of monopoly profits. Therefore, during the life of the first patent, which is 20 years from when the company filed the patent application, the patentee may develop a modified version of the prescription drug by (1) altering the dose to improve efficacy, (2) changing the absorption rate, or (3) switching the medication form, such as from tablets to capsules. Often, the manufacturer encourages physicians to prescribe a modified version of the drug instead of the original pioneer drug. To the extent that the newer version confers real therapeutic benefits, this practice may be unobjectionable. Product hopping may be anticompetitive, however, if the benefits to the patient from innovation are not greater than the harm to patients resulting from the delay in production of generic versions from competing drug manufacturers.

In some instances, a patentee may combine product hopping with conduct that prevents generic substitution. We will use the term *exclusionary product hopping* to describe product hopping that forecloses competition from generic substitutes. Arguably, this practice may be vulnerable to antitrust prosecution. But effectively distinguishing between general product hopping and exclusionary product hopping may be challenging. Exclusionary product hopping is a business practice that forces patients to switch from a prescription drug with an expiring patent to a newer version of the drug with a new patent. In this way, competition from generic equivalents is forestalled and monopoly profits continue to accrue. When product hopping works, it can mean hundreds of millions of dollars in economic profits for the pioneer firm. These profits come at the expense of patients, their insurers, and society.

When modified versions of pioneer drugs confer substantial benefits on patients due to improved safety and efficacy, these advances deserve patent protection. When a drug is switched from a capsule to a tablet simply to extend patent protection, the pioneer firm seems to be gaming the patent system. This conduct may be objectionable on social welfare grounds, but it may not violate Section 2 of the Sherman Act.

In Section 4.2, we spell out a few examples of product hopping to illustrate how this practice works and discuss the benefits to the patentee and the costs to patients and society. In Section 4.3, we review two legal challenges and an additional example of potential product hopping to illustrate the complexity of public policy. We then examine the possibility of antitrust remedies in Section 4.4. We close with some concluding observations in Section 4.5.

4.2 EXCLUSIONARY PRODUCT HOPPING

When the patent on a pioneer drug expires, generic equivalents can enter the market and compete with the pioneer drug. In most cases, the generic producers do little marketing. They simply make their products available. Pharmacies are able to supply patients with the generic drugs under state generic substitution laws that authorize, or even mandate, such substitution. Under these laws, the generic versions of the pioneer drug must be therapeutically equivalent.

State substitution laws were enacted in an effort to encourage the use of generic substitutes and thereby reduce costs to patients. Since all generic formulations would necessarily be therapeutically equivalent, they are all reasonable substitutes for the pioneer drug.

Consequently, no generic producer can engage in meaningful marketing of its particular version. To the extent that generic producers must rely on state substitution laws for sales, exclusionary product hopping thwarts legislative intent. Generic producers' reliance on the state substitution laws has been characterized in the literature as free riding on the developmental and promotional efforts of the pioneer drug.[1] But that has no bearing on whether a prescription drug manufacturer decides to engage in product hopping. After all, the patentee does enjoy a legally protected monopoly for the life of the patent, which should be a just reward for the patentee's efforts to develop and market the drug.

Therapeutic equivalence means a prescription drug must meet four criteria. First, of course, the active ingredient must be identical. This is necessary but not sufficient. Second, the dosage must be the same for the generic and the pioneer. If the pioneer brand drug is prescribed in 20 mg doses, the generic cannot be 15 mg or 25 mg; it must be 20 mg. Third, the absorption rate must be the same. If the pioneer drug is taken twice per day, the generic cannot be prescribed in three per day or one per day versions. Fourth, the form of the drug – tablet, capsule, powder, liquid – must be the same for both the pioneer drug and the generic. If there is any deviation between the generic and the pioneer drug, pharmacists will be unable to substitute the generic without a change in the prescription. Forbidding even the slightest deviation is the key to exclusionary product hopping.

The benefits of product hopping for the manufacturer are fairly obvious. Shortly after the patent's expiration, the pioneer firm will face substantial generic competition and the accompanying drop in profits.[2]

---

[1] Cheng (2008).

[2] Pioneer firms may also face generic entry in a different form. Generic firms may obtain a "skinny label," where the generic receives FDA approval for a nonpatented use. In other words, generic firms obtain FDA approval of a branded drug without any of the patented exclusive uses that the branded firm holds. Branded firms argue that this effectively ends their exclusivity with generics on the market, even if intended for different uses, whereas generic firms argue that the drug is distinct because it is marketed for nonoverlapping uses (Lopez 2021).

By replacing tablets with capsules or by altering the absorption rate, the pioneer firm may acquire a new patent and thereby extend its monopoly for another 20 years.[3] Unless its drug is displaced by another pioneer firm's product, the original producer will enjoy economic profits for the life of the new patent. Since the present value of these economic profits may amount to hundreds of millions of dollars, the incentive to engage in product hopping seems irresistible. Unfortunately, the costs of product hopping fall on patients who consume the prescription drugs, health insurers, and society at large.

In order to forestall the loss in profits from patent expiration, the pioneer firm may introduce a modified version of the original drug. If it discontinues production of the original drug before the patent expiration, physicians will be forced to switch their patients to the modified version because no generic substitute would be available at the time. This practice is called exclusionary product hopping,[4] and it is aimed at forestalling generic competition and extending the pioneer producer's monopoly.

The experience with the prescription drug Suboxone by Indivior provides a useful example.[5] Suboxone is a medication used to treat patients with opioid use disorder. It contains both buprenorphine, which treats the opioid dependence, and naloxone, which prevents abuse of the buprenorphine itself.[6] In 2002, Indivior received the exclusive right to sell Suboxone for seven years under orphan drug laws. At the end of that period, generic entry threatened to erode Indivior's $700 million profits, and Indivior took action. In 2010, it

---

[3] This investment may be large in absolute terms but modest relative to the sales volume of the pioneer drug.

[4] Once a patient has been switched to the new version of the pioneer drug, doctors may be reluctant to switch their patients to a generic version of the original pioneer drug.

[5] *Federal Trade Commission* v. *Indivior Inc.*, No. 1:20-cv-00036-JPJ-PMS (W.D. Vir. 2020).

[6] Naloxone is used broadly as an opioid antagonist, that is, a medication that can reverse the effects of an opioid overdose. In the case of Suboxone, if an individual were to intentionally misuse the Suboxone (e.g., snort or inject), the naloxone would protect against abuse by triggering immediate withdrawal symptoms.

introduced Suboxone Film, which was similar to the Suboxone tablets in all respects except for the delivery method.

Once Suboxone Film entered the market, Indivior raised the price of Suboxone tablets to induce patients to switch to Film, even though the cost of producing Film was higher. It later discontinued the tablets due to supposed safety concerns. Indivior claimed that the tablets were not tamper-safe for children, even though the FDA had already dismissed the claim and even indicated that Suboxone Film may be more likely to harm children. Indivior also submitted a citizen petition to the FDA with the goal of delaying generic abbreviated new drug applications (ANDAs). By switching to a new product, Indivior likely hoped to delay generic entry for Suboxone in order to maintain monopoly profits. In 2020, the FTC filed suit against Indivior for anticompetitive conduct, and later that year the FTC and Indivior reached a settlement agreement.

Exclusionary product hopping has not been confined to Suboxone.[7] Table 4.1 summarizes various product-hopping lawsuits.

4.3 LEGAL CHALLENGES TO PRODUCT HOPPING

There have been several legal challenges to product hopping, two of which have resulted in circuit court opinions. The first, in 2015, involved Namenda, which is used to treat patients with Alzheimer's disease. The second, in 2016, involved Doryx, which is used to treat acne. The diverging verdicts have created a split in the circuit courts that as of 2022 has not been resolved by the Supreme Court. The public policy dilemma created by what may amount to exclusionary product hopping can be appreciated more fully by examining the opinions in the Namenda and the Doryx cases. In each case, we

---

[7] For a recent example, see *King Drug Co. of Florence Inc.* v. *Abbott Labs*, No. 19-cv-3565 (E.D. Pa. 2019). According to the complaint, various tactics were employed to head off entry of a generic version of AndroGel. Allegedly, the purpose of the stall was to allow Abbott Laboratories to obtain a patent on a new version of AndroGel. The original product had a 1.0 percent solution, whereas the new and improved version had a 1.62 percent solution.

Table 4.1. *Product hopping litigation*

Case	Year	Drug	Purpose	Outcome
Abbot Laboratories v. Teva Pharmaceuticals	2006	Tricor	Lowers triglycerides, which may cause heart disease	Abbot Laboratories settled the case for $184 million.
Walgreen Co. v. Astrazeneca Pharmaceuticals	2008	Nexium	Stomach acid	The Court rejected a finding of product hopping.
In re Suboxone Antitrust Litigation	2014	Suboxone	Opioid dependence	The class action was certified in 2020 and Indivior settled for $600 million.
Teamsters Union 25 Health Services & Insurance Plan v. Allergan PLC	2015	Asacol	Ulcerative colitis	The class action was not certified, but Allergen later agreed to pay $2.7 million to settle the suit.
New York v. Actavis PLC et al.	2015	Namenda XR	Alzheimer's disease	The Court confirmed the injunction that forced Forest Laboratories to continue selling Namenda IR.

Table 4.1. (cont.)

Case	Year	Drug	Purpose	Outcome
Loestrin 24 FE Antitrust Litigation	2016	Loestrin	Contraceptive	Warner Chilcott settled the case for $300 million in 2020.
Hartig Drug Co. Inc. v. Senju Pharmaceutical, et al.	2016	Zymar or Zymaxid	Antimicrobial agent used to kill various types of bacteria used in ophthalmic solution for eye drops	The Third Circuit remanded the District Court's dismissal of the case in 2016.
Mylan Pharmaceuticals, Inc. v. Warner Chilcott Pub. Ltd.	2016	Doryx	Antibiotic	Warner's conduct was not condemned due to a number of substitutes for its product.
King Drug Co. of Florence Inc. v. Abbot Labs.	2019	AndroGel	Testosterone deficiency	AbbVie and Besins Healthcare Inc. were required by the FTC to disgorge $448 million in overcharges. They appealed.

examine the circuit court opinion. We also review OxyContin OP, which did not go to trial but provides another example of product hopping.

State of New York *v.* Actavis[8]

Forest Laboratories, which is a wholly owned subsidiary of Actavis, received FDA approval for Namenda IR in 2003 for the treatment of moderate to severe Alzheimer's disease. The drug was quite profitable and had a market valuation of $1.5 billion. With the threat of generic entry in 2015 due to patent expiration, Forest Laboratories had much to lose. Research has shown that once generics enter a market, the pioneer brand's market share rapidly falls from 100 percent to 10–20 percent.[9] One study found that a pioneer firm's market share fell to 16 percent on average after just one year.[10] Additionally, the retail price of a generic drug is estimated to be about 75 percent lower than the original brand price.[11]

Many states have drug substitution laws that permit or even mandate the substitution of a generic drug for the pioneer brand.[12] If a patient had a prescription for Namenda IR, a dispensing pharmacy would have the authority to substitute a generic equivalent if one were available. Consequently, generic drug manufacturers do little, if any, marketing. They simply make their products available and allow the state substitution laws to do their work. However, in all states, substitution is forbidden if the generic is not bioequivalent, which requires that the pioneer drug and the generic have the same active ingredient, dosage, form, strength, and route of administration. If a drug

---

[8] *State of New York* v. *Actavis*, 787 F.3d 638 (2d Cir. 2015). This decision provides an antitrust law and economics analysis of exclusionary product hopping in determining the likelihood of success at trial by the State of New York. Other private suits have been filed against the defendants, including *Sergeants Benevolent Association Health & Welfare Fund et al.* v. *Actavis PLC et al.*, No. 1:15-cv-06549 (S.D.N.Y. 2019), which settled with some of the defendants in 2019.

[9] This rapid decline in market share is called a patent cliff.

[10] Grabowski, Long, and Mortimer (2014).   [11] Sullivan (2018).

[12] National Conference of State Legislatures (2019).

manufacturer slightly modifies its drug, generics can no longer claim bioequivalency. Forest Laboratories took advantage of this loophole.

In 2010, the FDA approved Namenda XR, which contained the same active ingredient as Namenda IR. Both versions had the same therapeutic effect for patients with moderate to severe Alzheimer's disease. But the drugs were not therapeutically equivalent due to three key differences. First, the absorption rate was different. Namenda IR released its active ingredient immediately and had to be taken twice a day, whereas Namenda XR released its active ingredient gradually and was taken only once a day. This change would appear to be beneficial for the patient because it would improve compliance. Second, the delivery mechanism was different. Namenda IR came in tablets while Namenda XR came in capsules, which may be easier for patients to swallow. Third, the strength was different. Namenda IR therapy involved two 10 mg tablets, whereas Namenda XR involved one 28 mg capsule. This change may have improved the efficacy of the treatment.

Due to the differences between Namenda IR and Namenda XR, the drugs were not therapeutically equivalent. Five generic versions of Namenda IR were poised to enter the market in July 2015, with another seven that might have entered by October 2015. Although these generics could be substituted for Namenda IR, they could not be substituted for Namenda XR since they would not be therapeutically equivalent. Importantly, patent protection for Namenda XR would not expire until 2029.

It was obvious to Forest Laboratories that switching patients to Namenda XR before generic versions of Namenda IR hit the market could have substantial financial benefits. Ultimately, Forest Laboratories discontinued Namenda IR before the expiration of its patent and the entrance of generic versions. Physicians were forced to switch their Alzheimer's patients to Namenda XR.[13] When the

---

[13] Urging physicians to switch patients to a newer version while selling both versions is known as a soft switch. Discontinuing production of the older version before its

Namenda IR patent expired, generic substitutes could have appeared. Having recently switched their patients from Namenda IR to Namenda XR, there is some doubt that physicians would have switched their patients from Namenda XR to a generic substitute for Namenda IR.[14] Consequently, this strategy would exclude generic competition until 2029. The potential harm to consumers was in the billions of dollars.

The focus on profit is apparent in the following explanation by management: "[T]he core of our brand strategy with XR is to convert our existing IR business to Namenda XR as fast as we can and also gain new starts for Namenda XR. We need to transition volume to XR to protect our Namenda revenue from generic penetration in 2015 when we lose IR patent exclusivity."[15]

The antitrust question was simple: Does exclusionary product hopping constitute unlawful maintenance of monopoly in violation of Section 2 of the Sherman Act? The answer is not so simple because patentees are ordinarily free to produce a patented product or not produce it as they see fit. In this case, the court found that discontinuing the production of Namenda IR could only be explained as a strategy to extend its monopoly life and delay the expiration of the Namenda patent.

In spite of the usual deference to the rights of patentees, the Court of Appeals concluded "that the combination of withdrawing a successful drug from the market and introducing a reformulated

---

patent expiration and thereby forcing physicians to switch is a hard switch, which may be considered exclusionary.

[14] A quote from an executive indicated that physicians were likely to continue providing Namenda XR, even with generic entry of Namenda IR: "[I]f we do the hard switch and we convert patients and caregivers to once-a-day therapy versus twice a day, it's very difficult for the generics then to reverse-commute back, at least with the existing Rxs. They don't have the sales force. They don't have the capabilities to go do that. It doesn't mean that it can't happen, it just becomes very difficult and is an obstacle that will allow us to, I think, again go into a slow decline versus a complete cliff." *State of New York* v. *Actavis and Forest Laboratories*, No. 1:14-cv-07473-RWS (S.D.N.Y. 2014) at 51.

[15] *State of New York* v. *Actavis and Forest Laboratories*, No. 1:14-cv-07473-RWS (S.D.N.Y. 2014) at 51.

version of that drug, which has the dual effect of forcing patients to switch to the new version and impeding generic competition, without a legitimate business justification, violates Section 2 of the Sherman Act."[16]

Mylan Pharmaceuticals, Inc. *v.* Warner Chilcott Pub. Ltd. Co.[17]

Doryx is the brand name for an oral tetracycline-based drug for the treatment of acne, which is manufactured and sold by Warner Chilcott and Mayne Pharma (Warner/Mayne).[18] This product had been on the market in capsule form for many years, but it was not particularly successful. Doryx competed with generic versions, as well as with other reasonably substitutable tetracycline drugs.[19]

A new version of Doryx received FDA approval in 2005. Instead of capsule form, the newly introduced version was a delayed-release formulation in tablet form with a strength of 75 mg. The capsules were discontinued, and steps were taken to switch patients to the new tablet version. Note that generic Doryx capsules were already available and any generic could have entered the Doryx market. In fact, Mylan had attempted to create a generic Doryx capsule beginning in 2003, which failed. Beginning in 2007, Warner/Mayne began to make a series of relatively minor modifications to its 75 mg delayed-release tablet; specifically, the manufacturer introduced a 150 mg scored tablet that could be split into two 75 mg pieces. It replaced its 75 mg smooth tablet with a 75 mg scored tablet. It then scored the 150 mg smooth tablet so that it could be split into halves or thirds. As the modified versions were introduced, Warner/Mayne withdrew the

---

[16] *State of New York* v. *Actavis PLC, Forest Laboratories LLC, Co.*, No. 14-4624 (2d Cir. 2015) at 50.

[17] *Mylan Pharmaceuticals, Inc.* v. *Warner Chilcott Pub. Ltd. Co.*, No. 15-2236 (3d Cir. 2016).

[18] Doryx was originally produced by Mayne Pharma, an Australian firm, but Warner Chilcott was the distributor of branded Doryx in the United States.

[19] Mayne Pharma had sold a generic version in the US market. Poor sales for branded and generic Doryx prompted it to leave the market in 1997, leaving Warner Chilcott as the exclusive distributor in the United States.

older versions. Mylan asserted that this constituted a hard switch similar to the conduct at issue in the Namenda case. Allegedly, the aim of Warner/Mayne was to exclude generic competition in an effort to monopolize or attempt to monopolize the market for Doryx.

The facts in this case are substantially different from those in the Namenda case. Not surprisingly, therefore, the Court of Appeals reached a different conclusion. Along the way, however, the court recognized that the reasoning in the *Namenda* case was appropriate under the circumstances: "we do not rule out the possibility that certain insignificant design or formula changes, combined with other coercive conduct could present a closer call with respect to establishing liability in future cases." The court suggested that "courts might need to balance the important public interest in encouraging innovation in the pharmaceutical industry with [their] obligations to protect consumers and to ensure fair competition under the antitrust laws. At the same time, courts should also be wary both of second-guessing Congress's legislative judgement and of turning courts into tribunals over innovation sufficiency."[20]

In the present case, however, the evidence did not support a claim of exclusionary product hopping. In order to prove unlawful monopolization, a plaintiff must prove (1) that the defendant has monopoly power in the relevant market and (2) that its monopoly was due to predatory or exclusionary conduct.[21] For attempted monopolization, the plaintiff must prove that the defendant engaged in predatory or exclusionary conduct with the intent to monopolize the market, and the defendant's market share must be large enough to establish a reasonable probability that it will succeed.

For either claim, it would be necessary to define the market. Mylan alleged that the market encompassed sales of Doryx in the United States. Both the district court and the Court of Appeals

---

[20] *Mylan Pharmaceuticals, Inc.* v. *Warner Chilcott Pub. Ltd. Co.*, No. 15-2236 (3d Cir. 2016) at 40.

[21] These requirements are discussed in Section 2.4.

rejected this definition. They found that Doryx was part of the oral tetracycline market. Although neither the patient nor the pharmacist can substitute a rival product for Doryx once the prescription has been written, competition takes place elsewhere. Rival firms compete on the basis of being the drug of choice at the physician level because that is where the prescription is written. In the case of Doryx, the courts found that a variety of tetracycline-based acne medications were reasonably substitutable by physicians. Consequently, Warner/Mayne only held a market share of some 18 percent, which is too small to support a Section 2 allegation.

OxyContin

The prior two examples show the different ways in which courts have tried to determine the legality of exclusionary product hopping. In the literature, there is a debate about the use of the antitrust laws and treble damages to assess the appropriateness of product hopping. Some argue that the practice should be considered anticompetitive,[22] whereas others argue that the court is ill-equipped to weigh the benefits to consumers against the costs of reduced-price competition.[23] In this section, we consider the prescription drug OxyContin OP, which was not involved in product-hopping litigation but illustrates how difficult it can be to assess the competitive effects of product hopping.

In 1995, Purdue patented its opioid OxyContin, which was an oxycodone drug with an extended time release mechanism that granted pain relief for up to 12 hours. Purdue marketed it as more convenient and more abuse-resistant than previous opioids, and it soon became the drug of choice. Unfortunately, the addictive properties of the opioid led to rampant misuse of the drug. At this time, the United States saw increases in opioid prescriptions and later began to

[22] Burke (2018), Carrier and Shadowen (2016), Devlin (2007).
[23] Cheng (2008), Ginsburg, Wong-Ervin, and Wright (2015).

experience a severe opioid crisis that has claimed more than 840,000 lives from drug overdose since 1999.[24]

In 2010, Purdue received FDA approval for a reformulation of OxyContin, which culminated in Oxycontin OP, a more abuse-resistant opioid.[25] The company hardened the tablets, which made them difficult to misuse by crushing. Conveniently, this reformulation came on the market at a time when OxyContin was nearing the end of its patent, which had already been extended to 2013. The patents covering the reformulation extended patent protection until 2025. Citing concerns over drug misuse, Purdue asked the FDA to retract the patent for the original drug, which effectively removed all possibility for generics to offer a substitute for OxyContin. This example represents product hopping with a hard switch, but the net competitive effects are difficult to measure.

The benefit of OxyContin OP was its abuse-resistant formula. But patients who would not have misused the drug had to pay a premium for the same newly patented drug. Purdue profited from the FDA's decision through its continued patent exclusivity of OxyContin OP with no generic competition. From the perspective of public health authorities, however, the reformulation was useful in reducing misuse and diversion of OxyContin. It is difficult to weigh the public health benefits against the cost to individual patients and determine, on net, whether the product hopping requested by Purdue was privately or socially motivated. Lars Noah (2015) argues that Purdue's intention was to extend its monopoly. But one cannot discount the public health benefits the abuse-resistant formula had in

---

[24] Centers for Disease Control and Prevention (2021).

[25] The economics literature, however, has identified some unintended consequences of the OxyContin reformulation. Alpert, Powell, and Pacula (2018) study the effect of the supply-side disruption of the OxyContin reformulation, which significantly decreased access to abusable prescription opioids. Although the authors identify a decrease in prescription opioid deaths following the reformulation, they also find an increase in heroin overdose mortality, as individuals may have substituted away from OxyContin and toward illicit heroin.

reducing misuse of prescription opioids. Clearly, identifying the competitive effects of product hopping is complicated in practice.

4.4   SOLUTIONS, IF ANY

Product hopping and exclusionary product hopping raise public policy issues that warrant some serious thought. Should the patent system be amended by Congress? Is Section 2 of the Sherman Act robust enough to deal with exclusionary product hopping problems? Can we find relief in Section 5 of the FTC Act, which prohibits unfair methods of competition?

Reforming the Regulatory System

Under the patent system, our society rewards an inventor with patent protection for 20 years when he or she has discovered something "novel, useful, and non-obvious." If this discovery happens to be a pharmaceutical product, it may not be sold to patients until it has received FDA approval. The pharmaceutical producer must engage in extensive testing in order to establish the safety and efficacy of the new drug before the FDA will grant its approval.[26]

The changes to a successful drug that result in a new patent and an extended period of exclusivity may be significant or insignificant. If the changes are insignificant, the question is whether the government should issue a new patent with the same patent life. For example, if a manufacturer introduces a capsule version of precisely the same drug that is available in tablet form, does this not seem "obvious"? If so, the government should not issue a patent.

The FDA could help matters by rethinking its requirements for therapeutic equivalence and by reconsidering the exclusivity granted to firms making incremental innovation as opposed to the initial groundbreaking innovation.

---

[26] See Section 7.2 for a description of the approval process.

Antitrust Remedies

Traditionally, Section 2 of the Sherman Act deals with monopolization and attempts to monopolize. Both product hopping generally and exclusionary product hopping are means of maintaining monopoly power. Both practices, therefore, seem vulnerable to prosecution under Section 2 of the Sherman Act. The problem lies in identifying instances of product hopping that are objectionable. When an existing product is modified, it may well be a significant change that warrants patent protection and immunity from antitrust challenges. Exclusionary product hopping is more obviously anticompetitive. But requiring a manufacturer to continue producing older versions of the new and improved drug may be objectionable.

Cheng (2008) has little sympathy for generic producers that are frustrated by exclusionary product hopping, concluding that

> antitrust courts should not condemn product hopping for merely disrupting the ability of generic manufacturers to free ride on a brand name manufacturer's marketing and promotional expenditures, nor is antitrust law the proper vehicle for generic manufacturers to claim such an entitlement to free ride. Though requiring generic manufacturers to compete for prescriptions and incur advertising costs may negate some of the cost benefits that generic drugs offer and provide questionable social value, market antitrust concerns focus on promoting robust competition and do not "inquir[e] into the question [of] whether competition is good or bad."[27]

In this regard, Cheng seems to miss the point that the pioneer firms are trying to evade competition. Most other legal commentators view product hopping as a way for drug manufacturers to game the patent system.

---

[27] Cheng (2008, 1503); Nat'l Soc'y of Prof'l Eng'rs, 435 US 679, 695 (1978).

Some antitrust scholars contend that product hopping should only violate the antitrust laws if the patent extension involves fraud on the US Patent and Trademark Office.[28] In their view, a soft switch is simply competition on the merits. It is hard to disagree. Both the new version of the drug and the older version, along with generic equivalents, are available to patients. As long as physicians act in their patients' best interests, the new, more expensive version must compete with the older, less expensive option.

In our view, the hard switch is a different matter. Since the older pioneer drug is no longer available for physicians to prescribe, they must switch their patients to the new version. Following patent expiration on the pioneer drug, generics may enter. Whether physicians would switch their patients back to the original formulation is an empirical matter. In most cases, however, there is no incentive for them to do so. Thus, the hard switch may be exclusionary. With a hard switch, it is difficult for generics to compete on the merits. Since generic producers must compete with one another on price, a single firm may not be able to promote generic substitution. The benefits of doing so will be diffused across all generic producers while the costs are borne fully by the promoter. It is disingenuous to declare that generic producers can compete with the new brand on "advertising, promotion, cost competition, or superior product development."[29]

Many researchers question whether the courts have the expertise to determine whether a firm's reformulation is innovation for the benefit of consumers or innovation designed to maintain monopoly status. The courts do not have the expertise to determine the value of a reformulation. Even though a reformulation may seem trivial, it may produce a large benefit to patients. For example, compliance increases the fewer times that a medicine must be administered. In most markets, value is determined by the price that consumers are

---

[28] Ginsburg, Wong-Ervin, and Wright (2015).

[29] *Mylan Pharmaceuticals, Inc.* v. *Warner Chilcott Pub. Ltd. Co.*, No. 12-3824 WL 1736957 (E.D. Pa. 2015) at 14.

willing to pay. Yet, the pharmaceutical market is unique in that doctors prescribe drugs for which the patients and/or insurance companies pay. In other words, doctors are not subject to the same price incentives as their patients, which could bias them toward prescribing expensive drugs rather than less expensive generic equivalents. Even if pharmaceutical firms did not intend to monopolize markets with their reformulations, evidence shows that patients pay higher drug prices when formulations are changed and generic entry is delayed. If the FDA cannot implement changes to forestall this behavior, then the courts may alleviate the harm to patients by creating their own framework to evaluate the anticompetitive nature of product-hopping cases. This framework must maintain a delicate balance between forestalling monopolistic harm while encouraging innovation.

The pharmaceutical firm's actions can suggest whether the intent is to maintain monopoly or to innovate. If the firm patents its reformulated drug in the narrow window of time before patent expiration and subsequent generic entry, the case may be subject to antitrust scrutiny, especially if the firm discontinues production of the original drug. This would indicate an unwillingness to compete with generic firms. Aggressive marketing techniques that encourage doctors to switch to the reformulated drug before the expiration of the patent on the original drug may also arouse antitrust suspicion. Carrier and Shadowen (2016) suggest using a "no economic sense" test to further evaluate product-hopping behavior. If a firm's actions make no economic sense outside of increased profits from reduced competition, the product hopping should be objectionable.

Unfair Methods of Competition

If a firm engages in unfair methods of competition, that conduct can be challenged under Section 5 of the FTC Act, which provides that conduct that is anticompetitive but may not quite rise to an antitrust violation may be deemed "unfair." Exclusionary product hopping may fall into this category. The so-called hard switch certainly seems to be coercive when the pioneer drug has no reasonable substitutes that a physician could prescribe.

A bill proposed by Representative David Cicilline would make it easier for the Agencies to prosecute product hopping under Section 5 of the FTC Act. The Affordable Prescriptions for Patients through Promoting Competition Act of 2019 would allow the Federal Trade Commission to prosecute both "hard" and "soft" switches on the part of the pioneer firm.[30] Such a law would face the same identification problems as discussed in the Antitrust Remedies subsection, including difficulties by the FTC in determining the value of a modification to an original pharmaceutical drug.

4.5 CONCLUDING REMARKS

Does product hopping cause anticompetitive harm? The answer depends in part on distinguishing between product hopping that merely modifies existing versions of branded drugs that compete with generic substitutes and exclusionary product hopping. Arguably, product hopping without exclusion cannot harm consumers because generic substitutes are available to physicians to prescribe and to pharmacists for substitution under state substitution laws.

The competitive harm of exclusionary product hopping resides in the economic effects of excluding generic substitutes. In the case of prescription drugs, excluding generic competition allows unfettered monopoly pricing. Given the inelasticity of demand for such drugs, prices may soar. These higher prices turn consumer surplus into producer profit, lead to higher insurance premiums, and reduce social welfare.

If there is an antitrust remedy for exclusionary product hopping, it will be found in Section 2 of the Sherman Act, which condemns monopolization, attempts to monopolize, and conspiracies

---

[30] Affordable Prescriptions for Patients through Promoting Competition Act of 2019, H.R. 5133, 116th Congress (2019). The bill was introduced and passed between various committees, but no further action was taken.

to monopolize a market. Although the original patent monopoly is safe from prosecution, exclusionary product hopping may be seen as an unreasonable effort to maintain monopoly. Ordinarily, such a finding is unlikely unless the modification to the drug is trivial and the original version is withdrawn before its patent protection expires.

This sort of strategic behavior is not competition on the merits. Instead, it appears to be not much more than an effort to game the patent system. In dealing with what may be exclusionary product hopping, "[t]he challenge lies in fashioning a workable rule that preserves the ability of manufacturers to engage in beneficial product changes but also condemns product hopping strategies that only serve to impermissibly undermine generic competition."[31] So far, an ideal antitrust policy has not been found. The search goes on.

REFERENCES

Alpert, Abby, David Powell, and Rosalie Liccardo Pacula. (2018). Supply-Side Drug Policy in the Prescence of Substitutes: Evidence from the Introduction of Abuse-Deterrent Opioids. *American Economic Journal: Economic Policy* 10: 1–35.

Burke, Daniel. (2018). An Examination of Product Hopping by Brand-Name Prescription Drug Manufacturers: The Problem and a Proposed Solution. *Cleveland State Law Review* 66: 415–441.

Carrier, Michael, and Steve Shadowen. (2016). Product Hopping: A New Framework. *Notre Dame Law Review* 92: 167–230.

Centers for Disease Control and Prevention. (2021). *Drug Overdose Deaths*. www.cdc.gov/drugoverdose/data/statedeaths.html.

Cheng, Jessie. (2008). An Antitrust Analysis of Product Hopping in the Pharmaceutical Industry. *Columbia Law Review* 108: 1471–1515.

Devlin, Alan. (2007). Exclusionary Strategies in the Hatch-Waxman Context. *Michigan State Law Review* 2007: 631–681.

Ginsburg, Douglas H., Koren W. Wong-Ervin, and Joshua D. Wright. (2015). Product Hopping and the Limits of Antitrust: The Danger of Micromanaging Innovation. *CPI Antitrust Chronicle* 1: 2–4.

---

[31] Cheng (2008, 1495).

Grabowski, Henry, Genia Long, and Richard Mortimer. (2014). Recent Trends in Brand-Name and Generic Drug Competition. *Journal of Medical Economics* 17: 207–214.

Lopez, Ian. (2021). *Teva "Skinny Label" Ruling Comes amid Lawmaker Drug Fight*. Bloomberg Law. https://news.bloomberglaw.com/ip-law/teva-skinny-label-ruling-comes-amid-lawmaker-drug-cost-fight.

National Conference of State Legislatures. (2019). *Generic Drug Substitution Laws*. www.ncsl.org/portals/1/documents/health/Generic_Drug_Substitution_Laws_32193.pdf.

Noah, Lars. (2015). Product Hopping 2.0: Getting the FDA to Yank Your Original License Beats Stacking Patents. *Marquette Intellectual Property Law Review* 19: 161–179.

Sullivan, Thomas. (2018). *GAO Report Drug Pricing: Research on Savings from Generic Drug Use*. Policy & Medicine. www.policymed.com/2012/03/gao-report-drug-pricing-research-on-savings-from-generic-drug-use.html.

5 Bundled Discounts and PeaceHealth

5.1 INTRODUCTION

5.1 INTRODUCTION

Many input suppliers offer volume discounts that reduce the customer's costs.[1] In most circumstances, at least part of the cost reduction is passed on to the consumer. In this event, the discounts are procompetitive and consumer welfare increases. When a multiproduct firm bundles its discounts, the economic results are not always so positive.

Suppose that a multiproduct firm offers a 5 percent discount on its list prices if the customer buys all of its required latex gloves and surgical masks from the firm. If the customer buys any of the products from a second source, the discount falls to, say, 3 percent. The discounts are said to be *bundled* because the discount earned on gloves depends on the purchase of gloves *and* masks rather than just the purchase of gloves. Similarly, the discount on masks depends on the purchase of both products. In some instances, this apparently procompetitive discount schedule can foreclose an equally efficient producer of, say, surgical masks. In this event, the bundled discount schedule raises antitrust concerns. As we will see, however, formulating an economically sensible antitrust policy is not easy.

In the next section, we define bundled discounts and provide general examples. We continue this discussion in Section 5.3 by reviewing bundled discounts in health care settings. We also discuss the standard established in *PeaceHealth*, which dictates how the courts handle bundled discounts. In Section 5.4, we discuss a number of anomalies that can arise due to the discount attribution test, which

---

[1] This chapter relies heavily on Blair and Knight (2020).

has been used to evaluate bundled discounts. In Section 5.5, we discuss the antitrust treatment of bundled discounts. Finally, we close with some concluding remarks in Section 5.6.

5.2 BUNDLED DISCOUNTS

A *bundled discount* exists when a firm offers a lower price on a bundle of goods or services relative to the individual prices of the goods or services. For example, fast-food restaurants typically offer value meals that include a burger, fries, and a drink at a lower price than the sum of the prices of the individual items in the meal. These restaurants are motivated to use bundled discounts to increase sales and reduce transaction costs. Bundled discounts are extremely common and often procompetitive in many settings since they reduce the total price a consumer pays. This is certainly true in the short run. Antitrust questions arise if the price reductions exclude rivals, especially those that are at least as efficient as the bundler, which could reduce competition and raise prices in the long run.

Bundled discounts should not be confused with *predatory pricing*, where a monopolist faces rival entry and responds by reducing the price below its cost (and its rival's cost) with the intention of bankrupting that rival and regaining monopoly status. Such a strategy would require the monopolist to have market power and a high probability of recouping the losses sustained during the predation period if the rival was effectively excluded. Although predatory pricing is often discussed in the same space as bundled discounts, it is distinctly different in several ways. First, predatory pricing involves the pricing of one product as opposed to multiproduct bundled discounts. Second, a firm engaged in predatory pricing must have market power and be able to finance predation with prior earned profits. Third, predatory pricing (if successful) is clearly anticompetitive. Bundled discounts are in some ways more interesting since the antitrust concerns are not as clear-cut as with predatory pricing.

LePage's suit against 3M illustrates some of the antitrust concerns with bundled discounts.[2] The 3M Company is a conglomerate that sells an array of products that fall into six groups: health care products, home care products, home improvement products, stationery products, retail auto products, and leisure-time products. Its Scotch brand transparent tape fell into the stationery products group. LePage's Inc. produced a private label transparent tape that it sought to sell through retail outlets such as Walmart, Kmart, and Office Depot.

The 3M Company bundled discounts across all six product groups. The customer earned the maximum discount on purchases from 3M when it did not buy any rival products. If a customer bought transparent tape from LePage's, for example, that customer would receive lower discounts on all of its purchases from 3M.[3] LePage's complained that it could not compete with 3M since the discounts became exclusionary due to the breadth of 3M's offerings. The following numerical example reveals LePage's challenge.[4]

Suppose that 3M sold 50 products, including transparent tape, that fell into one product group or another. A multiproduct retailer like Walmart sells this array of products and enjoys 3M's full discount. Table 5.1 presents the hypothetical discount schedule.

Suppose that Walmart buys $1 million worth of each product at list prices. If it buys everything from 3M, it qualifies for a 5 percent discount and, therefore, pays a total of $47.5 million. If LePage's offers to sell its transparent tape to Walmart, it will face nearly impossible odds. If Walmart buys LePage's tape instead of 3M's tape, its discounts

---

[2] *LePage's, Inc.* v. *3M*, 324 F. 3d. 141 (3d Cir. 2003).

[3] Of course, buyer compliance may be an issue. Buyers will have an incentive to cheat by secretly purchasing from more than one source while claiming to exclusively buy products from the multiproduct firm in order to reap the benefits of the bundled discount. The multiproduct firm may need to monitor compliance or enforce fidelity with the bundled discount agreement terms.

[4] Although the names of the parties are real, the following example is purely hypothetical.

Table 5.1. *3M's discount schedule*

Percent of purchases	Percent discount
100	5
90–99	4
80–89	3
70–79	2
60–69	1
0–59	0

on the other products fall from 5 to 4 percent.[5] Consequently, Walmart will pay a net amount of $47.04 million to 3M. To make Walmart whole, LePage's can charge no more than $460,000 for its transparent tape. This amounts to a 54 percent discount off 3M's list price.

3M's net sales of Scotch tape would be $950,000, whereas the most that LePage's can realize is $460,000. Even if LePage's cost of supplying its tape were as low as $600,000, it would still be foreclosed from selling to Walmart. In this example, the bundled discount is exclusionary.[6]

The problem for LePage's was not in matching or beating 3M's discount on transparent tape. Since LePage's cost was only $600,000, a 5 percent discount would have left the company with $350,000 in profit. The problem was that LePage's was unable to provide a steep enough discount on its tape to offset Walmart's lost discounts on the other 49 items. In this example, LePage's could have been foreclosed even if it had been more efficient than 3M. Even if 3M's costs for its Scotch brand tape had been, say, $700,000 or $800,000, the bundled discount schedule would have excluded LePage's from earning Walmart's business.

---

[5] In this example, we assume that the transparent tape products manufactured by LePage's and 3M are of comparable quality and homogeneous. Other cases could be more complicated if the products are heterogeneous.

[6] The hypothetical discount schedule in the 3M example would be exclusionary if LePage's could not profitably offer a 54 percent discount.

An interesting characteristic of bundled discounts is that they need not be large if the number of products is large. Suppose that 3M offered a 1 percent discount if Walmart bought all of its requirements from 3M, but no discount if Walmart bought any of its requirements from a rival supplier. The net cost of the purchases would be $49.5 million if Walmart bought all its requirements from 3M. For a single-product supplier to sell its product to Walmart, it would have to make Walmart whole. Since Walmart would have to pay $49 million for the 3M products, LePage's could charge no more than $500,000 for its tape. Since LePage's costs for transparent tape exceed $500,000, the company is excluded even by a rather modest 1 percent bundled discount.

The Third Circuit affirmed the lower court findings, holding that the 3M rebate program violated Section 2 of the Sherman Act despite the fact that the prices effectively charged by 3M were not below cost. The Supreme Court declined to review this case.

5.3   BUNDLED DISCOUNTS IN HEALTH CARE SETTINGS

While *LePage's* provides a useful example of bundled discounts, we now review bundled discounts in health care settings by discussing several important court decisions.

Ortho Diagnostics *v.* Abbott Labs[7]

Ortho and Abbott are both producers of rival blood tests; Ortho offered three products, whereas Abbott offered five products. As part of its pricing scheme, Abbott offered bundled discounts based on the number of product offerings the buyer purchased. Specifically, Abbott offered discounts to buyers if they purchased four of the five products and a larger discount if they purchased all five of the products. The *Ortho* court rightly recognized that prices above average variable cost (AVC) could exclude an equally efficient rival. In its 1996 decision, the court held that to be successful with a bundled discount claim, a

---

[7] *Ortho Diagnostics* v. *Abbott Labs*, 926 F. Supp. 371 (S.D.N.Y. 1996).

plaintiff must prove that the discounted prices are below the firm's AVC or that the excluded plaintiff is at least as efficient as the defendant but was excluded by the defendant's pricing.[8]

Smith Kline v. Eli Lilly[9]

Both Smith Kline and Eli Lilly are pharmaceutical drug manufacturers that make cephalosporin antibiotics; Smith Kline had two products and Eli Lilly had five products. Eli Lilly offered a 3 percent bonus rebate if the buyer purchased three of five products. This bundled pricing scheme forced Smith Kline to reduce its price for antibiotics more than Eli Lilly to effectively compete. The court found that this conduct violated Section 2 of the Sherman Act.

Suture Express, Inc. v. Owen's & Minor Distribution Inc.[10]

Owens & Minor Distribution Inc. (O&M), Cardinal Health 200 LLC (Cardinal), and Suture Express, Inc. are suppliers of medical-surgical supplies. In 2012, Suture Express alleged that its rivals, Cardinal and O&M, bundled their prices in order to restrain competition. Specifically, customers who bought sutures and endomechanical products (i.e., products used during laparoscopic procedures) from Suture Express along with other medical-surgical products from O&M and Cardinal allegedly paid more than if they had bought all of their medical-surgical products from O&M and Cardinal, even though Suture Express sold its sutures and endomechnical products for less. The US Court of Appeals for the Tenth Circuit determined that Suture Express did not have enough evidence to support the

[8] Pfizer accused Johnson & Johnson of using bundled discounts for its anti-inflammatory drug Remicade to exclude Pfizer's generic version from the market. Johnson & Johnson allegedly used exclusionary conduct and bundled discounts to persuade insurers and other market participants to exclude Pfizer's generic from reimbursement. The case settled in July 2021. *Pfizer Inc.* v. *Johnson & Johnson*, No. 2:17-cv-4180 (E.D. Pa. 2017).

[9] *Smith Kline* v. *Eli Lilly*, 575 F. 2d. 1056 (3d Cir. 1978).

[10] *Suture Express, Inc.* v. *Owen's & Minor Distribution Inc.*, No. 16-3065 (10th Cir. 2017).

claim that O&M and Cardinal had enough market power to force customers to exclusively buy their products.

Sugartown Pediatrics, LLC *v.* Merck & Co., Inc. [11]

Merck is a major manufacturer of children's vaccines, and it was the only producer of the rotavirus vaccine until GlaxoSmithKline PLC (GSK) entered the market in 2009. Sugartown Pediatrics, LLC (Sugartown) is a member of a physician buying group that negotiated to buy vaccines from manufacturers. Sugartown sued Merck, on behalf of a class of plaintiffs, alleging that Merck used bundled discounts to monopolize the market for rotavirus vaccine. Merck offered a bundled discount on vaccines, including those for rotavirus, hepatitis A, hepatitis B, Hib, varicella, MMR, and HPV. GSK would have needed to offer a 40 percent discount on its rotavirus vaccine to effectively compete with Merck's bundled pricing. The plaintiffs argued that they overpaid for vaccines since the bundled discounts precluded price competition from GSK.

The PeaceHealth Standard

The Supreme Court has not ruled on the legality of bundled discounts. Consequently, we must rely on lower court decisions. At this time, the most influential decision for antitrust guidance appears to be the Ninth Circuit's opinion in *Cascade Health Solutions* v. *PeaceHealth*.[12]

McKenzie Willamette Hospital filed an antitrust suit against PeaceHealth. McKenzie was a 114-bed hospital offering primary and secondary acute care hospital services. PeaceHealth owned three acute care hospitals: a 432-bed hospital offering primary, secondary, and tertiary care; a 21-bed hospital; and an 11-bed hospital. Primary and secondary care services are relatively uncomplicated services,

---

[11] *Sugartown Pediatrics, LLC* v. *Merck & Co., Inc.*, No. 2:18-cv-01734 (E.D. Pa. 2018).

[12] *Cascade Health Solutions* v. *PeaceHealth*, 515 F. 3d 883 (3rd Cir. 2008). The McKenzie Willamette Hospital became part of Cascade Health Solutions during the litigation. In what follows, we refer to the plaintiff as McKenzie.

such as setting a broken bone or performing minor surgery (e.g., a tonsillectomy). Tertiary care is more complicated, such as open-heart surgery and intensive neonatal care.

McKenzie offered evidence that PeaceHealth bundled its discounts to health insurers and thereby foreclosed McKenzie from that business. In one case, PeaceHealth offered a 15 percent discount off its list prices to health insurers if it was the sole preferred provider for all acute care hospital services, but only a 10 percent discount if McKenzie was an alternative preferred provider of primary and secondary services. According to McKenzie, the bundling scheme made it impossible to compete with PeaceHealth for preferred provider status.

The Ninth Circuit recognized that it is possible for bundled discounts to foreclose an equally efficient, or even more efficient, rival and thereby be anticompetitive. It also recognized that bundled discounts reduce prices for consumers. Consequently, there was an obvious need for an operational standard that would condemn anticompetitive bundled discounts while allowing competitively benign bundled discounts. The Ninth Circuit applied the discount attribution test.

The Discount Attribution Test

In *PeaceHealth*, the court found that if the discounts on the uncontested business are attributed to the contested business and an equally efficient rival could not profitably compete for that business, then the bundled discount schedule would be deemed exclusionary and therefore anticompetitive. One nice feature of this test is that the firm offering the bundled discount has all the information it needs to determine whether its schedule is exclusionary. In other words, the discounter does not have to know the would-be rival's costs; the discounter only needs to know its own costs. Depending upon the details of the bundled discount schedule, applying this test is not too complicated and, therefore, is amenable to judicial administration. We use hypothetical examples from *LePage's* and *PeaceHealth* to demonstrate the test.

Returning to our previous example, suppose that LePage's and 3M were equally efficient; that is, the cost of supplying $1 million of tape was $600,000. At a 1 percent discount, the buyer would earn a $500,000 discount on its entire book of business if it bought products exclusively from 3M. By buying tape from LePage's, the buyer would lose its 3M discount and would only be willing to pay $500,000 for LePage's tape. Since only the tape business was being contested, the other $500,000 would be attributed to tape sales. This would amount to a 50 percent discount on the tape, which would exclude an equally efficient rival.

In one instance, PeaceHealth offered a 15 percent discount to the Blue Cross Blue Shield Association on all primary, secondary, and tertiary charges provided that PeaceHealth was the sole preferred provider for primary and secondary acute care hospital services. If Blue Cross included a second preferred provider, the discount on all three services dropped to 10 percent. On its face, this bundled discount plan is not necessarily exclusionary, but it may be.

Suppose that PeaceHealth and McKenzie are equally efficient and compete to offer Blue Cross primary and secondary services. Suppose that primary care and secondary care each amount to $10 million at list prices. If this were the end of the story, PeaceHealth could not foreclose McKenzie without offering predatory prices, that is, prices below its costs.[13] By hypothesis, the hospitals are equally efficient, so PeaceHealth cannot price McKenzie out of the market unless it reduces its prices below its costs. But this is not the whole story. Only PeaceHealth offers tertiary care, with a total book of business at a list price of, say, $40 million. If Blue Cross designates PeaceHealth as the only preferred provider, the net charges would be $8.5 million for primary care, $8.5 million for secondary care, and $34 million for tertiary care since Blue Cross is granted a 15 percent discount. The total is $51 million. If Blue Cross included McKenzie

---

[13] Predatory prices are unlawful. *Brooke Group Ltd.* v. *Brown and Williamson Tobacco Co.*, 509 US 209 (1993).

as an alternative preferred provider, PeaceHealth would reduce the discounts to 10 percent. If Blue Cross had done so and PeaceHealth and McKenzie split the primary and secondary business, Blue Cross would have had to pay PeaceHealth $9 million for primary and secondary services, plus $36 million for tertiary services, for a total of $45 million. As a result, McKenzie could charge no more than $6 million for the other half of the primary and secondary services. This amounts to a 40 percent discount! If the average cost to McKenzie is above $6 million, the discount schedule would have excluded McKenzie. Since we have assumed that the two hospital groups are equally efficient, PeaceHealth would also have lost money on this book of business. In other words, PeaceHealth would lose money on the contested business, which includes the primary and secondary care business.

Suppose, however, that McKenzie could take away all of the primary and secondary care business from PeaceHealth. Blue Cross would have had to pay $36 million for tertiary care. McKenzie could then charge $15 million for primary and secondary services, which would leave Blue Cross whole. McKenzie would have to offer a 25 percent discount rather than a 40 percent discount. If this offer is manageable, then the bundled discount schedule is no longer exclusionary. This conclusion raises an interesting feature of bundled discounts–the schedule may be exclusionary or not depending on how successful the competitor is in taking business from the discounter.

Now consider an altered example where the primary and secondary services are larger. As expected, the results change. Suppose that the primary and secondary services amount to $20 million each at list prices. Blue Cross would now have to pay a total of $68 million if PeaceHealth is the only preferred provider due to the 15 percent discount. If Blue Cross appoints McKenzie as an alternative preferred provider for primary and secondary care, the discount drops to 10 percent and Blue Cross will have to pay $36 million to PeaceHealth for tertiary care. If McKenzie and PeaceHealth split the primary and secondary business, Blue Cross will pay PeaceHealth $18 million, which means that McKenzie can charge no more than $14 million.

This is a 30 percent discount off the list price. Again, whether this is exclusionary depends on McKenzie's costs.

In contrast, if McKenzie could take all of the primary and secondary care business, Blue Cross would have to pay PeaceHealth $36 million. McKenzie could charge $32 million for the primary and secondary services, which would require only a 20 percent discount. This, of course, would be more manageable than a 30 percent discount. In the next section, we review a number of anomalies that arise from the discount attribution test.

5.4 ANOMALIES OF THE DISCOUNT ATTRIBUTION TEST

The discount attribution test for determining whether a bundled discount schedule is exclusionary appears to provide clear guidance to the court. The test does, however, provide some anomalous results. The same exact discount can be exclusionary or not exclusionary depending on the circumstances, such as the amount of product sold or the product breadth. In this section, we will examine a few of these anomalies using some hypothetical examples.

Anomaly 1: Whether a Discount Schedule Is Exclusionary Depends on the Book of Business

The pattern of business often determines the exclusionary nature of a discount. Therefore, a single-product rival may be excluded from some books of business but not others. Additionally, the multiproduct firm will generally receive positive profits on its business since it spreads out the discount across its product offerings, whereas other single-product rivals are excluded.

Suppose that Medical Equipment Co. produces latex gloves and masks. The list price of each is $10 per box. The per-unit cost of producing both gloves and masks is $7 each. Premier Protective Gear, Inc., also produces gloves at a per-unit cost of $7. The two rivals are clearly equally efficient in supplying latex gloves. Customers who buy all of their requirements of gloves and masks from Medical

Equipment are entitled to a 10 percent bundled discount. Otherwise, there is no discount.

Family Practice Associates, a physician group, buys latex gloves and masks for its staff. Suppose that Family Practice Associates buys 10,000 boxes of gloves and 10,000 boxes of masks from Medical Equipment at a net total cost of $180,000. If Family Practice Associates buys gloves from Premier Protective Gear, it will have to pay $100,000 for 10,000 boxes of masks, so Premier Protective Gear cannot charge more than $80,000 for 10,000 boxes of gloves. Since Premier's costs would amount to $70,000, it can charge that price and still earn a profit. The bundled discount is not exclusionary with respect to Family Practice Associates.

Now consider Internal Medicine Associates. Internal Medicine Associates buys 5,000 boxes of gloves and 15,000 boxes of masks. If it buys everything from Medical Equipment, it pays $180,000. In order for Premier Protective Gear to sell gloves to Internal Medicine Associates, it cannot charge more than $30,000 because Internal Medicine Associates will have to pay $150,000 for the masks. Premier's cost of producing 5,000 units is $35,000, so it cannot make the sale. As we can see, the bundled discount is exclusionary for Internal Medicine Associates.

This example illustrates two peculiarities of the discount attribution test. First, precisely the same bundled discount schedule forecloses a single-product rival from Internal Medicine's business, but not from Family Practice's business. To some extent, it is not the schedule that is exclusionary. Instead, it is the pattern of business.

Second, this example illustrates the Ninth Circuit's admonition in Peace Health that the bundled discount can be exclusionary even when the multiproduct seller earns positive profits on all products at the discounted price. The case of Internal Medicine Associates illustrates this proposition. Medical Equipment realizes sales revenues of $45,000 for its latex gloves while its costs are only $35,000, so the company earns a profit of $10,000 on its sale of gloves. On its sale of masks, the company receives $135,000 while incurring a cost of $105,000, for a profit of $30,000.

Anomaly 2: Small Bundled Discounts May Be Exclusionary

If a seller offers a broad product line, a relatively small discount – if bundled – can be exclusionary. The 3M discussion in Section 5.2 illustrates this proposition.

Anomaly 3: Discounts May Become Exclusionary When Product Breadth Increases

There are circumstances in which a bundled discount schedule is not exclusionary but becomes exclusionary when the firm expands its product line.

Suppose that Medical Equipment Co. sells surgical gowns and gloves. The SurgiCenter buys $100,000 worth of gowns and $100,000 worth of latex gloves at list prices. If SurgiCenter buys all its requirements from Medical Equipment, it receives a 10 percent discount. In that event, its net cost is $180,000. If SurgiCenter buys its gloves from Premier Protective Gear, which sells only gloves, SurgiCenter will have to pay the list price of $100,000 for its surgical gowns to Medical Equipment. If Premier Protective Gear's cost of supplying the gloves is $75,000, it can make the sale to SurgiCenter at a price of, say, $79,000 and still earn a profit of $4,000. SurgiCenter is better off because it pays $100,000 for the gowns and $79,000 for the gloves. In this case, the bundled discount is not exclusionary.

Suppose that Medical Equipment adds another product to its line, say, surgical masks. Assume that SurgiCenter buys $100,000 worth of each product at list prices, but the company earns a 10 percent discount only if it buys all three existing products from Medical Equipment. By adding a third product to its line, Medical Equipment's bundled discount schedule becomes exclusionary. If SurgiCenter pays a total of $200,000 for its gowns and masks, Premier Protective Gear cannot charge more than $70,000 for the gloves. Since its cost is $75,000, this is not economically feasible. Consequently, a non-exclusionary discount schedule may become exclusionary when the discounter expands its product offerings.

Anomaly 4: Discounts May Stop Being Exclusionary When an Excluded Rival Increases Its Product Breadth

An exclusionary bundled discount schedule may become non-exclusionary when the previously excluded rival expands its product offerings. In the previous example, the bundled discount schedule was exclusionary when Medical Equipment Co. offered three products and Premier Protective Gear offered only one. Suppose Premier Protective Gear adds gowns to its line. If Premier can take away all of Medical Equipment's gloves and gowns business, it will not be excluded.

SurgiCenter will have to pay full fare for the masks, which is $100,000. Premier Protective Gear can charge as much as $170,000 for the gowns and gloves and make SurgiCenter whole while still earning a profit of $20,000 since its costs are $150,000. Once again, a bundled discount schedule is exclusionary or not depending on the circumstances. Consequently, public policy cannot focus simply on the schedule itself.

Anomaly 5: Discounts May Exclude All Rivals Even When the Multiproduct Firm Makes Positive Profits

The discount attribution test may find that the discount excludes rivals on all products at the same time even though the company earns substantial profits on each product. The following example illustrates this point.

Suppose that SurgiCenter buys latex gloves, surgical masks, and gowns worth $100,000 each at the list price offered by Medical Equipment Co. The cost of each product is $75,000. If SurgiCenter buys all of its gloves, masks, and gowns from Medical Equipment, it earns a 10 percent discount. Otherwise, it receives no discount. If SurgiCenter buys everything from Medical Equipment, SurgiCenter pays a net amount of $270,000 and Medical Equipment earns profits of $15,000 on each product, for a total of $45,000.

If Premier Protective Gear is an equally efficient producer of latex gloves, it will be excluded because it would have to sell gloves to SurgiCenter for no more than $70,000 while its costs would amount to $75,000. If Masks R Us, an equally efficient producer of masks, attempts to sell surgical masks to SurgiCenter, it will not be able to charge more than $70,000 for the masks. But it cannot charge this amount since its costs are $75,000. The company is excluded from this book of business. Better Gowns, Inc., will find itself in the same boat as Premier Protective Gear and Masks R Us. Consequently, the bundled discount schedule may be deemed exclusionary with respect to each single product rival while Medical Equipment Co. earns positive profits of $15,000 on each of the three items.

Summary

These hypothetical examples demonstrate that the competitive effects of bundled discounts are not always procompetitive and not always anticompetitive. As such, any analysis of bundled discounts will necessarily require a rule-of-reason approach. Per se rules are only appropriate when a business practice is invariably anticompetitive. For example, a naked price-fixing agreement invariably results in higher prices, lower output, and consumer harm. These effects need not be proven over and over. Instead, they can be presumed. The economic consequences of bundled discounts are not so predictable. In some instances, bundled discounts will prove to be anticompetitive. In other cases, they will be ruled procompetitive. Antitrust challenges to bundled discounts must be considered on a case-by-case basis, that is, with a rule-of-reason approach.

5.5 ANTITRUST TREATMENT OF BUNDLED DISCOUNTS

A multiproduct firm that bundles its discounts is engaged in unilateral conduct. Consequently, a plaintiff must rely on Section 2 of the Sherman Act, which forbids monopolizing conduct and attempts to monopolize the market. The Supreme Court set out a two-prong test for illegal monopolization in its *Grinnell* decision:

> The offense of monopoly under § 2 of the Sherman Act has two elements: (1) the possession of monopoly power in the relevant market and (2) the willful acquisition or maintenance of that power as distinguished from growth or development as a consequence of a superior product, business acumen, or historic accident.[14]

According to the Supreme Court, the existence and possibly the exercise of monopoly power is a necessary but not sufficient condition for a Section 2 violation of the Sherman Act. Illegality also requires monopolizing conduct. Attempts to monopolize are unlawful if the defendant has engaged in exclusionary conduct and is close to achieving actual monopoly. In its *Spectrum Sports* decision, the Supreme Court explained:

> Consistent with our cases, it is generally required that to demonstrate attempted monopolization a plaintiff must prove (1) that the defendant has engaged in predatory or anticompetitive conduct with (2) a specific intent to monopolize and (3) a dangerous probability of achieving monopoly power. In order to determine whether there is a dangerous probability of monopolization, courts have found it necessary to consider the relevant market and the defendant's ability to lessen or destroy competition in that market.[15]

The conduct element of this test is the same as the monopolizing conduct element of the *Grinnell* test.[16]

In *PeaceHealth*, there were two markets: the market for tertiary care and the market for primary and secondary care. Since

---

[14] *United States* v. *Grinnell Corps.*, 384 US 563, 570–71 (1966).

[15] *Spectrum Sports, Inc.* v. *McQuillan*, 506 US 447, 456 (1993).

[16] Note that the same standard applies to predatory pricing. The Areeda-Turner test uses a standard comparing price relative to average variable cost to test whether the prices are predatory. This same comparison has arisen in the analysis of bundled discounts.

PeaceHealth was the only provider of tertiary care in the local market, an antitrust court would surely conclude that it was a monopolist. PeaceHealth, however, did not appear to have employed monopolizing conduct in the market for tertiary acute care hospital services. As a result, there was no antitrust problem in the market for tertiary care.

In contrast, PeaceHealth arguably engaged in exclusionary conduct in the market for primary and secondary acute care hospital services. By bundling its discounts, PeaceHealth arguably made it unprofitable for McKenzie to compete for certain books of business.

The Ninth Circuit's discount attribution test must be applied on a case-by-case basis (i.e., using a rule-of-reason approach) because the bundled discount schedule itself is not exclusionary in all circumstances. As we have seen in the examples above, the schedule may or may not be exclusionary depending upon the specific set of circumstances.

Unbundling the Discounts

If the seller is required to unbundle the discounts, an equally efficient rival cannot be excluded. Moreover, unbundling is apt to lead to lower net prices. To see this, return to the example involving Medical Equipment Co., which sold gowns, gloves, and masks pursuant to a 10 percent bundled discount schedule. Three specialized firms were excluded even though they were equally efficient (Anomaly 5). If the discounts were unbundled, the specialized producers would not be excluded. In addition, the net price for each item in the bundle would fall from $9.00 to $7.50 due to price competition.

Bundled discounts can be exclusionary because the lost discounts on the uncontested goods must be made up with additional discounts on the contested goods. Once the discounts are unbundled, there are no lost discounts. Thus, an equally efficient rival can match any non-predatory price.

But an antitrust rule that prohibits bundling seems a bit extreme. There are numerous examples of competitively innocent bundled discounts that benefit consumers by decreasing total costs.

Value meals at a fast-food restaurant cost less than the items in the meal purchased separately. The per-game cost of a season ticket may be below the sum of the ticket prices purchased individually. Buy-one-get-one offers at the grocery store involve implicit 50 percent discounts that are not available on an unbundled basis. An antitrust ban on such bundling seems unwarranted, so such a rule cannot be the answer. For the time being, the discount attribution test is the standard to evaluate bundled discounts. Even with its anomalies, the test is a useful tool for determining whether an equally efficient rival would be excluded.

5.6 CONCLUDING REMARKS

Bundled discounts are confusing. They have the appearance of being procompetitive since customers who buy all of their requirements from the seller offering a bundled discount schedule pay reduced prices for all of the items. As a result, the customer's production and distribution costs are reduced below the levels that would be incurred without the discounts. In most circumstances, the customer will pass on at least some of the cost savings to consumers. Consequently, consumer welfare rises.

In some – but not all – circumstances, the procompetitive benefits are a mirage. Bundling protects substantial profit margins from competition that would yield superior outcomes. Unfortunately, fashioning an antitrust remedy is not easy. A per se rule is obviously not appropriate. Instead, a rule-of-reason inquiry and the Ninth Circuit's discount attribution test may be better suited for analyzing bundled discounts.

REFERENCE

Blair, Roger D., and David T. Knight. (2020). Bundled Discounts, Loyalty Discounts, and Antitrust Policy. *Rutgers Business Law Review* 16: 123–139.

PART II Seller Cartels

In Part I, we introduced monopoly, which is a single seller of a good or service. We explained how a monopolist maximizes its profit by reducing its quantity below the competitive quantity so that it can increase prices. Consumers are worse off, deadweight welfare loss exists, and the monopolist earns profit. But the excess profit that the monopolist earns attracts competing firms. Unless protected by a patent or government regulation, a monopolist will soon see its profits eroded by entry of other firms into the market. In Part II, we discuss the interactions between multiple sellers in a market. We focus on collusion, which occurs when sellers cooperate, rather than compete, with one another to achieve monopoly profits, to the detriment of consumers.

When no collusion exists, sellers compete for customers by decreasing their prices to undercut their rivals. In a competitive market, this action drives prices to marginal cost, and the sellers in the market no longer make any economic profit. It is understandable that sellers would want to avoid this outcome. When firms collude, they form a seller cartel. Cooperating either overtly or tacitly, sellers cut their quantities in order to raise their prices to the profit-maximizing industry price – the monopoly price. Then the profits are shared among the sellers in the cartel. Unfortunately, this behavior leads to the familiar social welfare loss and consumer harm. But a legal remedy exists. Overt collusion is per se unlawful under Section 1 of the Sherman Act. Moreover, victims of collusion are entitled to recover compensation for the antitrust harm.

Chapter 6 provides an overview of collusion in health care industries and highlights various types of collusive activity. The most common form of collusion is price fixing, where firms agree to sell their products at a specific price. Naturally, this price is the monopoly price. This conduct has occurred among physician groups, hospitals, pharmaceutical manufacturers, and many others. But cartels also collude on other factors. For example, some hospitals have agreed not to compete on advertising.[1] Another form of collusion is market allocation, where firms allocate specific shares of the market. In other words, each firm becomes its own monopolist within its allotted market. The allocation may be geographic, as is often the case with health insurers, or product related.

In Chapter 7, we discuss an alleged price-fixing conspiracy in detail. Rather than competing to drive down prices of generic drugs, more than 26 generic drug producers allegedly colluded to raise the prices of more than 160 drugs. These price increases were quite substantial, with prices rising by an average of 448 percent![2] Some generic drug companies have already paid millions of dollars to settle criminal investigations by the Department of Justice. In this chapter, we discuss the incentives to collude and the mechanics of collusion, as well as antitrust remedies to minimize the frequency of collusive agreements.

Chapter 8 discusses a collusive strategy that is unique to the pharmaceutical industry. In attempting to lengthen the life of their patents, brand-name drug manufacturers (pioneer firms) have paid generic drug manufacturers (generic firms) to delay their entry into the drug market. Due to provisions in the Hatch-Waxman Act of 1984, these payments take the form of reverse payments. Pioneer firms sue generic firms for patent infringement and then settle in reverse; that is, the pioneer firm, who is the plaintiff, agrees to pay the generic firm, the defendant, to stay out of the market. The pioneer firm maintains its monopoly profits and the generic firm gets paid – to

---

[1] *U.S. and State of Michigan* v. *Hillsdale Community Health Center*, No. 2:15-cv-12311 (E.D. Mich. 2015).

[2] *State of Connecticut* v. *Teva Pharmaceuticals*, No. 3:19-cv-00710 (D.C. Conn. 2019), Complaint.

the detriment of consumers who pay higher prices. Fortunately, this practice has been condemned by the antitrust Agencies.

High prices in the pharmaceutical industry may not necessarily arise from collusion that is per se unlawful. Insulin prices have been rising at an alarming rate over the past two decades, and many diabetic patients struggle to afford these life-saving medications. We offer two explanations for this rise in prices in Chapter 9. First, the major insulin firms may be unilaterally pricing their insulin products to maximize profits. When firms act unilaterally, victims of anticompetitive harm have no recourse. Second, pharmaceutical benefit managers may be encouraging increased list prices in order to profit on higher rebates.

Firms can also collude by excluding their rivals. For example, official state licensing boards have substantial power to exclude competitors. These boards are presumably put in place by each individual state to ensure that charlatans cannot practice medicine. But the incentive to reduce competition by revoking licenses or preventing unlicensed competition may be too tempting for the board physicians to resist. In Chapter 10, we discuss this perverse incentive and consider whether state regulation through the state action doctrine is sufficient to mitigate anticompetitive harm.

In summary, collusion can be just as harmful as monopoly. Fortunately, however, victims of collusion among sellers are able to sue to recover antitrust damages. But deterring collusion is a much better solution. When enforcement is swift and severe, collusive behavior is disincentivized, thereby reducing the number of seller cartels and preventing new ones from forming.

6   Collusion in Health
     Care Markets

6.1   INTRODUCTION

In *The Wealth of Nations*, Adam Smith observed that "people of the same trade seldom meet together, even for merriment and diversion, but the conversation ends in a conspiracy against the public, or in some contrivance to raise prices."[1] As we will see, Smith's warning has stood the test of time. More than 240 years later, we find such conspiracies among physicians, hospitals, pharmaceutical manufacturers, medical device producers, health insurers, and many others. Their contrivances to raise prices add billions of dollars to US expenditures on health care.

We begin with a simple economic model of a price-fixing cartel. This model reveals the collusive impact on price, quantity, and social welfare while highlighting the effect on the distribution of wealth between health care consumers and the conspirators. In Section 6.3, we examine collusion among physicians and surgeons and look at staff privileges. In Section 6.4, we consider collusion among hospitals, which often takes the form of noncompete and exclusionary agreements. We then review collusion among pharmaceutical manufacturers in Section 6.5, among medical device manufacturers in Section 6.6, and among health insurers in Section 6.7. We close with concluding remarks in Section 6.8.

6.2   A BASIC CARTEL MODEL

A price-fixing cartel is a collection of legally independent economic entities that band together in order to emulate a multiplant

---

[1] Smith, Book 1, Chapter X (I.10.82) (1776).

monopoly.[2] The entities, or firms, must follow several steps to successfully accomplish this objective. First, the firms must agree to collude rather than compete. Since collusion is unlawful, this is a bold step for firms that have been (possibly) fierce competitors. Second, the cartel members must reach an agreement on the collusive price, the total output, and the output of each cartel member. In addition, the firms must agree on how to divide the economic profits that collusion yields. A third task is devising a plan for implementing the cartel agreement.[3] Fourth, the cartel will have to find a way to monitor the conduct of its members and punish those who cheat.[4] This final step is an extremely important one because cheating will appear to be profitable. If every firm cheats, however, there will be overproduction and losses rather than profits.

Cartel Profit Function

The cartel's profit function can be written as

$$\Pi = P(Q)Q - C_1(q_1) - C_2(q_2) - \cdots - C_n(q_n),$$

where Π denotes profit, $P(Q)$ is the inverse demand, Q is the total quantity, $C_i(q_i)$ is the ith firm's total cost function, and q_i is the output of firm i. Of course, $Q = q_1 + q_2 + \cdots + q_n$.

The first-order conditions for the maximum profit are

$$\frac{\partial \Pi}{\partial q_i} = \left(P(Q) + Q\frac{dP}{dQ} \right) \frac{\partial Q}{\partial q_i} - \frac{dC_i}{dq_i} = 0 \quad \text{for all } i = 1, 2, \ldots, n.$$

One solution to the cartel's problem is to solve these first-order conditions and instruct each cartel member to produce and sell the output where its marginal cost equals marginal revenue and keep whatever profit it earns. This is most likely to be satisfactory when

---

[2] Agreements among rivals to refrain from competing on any dimension are per se violations of Section 1 of the Sherman Act. Chapter 2 provides additional details.

[3] This is an oversimplification since quality, service, credit terms, location, ambiance, insurance coverage, and a multitude of other dimensions are important as well.

[4] For some useful insights, see Stigler (1964) and Ayres (1987).

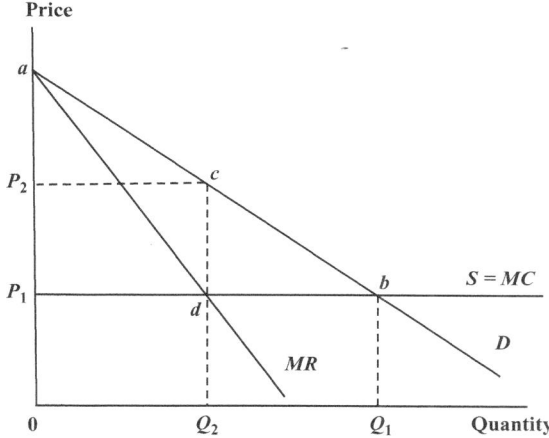

FIGURE 6.1 Competition and collusion

the cost functions are identical or nearly so. When this is not the case, some cartel members will earn more – perhaps much more – than others, which could result in dissatisfaction and cartel instability.[5]

Figures 6.1 and 6.2 illustrate the economic effects of the collusion for the cartel and for its individual members. If the preconspiracy market structure was competitive, market forces would have established a competitive price (P_1) and output (Q_1), where demand (D) and supply (S) are equal, as in Figure 6.1. In a competitive market, each economic entity proceeds as though its decision will have no discernible effect on price. Thus, individual firm demand appears to be perfectly elastic at the competitive price (P_1). Each firm will produce where marginal cost (MC) equals the equilibrium price. At this output, $P_1 = MC$ and $P_1 = AC$, where AC is average cost. Thus, economic profits will equal zero.

If the cartel maximizes profit, it will restrict output from Q_1 to Q_2 as depicted in Figure 6.1. As a result of the reduced output, the price will be bid up to P_2. In order to make this price stick, each

<hr />

[5] Even when the cost functions of the cartel members are identical, some members may still be dissatisfied. After all, one cannot have too much money.

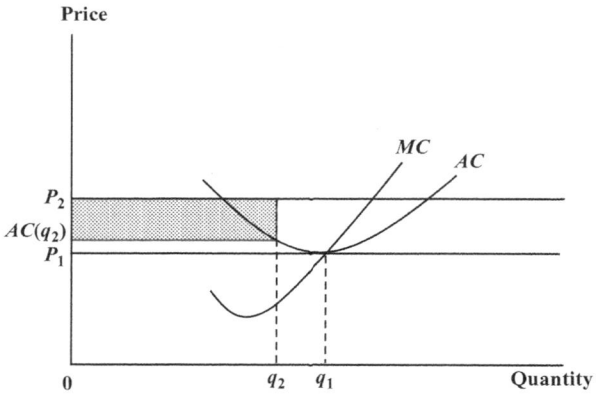

FIGURE 6.2 Profit of a colluding firm

member of the cartel will have to restrict its output from q_1 to q_2. At the
cartel price P_2, price exceeds average cost and the firm depicted in
Figure 6.2 will earn a positive economic profit: $\Pi = (P_2 - AC(q_2))q_2$,
which is shown as the shaded rectangle in Figure 6.2.

Welfare Loss of Collusion

Collusion in health care markets benefits the colluding health care
providers at the expense of patients and society as a whole. Recall that
social welfare is maximized at the competitive equilibrium. The
collusive output restriction leads to a deadweight social welfare loss.

In the absence of collusion, Figure 6.1 shows consumer surplus
is equal to the triangular area abP_1, which in this case is also equal to
total social welfare since there is no producer surplus. In the absence
of externalities, competition leads to the maximization of social welfare. In this example, the competitive output (Q_1) is sold at a competitive price (P_1) and social welfare is area abP_1. No other price and
output will lead to a larger measure of social welfare.

Since a price-fixing cartel acts like a monopolist, the welfare
consequences are similar. In Figure 6.1, we can see that the marginal
value of an additional unit of output at Q_2 (as measured by the height
of the demand curve) exceeds the marginal cost (as measured by the

height of the supply curve). Consequently, the firm should produce that additional unit. The same can be said for all units of output between Q_1 and Q_2. Thus, the welfare loss resulting from collusion is given by the triangular area cbd in Figure 6.1.

Not only does collusion shrink the total surplus due to allocative inefficiency, but it also redistributes the surplus away from patients and to the colluding providers. This can be seen in Figure 6.1. When the health care providers were competing, the consumer (the patient) surplus was equal to area abP_1. With collusion, consumer surplus shrinks to acP_2. Some of the reduction is lost due to the inefficiency, but area P_2cdP_1 is converted into health care provider surplus.

6.3   COLLUSION AMONG PHYSICIANS AND SURGEONS

There are numerous examples of collusion among physicians and/or surgeons. Some of those examples fit the cartel model in the preceding section quite well. In those cases, the colluders agree to raise the price with an attendant decrease in the services they provide. Allegations of collusion in staff privilege cases, however, are a bit different. In these cases, a rival is excluded from the market. With a reduced supply, the usual market forces lead to higher fees for the remaining physicians.

Physician Practice Groups[6]

Allegations of collusion among physicians often arise when independent practice groups and sole practitioners join forces to negotiate reimbursement rates with health insurers.[7] Health insurers and other

---

[6] In Chapter 12, we discuss situations where allowing physicians to bargain improves social welfare. Whether this collective bargaining is procompetitive depends on the monopsony power of the health insurers.

[7] In *FTC* v. *Indiana Federation of Dentists*, 476 US 447 (1986), a group of dentists tried to unionize so they could collectively refuse to accept oversight of their professional judgment by dental insurers. Since dentists are not employees, they do not enjoy antitrust immunity under the non-statutory labor exemption. Consequently, their horizontal agreement was found to be a violation of Section 1 of the Sherman Act.

managed care organizations try to negotiate the lowest possible reimbursement rates. Success in this regard reduces claims payments, thereby making the insurer more profitable and/or more competitive.[8] While these results benefit the insurance companies and their policyholders, the physicians are worse off. The reduction in their practice profits provides an incentive to take action. In *Carlsbad Physician Association (CPA)*, for example, independent physicians in the Carlsbad, New Mexico, area agreed among themselves to allow CPA to negotiate fees and other terms with third-party payers.[9] Since some 76 percent of all physicians in the Carlsbad area were members of CPA, the health insurers could not avoid dealing with CPA. According to the FTC, fees were elevated above non-collusive levels. This, of course, disadvantaged patients as their health care costs rose. This adverse impact also resulted in higher health insurance premiums since claims costs also rose.

When three independent orthopedic groups joined forces in an independent practice association called Professional Orthopedic Services, the economic issues were similar to those in *Carlsbad Physician Association*. Three practice groups – the Bone and Joint Clinic of Baton Rouge, the Baton Rouge Orthopedic Clinic, and Orthopedic Surgery Associates of Baton Rouge – accounted for some 70 percent of orthopedic services in the local Baton Rouge market. Consequently, third-party payers had to deal with Professional Orthopedic Services or forgo offering orthopedic services to their policyholders. In response to proposed price reductions for their services by United HealthCare, the group collectively decided to terminate their contracts with United HealthCare and negotiate for better rates. Reimbursement rates rose by 34 percent due to the conspiracy. According to the FTC, the price-fixing agreement

---

[8] Defendants often argue that they join forces only to create countervailing power to offset the monopsony (buying) power of large health insurers. See Chapter 12 for further analysis.

[9] *Carlsbad Physician Association Inc.*, Do. No. C-4081 (2003). In the Final Order, CPA settled and was dissolved.

caused health care costs for patients in Baton Rouge to rise above the non-collusive level.[10]

In most circumstances, collusion among health care providers has no redeeming virtues. The traditional economic objection to collusion rests on the allocative inefficiency that results in the deadweight social welfare losses. A related concern is the transfer of wealth (and welfare) from patients to the colluding health care providers. On either count, collusion is undesirable. Consequently, antitrust policy treats collusion with the hostility that it richly deserves. As explained in Chapter 2, collusion is a per se violation of Section 1 of the Sherman Act. Members of the price-fixing ring may face criminal sanctions – fines and prison sentences.

Staff Privileges[11]

Hospitals and physicians provide complementary services in treating patients. The hospital needs assurances that a physician is well qualified and, therefore, withholds the privilege of practicing at its facility until the physician's credentials have been reviewed by a hospital board generally comprised of currently employed physicians. Once a patient has been admitted to a hospital, he or she can be treated only by those physicians who have been granted *staff privileges*. For many specialties, physicians or surgeons must have staff privileges at a hospital in order to effectively practice. A cardiologist, for example, is apt to have patients who must be hospitalized. In order to treat his or her patients in the hospital, the cardiologist must have staff privileges. One way for a coalition of physicians to prevent or reduce competition is to deny staff privileges to a would-be competitor.[12] The costs and benefits of such collusion can be illustrated graphically.

---

[10] Federal Trade Commission (2003). The proposed consent order barred the members of Professional Orthopedic Services from negotiating jointly with health insurers.

[11] Chapter 10 examines occupational licensing, which involves similar economic concerns.

[12] The exclusion of rivals is not confined to physicians. In *Archer and White Sales, Inc.* v. *Henry Schein, Inc.*, No. 878 F.3d 488 (5th Cir. 2017), the plaintiff accused six distributors of dental supplies and equipment of excluding it from the market.

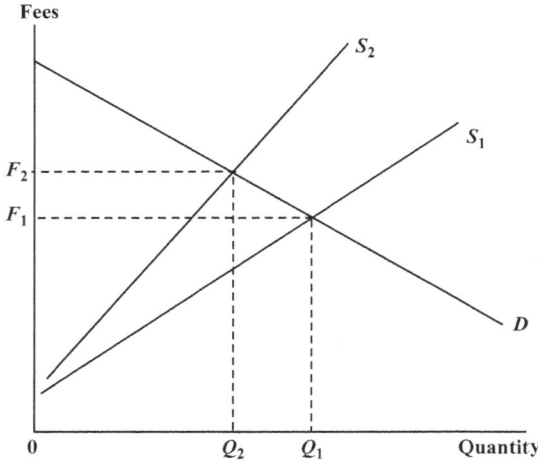

FIGURE 6.3 Eliminating rivals leads to higher prices and profits

In Figure 6.3, demand for physician services is D and the supply of such services, including all qualified physicians, is S_1. Competition results in a fee of F_1 and a quantity of services offered of Q_1. As usual, the competitive solution maximizes social welfare.

If a coalition of physicians can eliminate one or more rivals, the supply curve will rotate to S_2. Now, the interaction of demand and the new supply curve yields a higher fee equal to F_2 and a reduced quantity of services equal to Q_2. This higher fee, of course, improves the profits of the colluding physicians at the expense of the excluded physician(s). Patients suffer in two ways: (1) they pay higher fees and (2) they receive less medical care. Thus, we should be somewhat suspicious when staff privileges have been denied or withdrawn.

The case of *Boczar* v. *Manatee Memorial Hospital and Health System, Inc.* provides an illustrative example.[13] A number of obstetricians/gynecologists (OB/GYNs) who had been on staff at the Manatee Memorial Hospital defected to another local hospital. Since the

---

[13] 731 F. Supp. 1042 (M.D. Fla. 1990). To the extent that it is relevant, Roger Blair served as an economic expert on behalf of Dr. Boczar. For an antitrust analysis of collusive quality reduction, see Blair and Durrance (2014).

hospital revenue depended in part on the patients of OB/GYN providers, Manatee Memorial was concerned that it would experience a drop in business. Consequently, the hospital began a recruiting effort, which resulted in Dr. Linda Boczar's addition to the Manatee Memorial staff.

Linda Boczar was a successful OB/GYN in Sarasota, Florida, which is about 15 miles from Manatee Memorial. After agreeing to join the Manatee Memorial obstetrics staff, Dr. Boczar opened an office in Bradenton, Florida, and began practicing in both cities. Dr. Boczar posed a competitive threat to the other OB/GYNs on staff at Manatee Memorial for three reasons. First, Dr. Boczar was the only female OB/GYN in Manatee County, which may have been an important quality consideration for some patients. Second, Dr. Boczar's frequency of cesarean delivery was far below the average of her male competitors. In a very real sense, type of delivery is a matter of quality. Finally, when Dr. Boczar did perform a cesarean, she did not charge a premium for the delivery. This made her average prices lower than those of her male competitors, who typically charged more for a cesarean. Thus, Dr. Boczar provided (arguably) higher-quality service and charged lower (average) prices. Her male rivals could not have competed on gender grounds, but they certainly could have responded to the lower cesarean rate and to her lower prices. Instead, they simply excluded her from the market by having her staff privileges suspended.

For its part, the hospital also had an economic incentive to exclude Dr. Boczar. It had recruited her in the first place because a substantial number of OB/GYNs had defected to another hospital that competed directly with Manatee Memorial. It feared further defections since many of the remaining OB/GYNs openly opposed granting privileges to Dr. Boczar. In addition, Dr. Boczar clashed with the hospital shortly after joining its medical staff when she was critical of the hospital's emergency department. Even though Dr. Boczar brought business to the hospital, on balance, her presence became inconsistent with the hospital's economic interests. Ultimately,

Dr. Boczar's staff privileges were suspended and she resigned. Subsequently, Dr. Boczar filed an antitrust suit alleging a violation of Section 1 of the Sherman Act and claimed antitrust damages. At trial, the grounds for her suspension were found to be pretextual by the jury and she was awarded damages.[14]

6.4   COLLUSION AMONG HOSPITALS

Allegations of collusion among hospitals fall into two categories. In some cases, the colluding hospitals reach agreements that limit competition among themselves. In other cases, some hospitals agree with third parties to exclude a competing hospital or hospitals.

Agreements Not to Compete

US and State of Michigan v. *Hillsdale Community Health Center*[15] provides an example of an alleged agreement not to compete. In this case, the Department of Justice filed suit against four Michigan hospitals. In addition to Hillsdale Community Health Center, the defendants included Community Health Center of Branch County, Promedica Health System, Inc., and W. A. Foote Memorial Hospital, D/B/A Allegiance Health. These four hospitals were the only general acute care hospitals in their region.

The hospitals agreed not to advertise in one another's territory. The impact of such an agreement on prices for acute care hospital services is not as dramatic as a typical price-fixing agreement. Nonetheless, it is an agreement to refrain from competing for new business. To the extent that it is successful, each hospital would enjoy some pricing discretion and prices would rise, which would increase hospital profits.[16] But such an agreement harmed patients, who were

---

[14] This, of course, is not to say that all denials or suspensions of staff privileges are pretextual. Most are aimed at ensuring quality care for the patient, but some of them may be motivated by self-interest.

[15] No. 2:15-cv-12311 (E.D. Mich. 2015).

[16] The hospitals argued that no adverse competitive effects had materialized as a result of their collusion.

deprived of free health screenings and education along with information about the services offered at various hospitals, which would have allowed them to make more informed health care decisions. In this case, the hospitals settled and the parties agreed that they would no longer collude with one another.

Agreements to Exclude Rivals

In *Kissing Camels Surgery Center* v. *Centura Health Corporation*, the plaintiffs alleged that Centura conspired with health insurers to exclude the plaintiffs' ambulatory surgery centers from the Colorado market.[17] At Centura's request, insurers refused to directly negotiate network agreements with the plaintiffs. Additionally, they penalized physicians who referred patients to the plaintiffs.[18]

Similarly, in *Bristow Endeavor Health Center* v. *Blue Cross and Blue Shield Association et al.*, Bristow alleged that two of its largest medical center rivals had conspired with Blue Cross Blue Shield (BCBS) to fix prices and exclude Bristow's Center for Orthopedic Reconstruction and Excellence (CORE) from the Oklahoma market.[19] When Bristow wanted to add its newly opened CORE to its BCBS network, it was met with an alleged conspiracy between BCBS and its health care rivals to exclude CORE. Bristow claims that they performed fewer surgeries at lower reimbursement rates due to the conspiracy. To the extent that a rival is actively excluded from the market, prices are bound to rise at the patient's expense at the

---

[17] *Kissing Camels Surgery Center* v. *Centura Health Corporation et al.*, No. 1:2012-cv-3012, Document 295 (D. Colo. 2015).

[18] In a similar case, Indiana University was alleged to have excluded Dr. Ricardo Vasquez, an independent vascular surgeon, through the use of its internal referral program. Any physician affiliated with Indiana University must refer his or her patients to other physicians in the Indiana University system. Since Indiana Health allegedly had a monopoly in primary care for the region, this could prove quite detrimental for independent doctors looking to serve the market. This independent behavior by Indiana University Health System was challenged under Section 2 of the Sherman Act. *Vasquez* v. *Indiana University Health Inc.*, No. 21-cv-1693 (S.D. Ind. 2021).

[19] No. 16-cv-0057-cve-pjc (N.D. Okla. 2016).

hospitals that have not been excluded.[20] The district court decided the case on behalf of the defendants since they argued that Bristow had not sufficiently proved antitrust injury or the existence of a cartel.

6.5 COLLUSION AMONG PHARMACEUTICAL MANUFACTURERS[21]

Generic drugs are unbranded therapeutically equivalent versions of pioneer drugs whose patent life has expired. Generic drugs must be approved by the Food and Drug Administration, but they do not require the extensive and expensive testing that is required for pioneer drugs.[22] In many cases, the production cost of pharmaceutical drugs is quite low. Consequently, the price of a generic drug may be substantially below the price of the pioneer drug prior to the patent expiration. Demand for the generic version of some drugs remains quite high and thereby provides an incentive for generic drug producers to collude and avoid competition.

This can be seen in Figure 6.4, where D represents demand, MR is the associated marginal revenue, and MC is the marginal cost of production. With competition, price will be P_1, which is equal to marginal cost, and the quantity sold will be Q_1. If the generic producers collude, the profit-maximizing price will soar to P_2 and the quantity will fall to Q_2. The colluding producers will share the economic profit of $(P_2 - MC)Q_2$.

Note, however, that this profit is made possible by restricting output from Q_1 to Q_2. This difference represents medication that was not taken; thus, the profits come at the expense of pain and suffering.

---

[20] It is not clear how the health insurance company benefits from reduced competition among the hospitals.

[21] Chapter 7 has a more detailed account of generic price-fixing cartels. Chapter 9 has a more detailed account of the alleged insulin cartel.

[22] See Chapter 8 for an explanation.

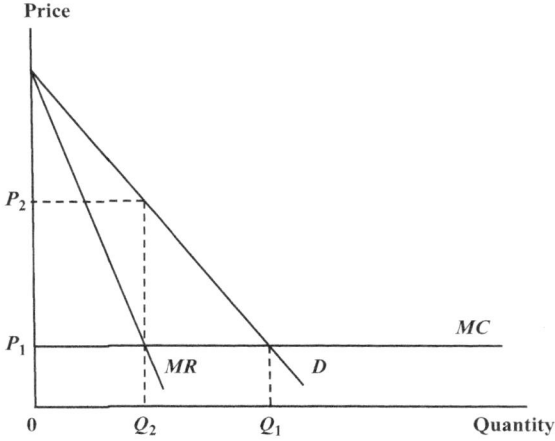

FIGURE 6.4 Collusion results in higher prices and profits

Numerical Example

Suppose that the demand for a pharmaceutical product can be written as

$$P = 1010 - 4Q,$$

where P is price and Q is quantity measured in hundred thousands. In addition, suppose that the marginal and average cost of production is $10. Competition results in marginal cost pricing, so price will be equal to $10 and quantity will be 25 million doses. Each seller earns a competitive return on its investment but earns no economic profit. If the sellers collude, they will reduce output to the point where marginal revenue equals marginal cost:

$$1010 - 8Q = 10.$$

In this case, they will produce 12.5 million doses. At that quantity, the collusive price will be $510. Now, the colluding firms enjoy profits of

$$\Pi = (P - MC)Q = \$62,500;$$

that is, the cartel members will split up $6.25 billion.

The lure of substantial economic profits proved irresistible for many generic drug producers. In 2016–2017, the DOJ conducted a criminal investigation of price fixing by major generic drug firms. The investigation involved about a dozen manufacturers and several dozen drugs. At the same time, private suits were multiplying rapidly. By June 2017, there were 70 private actions filed in four district courts. For reasons of consistency and judicial economy, cases began to be consolidated in MDL (2724), which was named *In re Generic Pharmaceuticals Pricing Litigation*. We discuss this cartel in more detail in Chapter 7.

Collusion in the Market for Diabetes Care

Another interesting example of generic drug producer collusion involves insulin, which is vital to patients with diabetes. Three major producers of insulin – Eli Lilly, Sanofi Aventis, and Novo Nordisk – allegedly conspired with three major pharmacy benefit managers (PBMs) – CVS Health, Express Scripts, and OptumRx.[23] A class of plaintiffs alleged that the PBMs allowed the producers to inflate insulin prices and then shared in the increased profits by taking a percentage of the higher rebates that they negotiated from the producers.[24] We discuss this in more detail in Chapter 9.

Another case of collusion involved glucose test strips, which diabetics use to maintain the glucose levels in their blood. Some 30 million people suffer from diabetes and spend about $4 billion per year on glucose strips. A class action suit was filed in 2017 against the three largest PBMs and the four leading producers of glucose test strips.[25] The complaint alleged that CVS Health Corporation, Express Scripts Holding, and OptumRx colluded to extort enlarged rebates from Roche Diagnostics, Bayer HealthCare, Abbott Laboratories, and Johnson & Johnson. The manufacturers inflated

---

[23] Chapter 9 explains one potential interpretation of the alleged insulin conspiracy, that is, the role of PBMs in the high price of insulin.

[24] *Boss* v. *CVS Health, Inc. et al.*, No. 3:17-cv-01823 (D. N.J. 2017).

[25] *Prescott* v. *CVS Health Corp.*, No. 2:17-cv-00803 (W.D. Wash. 2017).

the list prices to cover the rebates that were paid to the PBMs. The higher the list price, the higher the rebates and thus the higher the profits to the PBMs. But consumers, especially the uninsured, paid higher prices. The suspicion is that the PBMs encouraged the producers to raise their list prices so the PBMs could earn increased profits from the percentages they take from the higher rebates.

Refusal to Deal

Similar to hospital agreements to exclude rivals, manufacturing firms can also collude to restrict access to necessary components in the supply chain and thereby preclude rivals from producing or selling their product. In *Sandoz* v. *United Therapeutics*,[26] Sandoz alleged that Smiths Medical ASD Inc. and United Therapeutics agreed to withhold access to injection cartridges necessary to sell Sandoz's generic version of Remodulin, which treats pulmonary arterial hypertension. To limit competition for generic Remodulin, the firms used contract clauses that restricted a pharmacy's ability to deliver generic Remodulin with Smiths injection cartridges. Pharmacies would presumably be forced to sell branded Remodulin, which was marketed by United Therapeutics. In this way, Sandoz's generic Remodulin was excluded from the market.

6.6 COLLUSION AMONG MEDICAL DEVICE MANUFACTURERS

The distribution of dental supplies and equipment is highly concentrated. Three distributors, Patterson Cos, Inc., Henry Schein, Inc., and Benco Dental Supply Co., account for more than 80 percent of the dental supply market in the United States. This market structure is conducive to collusion since a cartel is easier to coordinate when fewer firms exist in a market. Not surprisingly, charges of collusion have surfaced. Dentists have filed class action suits accusing the major distributors of dental supplies and equipment of collusion.

---

[26] No. 19-cv-10170 (D. N.J. 2020).

Allegations include price fixing, anti-poaching agreements, and punishment of entities that turned to lower-cost distributors.[27] First, the plaintiffs alleged that the major dental suppliers had agreed to fix profit margins at 35 percent. Second, the defendants agreed not to poach each other's sales employees. Finally, the defendants allegedly threatened dental supply manufacturers if they offered supplies to other entrants into the dental supplies market. Thus, the defendants were allegedly able to prevent entry into the dental supplies market and maintain supra-competitive prices. Collusion has also been observed among other medical device manufacturers.[28]

6.7 COLLUSION AMONG HEALTH INSURERS

The business of insurance, including health insurance, is regulated at the state level. A major concern of the regulators is ensuring that the insurance company has the ability to pay the claims of its policyholders. To that end, insurance rates are filed with the regulator for approval and, once approved, are somewhat immune from allegations of unlawful overcharges. There is, however, mounting concern that health insurance markets are highly concentrated and, therefore, vulnerable to decidedly noncompetitive prices.[29]

Although health insurers may be protected by the "filed-rate" doctrine,[30] they do not have carte blanche to divide markets and thereby create local monopolies. Market allocation, or market

---

[27] *In re Dental Supplies Antitrust Litigation*, No. 16-696 (E.D.N.Y. 2016). The case settled in June 2019 for $80 million.

[28] In China, the antitrust authorities fined Medtronic, PLC, $17.2 million for price fixing. The medical devices at issue involved cardiovascular restorative therapy and diabetes treatments (Reuters 2016).

[29] In an issue brief written for the Commonwealth Fund, Frank and McGuire (2019) find high concentration in nearly all local markets for private Medicare Advantage insurance, which are plans created by private companies that contract with Medicare.

[30] In industries such as insurance, energy, and shipping, firms must file and obtain approval of their rates from a government agency, which is known as the filed-rate doctrine. Presumably, since these rates were approved by a third party, the firm should not face antitrust scrutiny. *Square D Co.* v. *Niagara Frontier Tariff Bureau, Inc.*, 476 US 409 (1986).

division, is at the heart of the *In re Blue Cross Blue Shield Antitrust Litigation*.[31] Independent health insurers operating under the BCBS label allegedly divided health insurance markets in an effort to refrain from competing with one another. In 2020, the parties settled for the class action fee of $2.67 billion. The deal also called for a payment of $100 million to the class attorneys who planned to request some 25 percent of the damage award.

As a collusive mechanism, there are some real benefits of market division. First, market division creates local monopolies in each market, meaning that there will be no cheating on the price. Second, since the cartel members cannot compete for the same policyholders, there will be no need for non-price competition that could erode the profits.[32] Third, to the extent that the cartel members do not have the same cost functions, dividing markets will not destabilize the cartel, which is illustrated in Figure 6.5.

Panel (a) of Figure 6.5 shows that the lower-cost insurers would prefer to sell a quantity of Q_1 at a price of P_1. In panel (b), the local demand is the same as that in panel (a), but the insurer's cost of doing business is higher. Consequently, this insurer prefers the higher price, P_2, and a lower quantity, Q_2. If the two insurers considered a price-fixing arrangement, it would be difficult for the firms to agree on the best price–quantity combination. By dividing the market, the two insurers can proceed independently.

So far, we have considered market division based on geographic location, but markets can also be divided by product. A recent example of such market division involved Florida Cancer Specialists (FCS) and one of its rivals. The firms agreed to split the market for cancer treatment in Southwest Florida. FCS would provide medical oncology treatment and refrain from supplying radiation therapy. The rival agreed to refrain from providing medical therapy, but would provide radiation

---

[31] *In re Blue Cross Blue Shield Antitrust Litigation*, No. 2:13-cv-20000 (11th Cir. 2018).

[32] Stigler (1968).

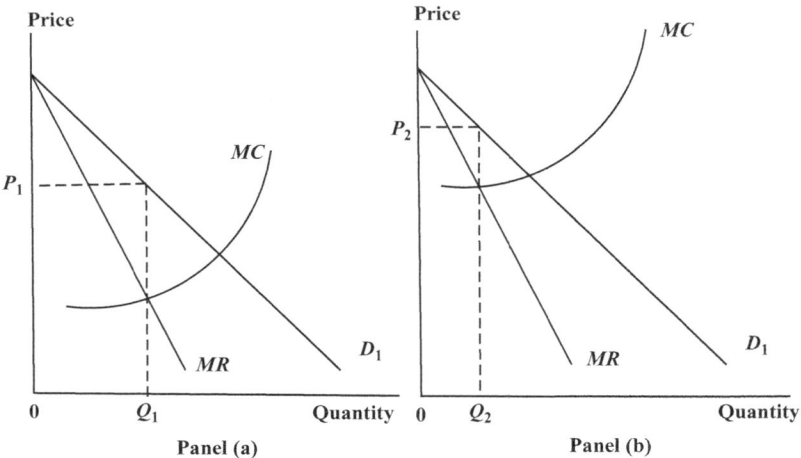

FIGURE 6.5 The effects of marginal cost on price and quantity

therapy. In exchange for deferred prosecution, FCS agreed to pay a $100 million fine. The State of Florida also settled with FCS for $20 million.[33]

6.8   CONCLUDING REMARKS

When otherwise independent firms make joint pricing decisions, those firms are engaged in price fixing, which is a violation of Section 1 of the Sherman Act. Firms can also conspire to make joint decisions on other factors that are similarly anticompetitive, such as decisions about quality or advertising. They can also conspire by dividing markets. Collusive activity in health care markets directly harms health care consumers by raising prices and reducing output relative to the non-collusive outcome. Consumers and society as a whole are worse off in the form of reduced consumer welfare and deadweight social welfare loss. But such harm can be mitigated by effective antitrust enforcement since overt collusion is a per se violation of Section 1 of the Sherman Act. In the next two chapters, we take a closer look at collusive behavior in the generic drugs market and the insulin market.

---

[33] Bolado (2020).

REFERENCES

Ayres, Ian. (1987). How Cartels Punish: A Structural Theory of Self-Enforcing Collusion. *Columbia Law Review* 87: 295–325.

Blair, Roger D., and Christine Piette Durrance. (2014). Restraints on Quality Competition, *Journal of Competition Law and Economics* 10: 27–46.

Bolado, Carolina. (2020). *Fla. Cancer Group Nabs Partial Win in Adventist Antitrust Suit*. Law360. www.law360.com/articles/1316731/fla-cancer-group-nabs-partial-win-in-adventist-antitrust-suit.

Federal Trade Commission. (2003). *FTC Settles Price-Fixing Charges Brought against Baton Rouge Physician Groups and Their Agent*. FTC. www.ftc.gov/news-events/press-releases/2003/07/ftc-settles-price-fixing-charges-brought-against-baton-rouge.

Frank, Richard G., and Thomas G. McGuire. (2019). *Market Concentration and Potential Competition in Medicare Advantage*. Commonwealth Fund. www.commonwealthfund.org/sites/default/files/2019-02/Frank_market_concentration_medicare_advantage_ib_0.pdf.

Reuters. (2016). *China Says Fines Medtronic Local Unit $17.2 Million for Price Fixing*. Reuters. www.reuters.com/article/us-china-antitrust-medtronic-idUSKBN13W2YN.

Smith, Adam. (1776). *The Wealth of Nations*. London: W. Strahan and T. Cadell.

Stigler, George. (1964). A Theory of Oligopoly. *Journal of Political Economy* 72: 44–61.

Stigler, George. (1968). Price and Non-Price Competition. *Journal of Political Economy* 74: 149–154.

7 Collusion in Generic Drug Markets

7.1 INTRODUCTION

When a patent on a pharmaceutical product expires, therapeutically equivalent generic versions of the drug rapidly enter the market, providing consumers with a less expensive alternative. For most generic drugs, the marginal cost of production is quite low and distribution costs are minimal. Consequently, competition among the generic producers ordinarily causes the price of drugs to plummet.[1] This, of course, is socially beneficial as consumers, both insured and uninsured, are considerably better off.[2] Health insurers are also better off because the cost of insurance claims falls. Employers that offer health insurance plans to their employees also benefit as the insurance premiums fall. Nearly everyone gains – except for the pioneer firm whose patent monopoly has expired.

For many generic drugs, however, this scenario has failed to materialize because the generic producers allegedly decided to collude rather than compete. Various state attorneys general have filed complaints against 30 well-known generic drug manufacturers for their alleged collusion involving more than 160 pharmaceutical drugs. Moreover, the Department of Justice has sued some of the same generic manufacturers. The complaints allege a large-scale cartel that engaged in price fixing, customer allocation, and bid rigging in the market for generic drugs. As a result of this conspiracy, prices did not

---

[1] We refer to producers of patented drugs as *pioneer* firms and the producers of generic equivalents as *generic* firms.

[2] The 2019 savings to US consumers due to generic drugs were estimated to be more than $313 billion, an amount close to what was spent on prescription drugs in 2019 ($370 billion; Centers for Medicare & Medicaid Services 2021; Mikulic 2020).

fall, sales did not rise, and the ensuing benefits of competition went up in smoke.

In this chapter, we will examine the alleged price-fixing conspiracies found in a number of generic drug markets. Although litigation is ongoing at the time of this writing, much can be understood about this alleged cartel activity from the filings in this litigation. We will begin in Section 7.2 by describing the benefits provided by generic drugs and their role in the health care industry. In Section 7.3, we examine the incentives for collusion. In Section 7.4, we provide details about the alleged cartel among generic pharmaceutical firms. Section 7.5 discusses the economic consequences of collusion, and Section 7.6 discusses ways of deterring price-fixing behavior. Finally, Section 7.7 provides some concluding remarks.

7.2   THE COMPETITIVE PROMISE
OF GENERIC PHARMACEUTICALS

A pioneer firm's branded drug is insulated from competition for the life of its patent since the patent blocks the entry of imitations. As the patent nears expiration, generic producers often formulate therapeutically equivalent versions of the pioneer brand. According to FDA regulations, for a generic drug to be therapeutically equivalent, the following features must be identical to those of the pioneer drug: active ingredients, route of administration, dosage form, strength, and intended use. The only difference between a pioneer brand and a generic brand should be the name on the label.

Some 35 years ago, generic drugs accounted for only 18.6 percent of all prescriptions, but by 2019, generic drugs accounted for about 90 percent of all prescription drugs sold in the United States.[3] This dramatic change can, in large part, be attributed to the Hatch-Waxman Act of 1984. Prior to the Act, a generic producer would have had to file a New Drug Application (NDA), which required time-

---

[3] *State of Connecticut* v. *Teva Pharmaceuticals*, No. 3:19-cv-00710 (D.C. Conn. 2019), Complaint. See also Berndt and Aiken (2011).

consuming and expensive clinical trials. Under provisions of the Hatch-Waxman Act, generic producers can now file an Abbreviated New Drug Application (ANDA) with the FDA. Generic firms can rely on the pioneer brand's demonstration of the safety and efficacy of the drug, thereby eliminating the need for expensive clinical trials, but those firms must convince the FDA that their products are therapeutically equivalent to those of the pioneer firm. The introduction of ANDAs led to an increase in the number of generic firms entering the market as well as their speed of entry.

The Competitive Promise

All generic versions of a pioneer drug are homogenous. That is, they are precisely the same drug. Therefore, generic firms have no incentive to invest in marketing their products since marketing would raise their costs while benefiting their rivals.[4] Instead, generic firms compete on price. As one would suspect, increased generic entry leads to lower average prices. In general, the more generic firms that enter a market, the lower the price of the generic drug. Figure 7.1 shows how the price ratio of the generic to the pre-entry brand price plummets as firms enter the market.[5] On average, the price of a generic drug is approximately 20 percent of the price of the corresponding pioneer brand, leading to substantial cost savings for patients, health insurers, employers, and even the uninsured.[6]

Competition leads to remarkable cost savings for consumers. In Chapter 3, we considered the drug Sovaldi, which treats hepatitis C. The brand price for this drug was $1,000, and the marginal cost of

---

[4] *State of Connecticut* v. *Teva Pharmaceuticals*, No. 3:19-cv-00710 (D.C. Conn. 2019), Complaint.

[5] Conrad and Lutter (2019) examined pricing for drugs with initial generic entry from 2015 to 2017. There may be some bias due to the alleged cartel, but many of the alleged conspiracies were abandoned after 2014 since the generic firms were being investigated by the government. Note that other studies, such as Dave, Hartzema, and Kesselheim (2017), find a similar trend but different price ratios.

[6] *State of Connecticut* v. *Sandoz Inc.*, No. 3:20-cv-00802 (D.C. Conn. 2020), Complaint.

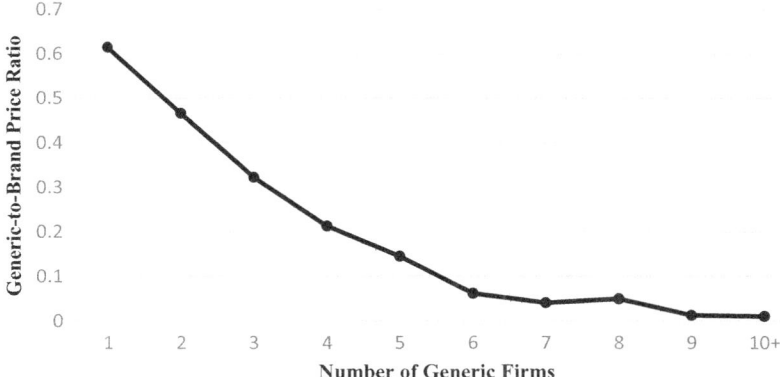

FIGURE 7.1 The influence of generic competition on drug prices
The graph captures prices for drugs with initial entry from 2015 to 2017.
Source: Conrad and Lutter (2019).

the drug may have been approximately $2. In a competitive market, goods are sold at marginal cost. Introducing generic competition could therefore lead to a $998 discount on Sovaldi. Even if the generic market for Sovaldi included only a few competitors, Figure 7.1 suggests that consumers would see substantial discounts.

Based on this competitive promise, states and insurers have implemented policies that incentivize consumers to adopt generic drugs. Some states have introduced mandatory substitution laws, which compel pharmacies to substitute generic drugs for branded drugs when they are less expensive.[7] Presumed consent laws are a complementary state policy allowing pharmacies to make a generic substitution without explicit permission from consumers. Health insurers also want to take advantage of cheaper generic drugs. In many health insurance plans, a policyholder must pay a higher copay with higher cost sharing for a branded drug if an equivalent generic is available.[8] These laws and policies encourage generic substitution,

---

[7] In Florida, for example, "[a] pharmacist who receives a prescription for a brand name drug shall, unless requested otherwise by the purchaser, substitute a less expensive, generically equivalent drug product." FL Stat Section 465.025 (2016).

[8] Frakt (2017).

but they only benefit consumers when the generic drug market works as it is supposed to work.

In the early 2010s, generic drug prices seemed to rise inexplicably. For hundreds of drugs, competition no longer seemed to work. Prices of more than 1,200 drugs increased by an average of 448 percent from 2013 to 2014.[9] Many of these drugs were quite popular; for example, the price of pravastatin, which reduces high cholesterol levels, rose from $27.20 in 2013 to $196 in 2014.[10] In that same year, pravastatin was prescribed about 33 million times, ranking 15th for the most frequently prescribed prescription drug.[11] These price increases may be attributed to price collusion among a cartel of generic manufacturers.[12]

7.3   THE INCENTIVE TO COLLUDE

If a pioneer brand is successful in the market, generic producers will enter once the pioneer firm's patent protection ends. Relative to the pioneer firm's monopoly price, the price of the generic falls precipitously as generic producers enter. As we can see in Figure 7.1, with 10 or more generic rivals, the price approaches marginal and average cost. Eventually, as more firms enter the market, generic firms earn only a competitive return. According to various complaints, many generic producers appear to have been dissatisfied with competitive returns and elected to collude rather than compete.

Collusion on Price

People value their health and allocate large portions of their income to drugs that promote health. Some pharmaceutical drugs are so

---

[9] *State of Connecticut* v. *Teva Pharmaceuticals*, No. 3:19-cv-00710 (D.C. Conn. 2019), Complaint.

[10] Poitras (2019).

[11] In 2014, prescription rates for pravastatin decreased, most likely due to the higher prices. Higher prices and lower quantity go hand in hand, which is corroborated by this example. Statistics were derived from Clincalc (2021).

[12] Apotex, a maker of pravastatin, admitted to conspiring with other generic drug manufacturers to inflate the price of pravastatin and settled with the DOJ for $24.1 million (Benner 2020).

essential that consumer demand is relatively inelastic for those products. As a result, pharmaceutical companies can substantially raise the price of their drugs without seeing a large drop in the quantity that consumers purchase. This implies that firms can profitably charge a price (P) that is generally much greater than the average cost (AC) of producing the product.[13] In other words, the markups can be quite high since consumers are not very price-sensitive when a product benefits their health and well-being.[14] For example, as referenced in Section 7.2, Gilead Sciences could profitably charge a \$998 markup for its drug Sovaldi. By competing, the generic firms lose out on substantial profit. By colluding, however, the generic firms would stand to gain a substantial profit – provided that they are not caught and prosecuted.

The substantial return to collusion is illustrated in Figure 7.2, where D represents the demand for a specific generic drug and MR is the associated marginal revenue. The marginal and average costs are MC and AC. If the generic producers compete on price, Q_1 units will be sold at a price of P_1, which will equal average cost. The firms will earn a competitive return, but no more.

If the producers collude, they will behave like a multiplant monopolist in the short run. Consequently, they will reduce total production from Q_1 to Q_2 and prices will rise from P_1 to P_2. As a result, the firms will split the economic profit equal to $(P_2 - AC)Q_2$. Of course, the details of the cartel operation and the division of the spoils may be complicated, but the collusive pot of gold provides these generic firms with ample incentive to collude rather than compete. There is reason to believe that these illicit profits were irresistible in the markets for generic drugs.

---

[13] Here, we assume that average cost is equal to marginal cost.

[14] In Chapter 3, we discuss how insurance can further blunt a consumer's sensitivity to price changes. If the price of a prescription drug increases, the insurer will absorb a portion of the increase, which lessens the impact that price changes have on the consumer.

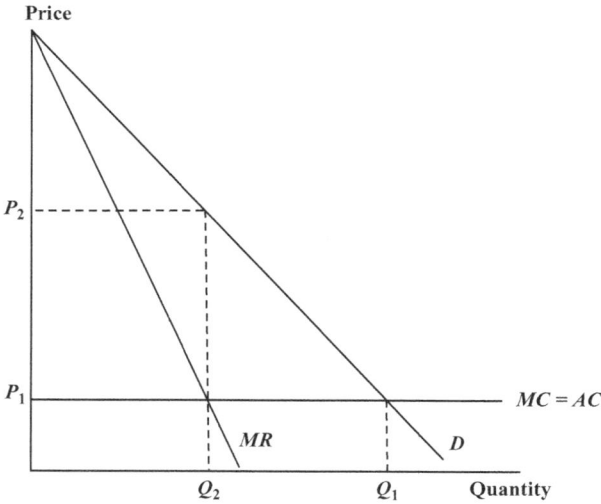

FIGURE 7.2 Collusion results in higher prices and economic profits

7.4   THE ALLEGED CONSPIRACIES

In 2014, Connecticut's Attorney General William Tong and his staff began to investigate inexplicably high price increases in the generic drug markets. They uncovered what is thought to be a multibillion-dollar cartel that involves 30 corporate defendants, many of which are well-known pharmaceutical firms, and more than 160 drugs. From approximately 2016 to 2020, numerous state attorneys general filed three complementary private complaints in connection with the alleged generic drug cartel based on copious amounts of direct and circumstantial evidence.[15] Defendants were alleged to have conspired through phone calls, meetings, and social gatherings. The complaints differ in the targeted generic manufacturers, individual defendants, and generic drugs. Additionally, the US Department of Justice has sued seven generic manufacturers. Five of these firms have settled

---

[15] *In re: Generic Pharmaceuticals Pricing Antitrust Litigation*, No. 16-AG-27240 (D.C.E. Penn. 2017), Complaint; *State of Connecticut v. Teva Pharmaceuticals*, No. 3:19-cv-00710 (D.C. Conn. 2019), Complaint; *State of Connecticut v. Sandoz Inc.*, No. 3:20-cv-00802 (D.C. Conn. 2020), Complaint.

for millions of dollars through the process of deferred prosecution, whereby the firms admit guilt and pay a fine in exchange for the DOJ dropping the case.[16]

We focus on the allegations and evidence contained in the private complaints filed by more than 45 state attorneys general and US territories, which together involve 30 corporate defendants. Table 7.1 lists these defendants, and the Appendix lists 166 of the drugs involved. The complaint alleges that the generic manufacturers colluded in two main ways. First, they agreed to not compete with one another by accommodating the entry of new firms and by allowing every firm to get its "fair share."[17] Second, the firms colluded with one another to fix prices. As evidenced by the sheer number of drugs involved in the complaints, one would be hard-pressed to find any US citizen who was not affected by the alleged conspiracy. In what follows, we detail the allegations set forth in the complaints and provide some economic context.

Fair-Share Agreement

Generic manufacturers sell their drugs to wholesalers, large pharmacies, and large hospital systems, which distribute the drugs to retailers and patients. In a competitive market, an entering generic firm would compete for market share by offering lower prices to the incumbent's customers. Then the incumbent could offer to meet or beat the entrant's offer. In either event, prices would fall and the quantity of the drug produced would rise. As entrants continue to compete for market share, prices would continue to fall. Prices bottom out at the competitive level. For the generic producers, this is an unsatisfactory

---

[16] Heritage Pharmaceuticals paid $7.1 million, Rising Pharmaceuticals paid more than $3 million, Apotex Corp. paid $24.1 million, Sandoz Inc. paid $195 million, and Taro Pharmaceuticals paid $205.7 million to settle the DOJ's claims. Teva Pharmaceuticals and Glenmark Pharmaceuticals were also charged, but they have not admitted guilt for the time being (Department of Justice 2019a, 2019b, 2020, 2021).

[17] *In re Generic Pharmaceuticals Pricing Antitrust Litigation*, No. 16-AG-27240 (D.C.E. Penn. 2017), Complaint.

Table 7.1. *Alleged cartel members*

	Number of drugs by complaint		
Defendant-company	2017[a]	2019[b]	2021[c]
Actavis Pharma, Inc.	2	20	11
Amneal Pharmaceuticals, Inc.	0	3	1
Apotex Corp.*	1	5	0
Ascend Laboratories, LLC	1	0	0
Aurobindo Pharma USA, Inc.	3	3	4
Breckenridge Pharmaceutical, Inc.	0	2	0
Citron Pharma, LLC	1	0	0
Dr. Reddy's Laboratories, Inc.	2	5	0
Emcure Pharmaceuticals, LTD	1	0	0
G & W	0	0	13
Glenmark Pharmaceuticals, Inc.	1	9	6
Greenstone LLC (Pfizer)	0	6	3
Heritage Pharmaceuticals, Inc.*	15	0	0
Lannett Company, Inc.	1	2	1
Lupin Pharmaceuticals, Inc.	0	10	1
Mallinckrodt	0	0	1
Mayne Pharma, Inc.	1	0	0
Mylan Pharmaceuticals, Inc.	4	33	3
Par Pharmaceutical Companies, Inc.	1	7	0
Perrigo	0	0	21
Pfizer, Inc.	0	8	3
Sandoz, Inc.*	1	28	42
Sun Pharmaceutical Industries, Inc.	3	0	2
Taro Pharmaceuticals USA, Inc.*	1	9	24
Teligent	0	0	1
Teva Pharmaceuticals USA, Inc.	7	90	0
Upsher-Smith Laboratories, LLC	0	2	0
Valeant	0	0	2
Wockhardt USA LLC	2	1	2
Zydus Pharmaceuticals (USA) Inc.	1	9	0

[a] *In re Generic Pharmaceuticals Pricing Antitrust Litigation*, No. 16-AG-27240 (D.C.E. Penn. 2017), Complaint.
[b] *State of Connecticut* v. *Teva Pharmaceuticals* (D.C. Conn. 2019), Complaint.
[c] *State of Connecticut* v. *Sandoz Inc.* (D.C. Conn. 2020), Complaint.
* These firms were sued by the Department of Justice for price fixing. They admitted guilt through a deferred prosecution agreement and paid a settlement.

state of affairs. One way to avoid this outcome is the so-called fair-share agreement.

From our economic models, we know that the profit-maximizing price in any industry is the monopoly price. Consequently, firms want to charge a price as close to the monopoly price as possible to maximize industry profits. But when new firms enter the market, the productive capacity increases generally lead to higher quantities and lower prices. In order to maintain high prices, existing firms must curb their own production to accommodate the entry. Curbing production would reduce profits, but profits would be higher than in a competitive market where prices would be driven down to marginal cost and profits would be zero.

According to the initial complaint by the attorneys general, since at least 2006, generic firms have maintained fair-share agreements in which they agreed not to compete for market share.[18] Each firm's share depended on the number of firms in the market and the order of entry. Generally, first movers would supply a higher share of the market. For example, a market with two firms could be split 60-40, with the first firm to enter receiving 60 percent. If two firms entered at the same time, the market would be split equally.[19]

The existing firms would accommodate new entrants because they recognized the necessity of conceding some market share to ensure that entering firms would not drive prices down. Thus, they engaged in customer allocation by dividing customers among themselves. When a new firm entered, existing firms would give up some of their lucrative contracts to the entrant. When asked for a counterbid

---

[18] *In re Generic Pharmaceuticals Pricing Antitrust Litigation*, No. 16-AG-27240 (D.C.E. Penn. 2017), Complaint.

[19] *In re Generic Pharmaceuticals Pricing Antitrust Litigation*, No. 16-AG-27240 (D.C.E. Penn. 2017), Complaint. For example, the vice president of sales and marketing at Dr. Reddy's said the following when Dr. Reddy's was preparing to enter a drug market: "If they [Dr. Reddy's] are first and others come out after, he deserves 60%. If he launches with others on day [one], he considers fair share 2–50%, 3–33%, 4–25%, etc." *State of Connecticut* v. *Teva Pharmaceuticals*, No. 3:19-cv-00710 (D.C. Conn. 2019), Complaint p. 38.

by the entrant's prospective customer, the incumbent would refuse to bid or would offer slightly higher prices to ensure that the new entrant would get the contract. This is a form of bid rigging. For example, Mylan Pharmaceuticals, Inc. (Mylan) walked away from at least one large wholesaler and one large pharmacy chain so that Heritage Pharmaceuticals Inc. (Heritage) could claim the contracts for selling doxycycline hyclate delayed response (doxycycline), which treats acne.[20] In this way, the quantity of doxycycline sold stayed roughly the same, and prices remained the same.

Once a firm had its fair share of the market, it would not compete with its rivals by undercutting their deals with drug wholesalers or large pharmacies.[21] The firms also had procedures set in place for supply disruptions. If one firm had a temporary issue with its supply, the other firms would not interfere with its contracts. If, however, the firm exited the market, its customers would be divided equally among the remaining firms. If the firm were to reenter, the existing firms would allow it to seamlessly regain its market share. In this way, prices stayed remarkably stable with entry.

Prices would often rise when a firm exited the market. Teva Pharmaceuticals USA, Inc. (Teva) and Mylan produced clonidine TTS patches, which are used to treat high blood pressure. In 2012, Mylan was forced to exit the market due to supply chain issues and Teva immediately increased its prices. Soon thereafter, Mylan reentered the market and sold clonidine TTS patches at the new higher price.[22] Presumably, Teva and Mylan were still searching for the joint profit-maximizing price when Mylan left the market. Apparently, Teva found that price just as Mylan was exiting the market. When it reentered, Mylan also charged the higher price. The higher profits

---

[20] *In re Generic Pharmaceuticals Pricing Antitrust Litigation*, No. 16-AG-27240 (D.C.E. Penn. 2017), Complaint.

[21] *State of Connecticut v. Teva Pharmaceuticals*, No. 3:19-cv-00710 (D.C. Conn. 2019), Complaint.

[22] *State of Connecticut v. Teva Pharmaceuticals*, No. 3:19-cv-00710 (D.C. Conn. 2019), Complaint.

were split equally due to the fair-share agreement that allowed the firms to divide the market.[23]

Sometimes, prices would increase before entry. For example, Teva had a virtual monopoly on the market for generic budesonide inhalation, a steroid to control asthma. When Teva learned that Actavis Pharma, Inc. (Actavis) would enter the market for budesonide inhalation, Teva increased the price by 9 percent. When Actavis entered shortly thereafter, it charged the same higher price.[24] These price increases were not uncommon. For example, Teva also increased the price for niacin ER, which treats high cholesterol, before Lupin Pharmaceuticals, Inc. and Zydus Pharmaceuticals Inc. entered the market.

In general, we assume that firms are always maximizing profit. Any change in price, therefore, would indicate that a firm was not previously producing at the profit-maximizing level. Frequent adjustments to price are necessary since it can be difficult to pinpoint the exact profit-maximizing price, which fluctuates with changes in demand. Finding the best price is often an iterative process, so increasing prices, as Teva did with budesonide inhalation, could merely indicate that Teva was adjusting its price in an effort to maximize profit, either because it had not hit the sweet spot or because changes in demand caused the profit-maximizing price to change. The firm's timing could be either a coincidence or collusion. More evidence is necessary to determine whether these price increases were collusive.

The plaintiffs claim that the drug industry's fair-share agreement "was a direct result of specific discussion, negotiation and collusion among industry participants over the course of many years."[25] Executives often exchanged emails and phone calls to

---

[23] Unilateral price increases are not illegal. Teva's and Mylan's behavior would only be objectionable if they overtly colluded in some way.

[24] *State of Connecticut* v. *Teva Pharmaceuticals*, No. 3:19-cv-00710 (D.C. Conn. 2019), Complaint.

[25] *State of Connecticut* v. *Teva Pharmaceuticals*, No. 3:19-cv-00710 (D.C. Conn. 2019), Complaint.

coordinate their allocation of market shares according to the fair-share agreement.[26] Because this collusion was overt, the market allocation scheme would be considered per se unlawful.[27]

Price Fixing

In addition to evidence on unlawful fair-share agreements, the complaints point to direct price-fixing agreements, which have been per se unlawful for more than 100 years. The attorneys general alleged that once each firm had its "fair share," the firms coordinated with each other through phone calls and communication at trade shows to increase the prices on select drugs. This conspiracy was quite profitable. Between 2008 and 2016, for example, profits on generic topical products increased by more than 1,300 percent for Taro Pharmaceuticals Inc. and Perrigo New York, Inc.[28] Additionally, an executive at Teva estimated that the set of price increases it implemented on July 3, 2013, and its price increases for two other drugs would together increase revenue by more than $937 million in just one quarter.[29]

According to one complaint, the price-fixing agreement commenced as follows.[30] A sales executive at Teva or another generic firm compiled a list of generic drugs amenable to increased prices based on market research and the quality of their relationship with other competitors. Essentially, they looked for drugs that were not being sold at the joint profit-maximizing level. The pricing list would be disseminated to the relevant competitors, and the competitors discussed and agreed upon the price increases. Once a price was agreed upon, one firm

---

[26] Although the plaintiffs did not have a record of what was said on the phone calls, the timing of the phone calls suspiciously coincided with price increases and market share allocations.

[27] If this scheme were tacit and the generic drug manufacturers did not discuss the agreement among themselves, the attorneys general would find it difficult to sue the defendants. Unilateral pricing decisions are not illegal, even if a collusive outcome is reached. We discuss tacit collusion in Chapter 9.

[28] *State of Connecticut* v. *Sandoz Inc.*, No. 3:20-cv-00802 (D.C. Conn. 2020), Complaint.

[29] *State of Connecticut* v. *Teva Pharmaceuticals*, No. 3:19-cv-00710 (D.C. Conn. 2019), Complaint.

[30] *State of Connecticut* v. *Teva Pharmaceuticals*, No. 3:19-cv-00710 (D.C. Conn. 2019), Complaint.

would increase its price with the other firms following suit. Each firm would agree not to poach another's customers after a price increase. If any firm began to poach customers, the firm that increased its price first could lose substantial profit, making this concession very important. Finally, the generic firms would claim that the price increases were due to other lawful factors, such as industry consolidation, FDA-mandated plant closures, or elimination of unprofitable product lines.[31]

The generic firms also took advantage of changes in input costs and firm structure to hide their collusion. If input costs increased, the firms would increase prices disproportionately and then blame it on the increased input costs. If one firm left the market, prices would increase immediately thereafter.[32]

Price fixing is per se unlawful. In this case, the states seem to have ample evidence of overt collusion in the form of email correspondence and phone records for many of the alleged drug conspiracies. Although the complaints do not include all the drugs that saw price increases, the generic drug industry will face a day of reckoning if the courts side with the states.

Other Private Cases

The generic firms' antitrust troubles do not end with the state cases. A number of private parties have also sued the generic firms for price fixing. Both Humana Care and United HealthCare Services, Inc. filed suit against Teva, Mylan, and a number of other defendants for their roles in fixing prices for more than 100 generic drugs.[33] Health insurers were harmed by the collusion since they had to pay more for the drugs that their policyholders required. Another health insurer, Cigna Corp., also filed suit in 2020.[34] Rite Aid Corp., a pharmaceutical benefit

---

[31] *In re Generic Pharmaceuticals Pricing Antitrust Litigation*, No. 16-AG-27240 (D.C.E. Penn. 2017), Complaint.

[32] This scenario can also be explained by an oligopoly model. We discuss oligopoly in Chapter 9.

[33] *United HealthCare Services, Inc.* v. *Teva Pharmaceuticals USA, Inc.*, No. 0:19-cv-02696 (D. Minn 2019) and *Humana Inc.* v. *Actavis Elizabeth LLC*, No. 2:19-cv-4862 (E.D. Pa. 2019).

[34] *Cigna Corp.* v. *Actavis Holdco US Inc.*, No. 2:20-cv-02711 (E.D. Pa. 2020).

manager that negotiates drug prices between manufacturers and pharmacies, also sued the generic drug manufacturers on similar grounds.[35] Even investors are suing for damages. In 2019, the Ontario Teachers' Pension Plan Board and the Anchorage Police & Fire Retirement System filed suit against Teva for misleading investors about their pricing strategy.[36] The generic firms are likely to face other private suits in the future as new details about the alleged cartel continue to emerge.

7.5 ECONOMIC CONSEQUENCES OF COLLUSION

In this section, we describe the economic consequences of collusion, including the social welfare loss, private damages, and settlements. For purposes of this discussion, we assume that the plaintiffs have prevailed on liability.[37]

Social Welfare

The welfare losses of collusion are well known. Prices are above the competitive, welfare-maximizing level. There are several concerns resulting from price fixing. First, collusion leads to a loss in social welfare or deadweight welfare loss. Second, some consumer surplus is unlawfully transferred from patients to the colluding pharmaceutical firms. From an economic perspective, this transfer may be a wash, but it is significant. The colluding producers have essentially stolen wealth from consumers. This should not be tolerated. The firms should be fined as heavily as the law permits, and the decision makers responsible for the collusion should also be fined and sent to prison. Third, consumers who have been priced out of the market are particularly hard hit by the conspiracy. They are unable to take medications that are necessary for their health. Some people may have suffered or died as a result of corporate greed.

---

[35] *Rite Aid Corp.* v. *Actavis Holdco US Inc.*, No. 2:20-cv-03367 (E.D. Pa. 2020).

[36] *Ontario Teachers' Pension Plan Bd.* v. *Teva Pharm. Indus. Ltd.*, No. 3:17-cv-00558 (D. Conn. 2019).

[37] At this writing, the litigation is ongoing and, therefore, liability has not yet been determined.

Antitrust Damages

The economic effects of collusion in many generic drug markets ripple through the economy. At a minimum, taxpayers, employers, health insurers, policyholders, government agencies, and patients have all suffered to some extent. Some, but not necessarily all, of these groups will have standing to sue the guilty parties for treble damages pursuant to Section 4 of the Clayton Act, which states:

> Any person who shall be injured in his business or property by reason of anything forbidden in the antitrust laws may sue therefor ... and shall recover threefold the damages by him sustained, and the cost of suit, including a reasonable attorney's fee.[38]

Under *Illinois Brick* precedent, only the direct buyers have standing to sue for antitrust damages.[39] For those direct buyers who have standing, antitrust damages are fairly clear. According to the Supreme Court's opinion in *Bigelow* v. *RKO Radio Pictures*,[40] antitrust damages should be calculated "by a comparison of profits, prices and values as affected by the [antitrust violation], with what they would have been in its absence under freely competitive conditions."[41]

In a price-fixing case, the total damages (Δ) are

$$\Delta = (P_a - P_{bf})Q_a,$$

where P_{bf} is the but-for price that would have prevailed in the absence of the unlawful collusion. This price is not necessarily the competitive price, but it is the non-collusive price. The actual (unlawful) price and actual quantity sold are P_a and Q_a, respectively. If the court or the jury finds that the damage is Δ, the award will be 3Δ, as damages are automatically trebled (or tripled) under Section 4 of the Clayton Act.

---

[38] 15 USC §15.   [39] *Illinois Brick Co.* v. *Illinois*, 431 US 720 (1977).
[40] 327 US 251, 264 (1946).
[41] *Bigelow* v. *RKO Radio Pictures*, 327 US 251, 264 (1946).

Settlements

Nearly all private damage suits are settled before a final judicial resolution. Settlements are efficient because the expected value of the suit to the plaintiff is lower than the expected cost to the defendant. In effect, the defendant "buys" the suit from the plaintiff. Both parties are better off settling than going forward with the litigation.

In most instances, the settlement amount is some fraction of the single damages, rather than treble damages.[42] Settlement benefits the defendants but substantially weakens both the compensatory and deterrent roles of private enforcement to the detriment of consumers.

7.6   DETERRING PRICE FIXING

Price fixing is risky since it is unlawful per se. If the collusion is not detected, there is a substantial upside. On the other hand, if the price fixing is detected and the parties are convicted, the punishment involves substantial monetary penalties and even prison sentences. Consequently, the benefits of collusion are not certain. The value of a price-fixing conspiracy, therefore, is a probability-weighted average or expected value.

In general, public policy should be aimed at deterring undesirable conduct rather than punishing that conduct. Ideally, the punishment should deter the conduct. When it comes to price fixing, however, the per se illegality of price fixing and the associated sanctions do not seem to have worked since price fixing continues to exist. In an expectation sense, public policy has failed to make price fixing unprofitable. But public policy, either by increasing the probability of detection or magnitude of sanctions, can negatively affect the expected profitability of price fixing going forward.

The Deterrent Function

The deterrent function (Δ) is

$$\Delta = \Pi_o - E[\Pi],$$

---

[42] See Lande (1993) for some thoughts on this issue.

where Π_o is the potential conspirator's profit without price fixing and $E[\Pi]$ is the firm's expected profit if it joins a price-fixing cartel. If Δ is positive, then the firm is better off by not colluding and, therefore, collusion is deterred. This, of course, is the ideal outcome since consumers are not harmed and scarce resources are not used to prosecute and punish the guilty. The question is how public policy can make Δ positive. To find the solution, we examine the expected profit.

The expected profit is $E[\Pi] = p(\Pi_C - S) + (1 - p)\Pi_C$, where p is the probability of detection and conviction; $(1 - p)$ is the probability of not getting caught or convicted; S is the sanction imposed on the firm after conviction; and Π_C is the collusive profit. Consequently, the deterrent function is

$$\Delta = \Pi_o - [-p(S) + \Pi_C].$$

It can be seen that Δ increases with an increase in the probability of detection and/or an increase in the sanction. These are the public policy variables at our disposal. If the current values of p and S do not deter price fixing, then one or both should be increased.

Current sanctions appear to be substantial in a price-fixing case. For the firm, the maximum fine per offense is \$100 million, or twice the gain of the criminal behavior or twice the loss to the victims, whichever is greater. The decision makers face maximum fines of \$1 million and prison sentences of up to 10 years. However, executives are seldom fined substantially and never receive the maximum prison sentence. The longest prison sentence for a price fixer was five years, and many prison sentences are much less. Putting more sales executives in prison for price fixing may be a wake-up call for those who are engaging in such illegal behavior.

Private damage suits under Section 4 of the Clayton Act supplement public enforcement in deterring price fixing. But as we discussed previously, private cases often settle for much less than treble damages – making private suits less effective at deterring price-fixing behavior.

By putting laws in place that increase p, the antitrust agencies should be able to deter some price-fixing cartels. In general, the Agencies discover price fixing by investigating suspicious pricing patterns or through a whistleblower, who is generally an employee of the colluding firm that decides to come forward and report the illegal behavior. For example, the State of Connecticut began investigating the generic drug companies due to unusually high prices. Thereafter, whistleblowers came forward and provided more details about the conspiracy. In the future, the Agencies could use computer programs and artificial intelligence to identify suspicious pricing patterns, which would require further investigation. Additionally, the Agencies could introduce greater incentives and protections for whistleblowers, which could incentivize more whistleblowers to come forward.

7.7 CONCLUDING REMARKS

Generic drugs should be one of the greatest bargains in the US health care system since competition makes life-saving drugs affordable. Price-fixing agreements in generic markets break this competitive promise and harm consumers who rely on generic drugs to maintain their health and well-being. If the plaintiffs prevail in their suits against the generic drug companies, there will be a truly significant day of reckoning in the generic drug sector. The producers will be hit with enormous damage awards that may bankrupt some of them. One will hope that this can serve as a warning to other prospective price-fixing cartels and thereby protect competition in the health care sector.

APPENDIX: ALLEGED PARTICIPANTS IN GENERIC PHARMACEUTICAL DRUG CONSPIRACY

In 2014, Connecticut's Attorney General William Tong and his staff began to investigate inexplicably high price increases in generic drug markets. Through their investigation, they pinpointed at least 166 drugs that were suspected to have been involved in an alleged price-fixing conspiracy. Table 7.2 presents those drugs.

Table 7.2. Drugs in the alleged conspiracy

	Drugs	Complaint[a]	Use	Firms
1	Acetazolamide	3	Glaucoma, epilepsy, mountain sickness, and edema	Taro/Lannett
2	Acetazolamide ER	1	Glaucoma, epilepsy, altitude sickness, perioidic paralysis, and heart failure	Heritage/Teva/Zydus
3	Adapalene	2, 3	Acne	Teva/Glenmark/Taro; Sandoz/Perrigo
4	Adderall IR or MAS-IR	2	ADHD	Teva/Actavis/Aurobindo
5	Adderall XR or Mixed Amphetamine Salts or MAS	2	ADHD	Teva/Actavis
6	Alclometasone Dipropionate	3	Skin inflammation and itching	Sandoz/Taro/Glenmark
7	Amiloride Hydrochloride	2	High blood pressure	Teva/Mylan
8	Ammonium Lactate	3	Xerosis and ichthyosis vulgaris	Taro/Perrigo/Actavis
9	Amoxicillin	2	Infections and stomach ulcers	Teva/Sandoz
10	Azithromycin	2	Bacterial infection (pink eye)	Teva/Greenstone/Pfizer
11	Baclofen	2	Muscle relaxer	Teva/Lannett/Upsher-Smith
12	Balziva	2	Contraception	Teva/Lupin
13	Benazepril HCTZ	2	High blood pressure	Mylan/Sandoz/Rising
14	Betamethasone Dipropianate	3	Skin inflammation, itching, and redness	Sandoz/Taro/Perrigo

Table 7.2. (cont.)

	Drugs	Complaint[a]	Use	Firms
15	Betamethasone Valerate	3	Skin inflammation, itching, and redness	Sandoz/Taro/G&W/Actavis
16	Bethanechol Chloride	2	Urinary and bladder issues	Teva/Amneal
17	Bromocriptine Mesylate	3	Hyperprolactinemia-associated dysfunctions, Parkinson's disease, and acromegaly	Sandoz/Perrigo/Mylan
18	Budesonide DR Capsules	2	Chron's disease and ulcerative colitis	Teva/Par/Mylan
19	Budesonide Inhalation	2	Steroid for asthma	Teva/Actavis
20	Bumetanide	2	Edema and high blood pressure	Teva/Sandoz
21	Buspirone HCL	2	Anxiety	Teva/Mylan
22	Cabergoline	2	Hormone treatment	Teva/Greenstone/Pfizer
23	Calcipotriene Betamethasone Dipropionate	3	Psoriasis	Sandoz/Perrigo
24	Calcipotriene	3	Plaque psoriasis	Sandoz/G&W
25	Capecitabine	2	Anti-cancer chemotherapy	Teva/Mylan
26	Carbamazepine	2	Seizures	Teva/Taro/Apotex
27	Carbamazepine ER	3	Seizures	Sandoz/Taro
28	Cefdinir	2	Bacterial infection	Teva/Lupin/Sandoz
29	Cefpodoxime Proxetil	3	Bacterial infection	Sandoz/Aurobindo
30	Cefprozil	2	Bacterial infection	Teva/Lupin/Sandoz

31	Celecoxib	2	NSAID for arthritis	Teva/Actavis
32	Cephalexin Oral Suspension	2	Bacterial infection	Teva/Lupin
33	Chlorpromazine HCL	3	Mental illness, behavorial disorder, tetanus, and blood disorder	Sandoz
34	Cholestyramine	3	Cholesterol	Sandoz
35	Cholestyramine/Aspartame	3	Cholesterol	Sandoz
36	Ciclopirox	3	Fungal skin infection	Sandoz/Perrigo/G&W/Actavis/Glenmark
37	Cimetidine	2	Stomach ulcers and acid reflux	Teva/Mylan
38	Ciprofloxacin HCL	2	Bacterial infections	Teva/Dr. Reddy's/Actavis
39	Clarithromycin	2	Infection and ulcers	Teva/Actavis/Zydus
40	Clemastine Fumarate	2	Allergies	Teva/Sandoz
41	Clindamycin Phosphate	3	Acne	Sandoz/Taro/Perrigo/Greenstone/Pfizer
42	Clobetasol Propionate	3	Eczema, contact dermatitis, seborrheic dermatitis, and psoriasis	Sandoz/Taro/Wockhardt
43	Clomipramine HCL	2	OCD, panic disorder, depression, and chronic pain	Mylan/Sandoz/Taro
44	Clonidine-TTS Patch	2	High blood pressure	Teva/Mylan/Actavis
45	Clotrimazole	2, 3	Fungal infection	Teva/Taro; Sandoz/Taro
46	Clotrimazole Betamethasone Dipropionate	3	Fungal skin infection	Sandoz/Actavis

Table 7.2. (cont.)

	Drugs	Complaint[a]	Use	Firms
47	Cyproheptadine	2	Allergies	Teva/Breckenridge
48	Desmopression Acetate	2	Diabetes insipidus	Teva/Actavis
49	Desogestrel and Ethinyl Estradiol	2	Contraception	Teva/Glenmark
50	Desonide	3	Atopic dermatitis and other skin conditions	Sandoz/Taro/Perrigo/Actavis
51	Desoximetasone	3	Skin irritation, allergic reactions, and plaque psoriasis	Sandoz/Taro/Glenmark
52	Dexmethylphenidate HCL ER	2	ADHD	Teva/Sandoz
53	Dextroamphetamine sulfate XR	2	Hyperactivity and impulse control	Teva/Actavis
54	Diclofenac Potassium	2	Muscle aches and swelling	Teva/Mylan/Sandoz
55	Dicloxacillin Sodium	2	Infections	Sandoz
56	Diflunisal	2	NSAID	Teva/Rising
57	Diltiazim HCL	2	High blood pressure and angina	Teva/Mylan
58	Disopyramide Phosphate	2	Heart arrhythmia	Teva/Actavis
59	Drospirenone and Ethinyl estradiol	2	Combination for contraception	Teva/Lupin/Actavis
60	Doxazosin Mesylate	2	Antihypertensive	Teva/Apotex/Mylan

61	Doxycycline Hyclate DR	1	Severe acne	Heritage/Mylan/Mayne/Emcure
62	Doxycycline Monohydrate	1	Bacterial infection (acne) and malaria	Heritage/Lannett/Mylan/Par
63	Econazole Nitrate	3	Fungal skin infection	Sandoz/Taro/Perrigo/Teligent
64	Enalapril Maleate	2	High blood pressure and congestive heart failure	Teva/Taro/Mylan/Wockhardt
65	Entecavir	2	Chronic hepatitis B	Teva/Par
66	Eplerenone	3	High blood pressure	Sandoz/Greenstone/Pfizer
67	Erythromycin Base/ Ethyl Alcohol	3	Acne	Sandoz/Perrigo/Wockhardt
68	Estazolam	2	Insomnia	Teva/Actavis
69	Estradiol/ Norethindrone Acetate	2	Menopause	Teva/Breckenridge/Mylan/ Actavis
70	Ethambutol HCL	3	Tuberculosis	G&W/Lupin
71	Ethinyl Estradiol	2	Birth control	Teva/Sandoz
72	Ethosuximide	2	Seisures	Teva
73	Etodolac/Etodolac ER	2	NSAID for arthritis	Teva/Taro/Zydus/ Sandoz
74	Fenofibrate	2	Cholesterol	Teva/Mylan/Lupin/Zydus
75	Flucanazole	2	Fungal infections	Teva/Greenstone/Glenmark/ Pfizer
76	Fluocinolone Acetonide	3	Eczema, dermatitis, allergies, and rash	Sandoz/G&W
77	Fluocinonide	2, 3	Eczema and other skin conditions	Teva/Taro/Sandoz/Actavis; Sandoz/Taro/Perrigo/G&W/ Actavis/ Glenmark/Valeant

Table 7.2. (cont.)

	Drugs	Complaint[a]	Use	Firms
78	Fluoxetine	2	Depression and OCD	Teva/Mylan/Par
79	Flurbiprofen	2	NSAID	Teva/Mylan
80	Flutamide	2	Prostate cancer	Teva/Actavis/Par
81	Fluticasone Propionate	3	Seasonal allergies	Sandoz/Perrigo/Glenmark
82	Fluvastatin	2	High cholesterol	Teva/Mylan
83	Fosinopril-Hydrochlorothiazide	1	Hypertension	Heritage/Aurobindo/Glenmark/Sandoz
84	Gabapentin	2	Epilepsy and neuropathic pain	Teva/Glenmark
85	Glimepiride	2	High blood sugar	Teva/Dr. Reddy's
86	Glipizide-Metformin	1	High blood sugar due to diabetes	Heritage/Teva/Mylan
87	Glyburide	1	Type 2 diabetes	Heritage/Teva/Aurobindo/Citron
88	Glyburide-Metformin	1	Type 2 diabetes	Heritage/Teva/Aurobindo/Actavis
89	Griseofulvin	2, 3	Fungal infections of the skin, hair, and nails	Teva/Actavis; Sandoz
90	Halobetasol Propionate	3	Eczema, dermatitis, psoriasis, and rash	Sandoz/Taro/Perrigo/G&W
91	Haloperidol	2	Tourette's syndrome	Mylan/Sandoz
92	Hydrocortisone Acetate	3	Hemorrhoids	Perrigo/G&W
93	Hydrocortisone Valerate	3	Eczema, dermatitis, allergies, and rash	Taro/Perrigo

#	Drug	Indication	Note	Manufacturers
94	Hydroxyurea	Leukemia and head and neck cancer	2	Teva/Par
95	Hydroxyzine Pamoate	Itching due to allergies	2	Teva/Rising/Sandoz/ Actavis
96	Imiquimod	Actinic keratosis	3	Sandoz/Taro/Perrigo
97	Irbesartan	Hypertension	2	Teva/Lupin
98	Isoniazid	Tuberculosis	2	Teva/Sandoz
99	Ketoconazole Cream	Fungal infections	2, 3	Teva/Taro/Sandoz; Sandoz/ Taro/G&W
100	Ketoconazole Tablet	Fungal infections	2	Teva/Mylan/Taro
101	Ketoprofen	NSAID for arthritis	2	Teva/Mylan
102	Ketorolac	NSAID for pain	2	Teva/Mylan
103	Labetalol	High blood pressure	2	Teva/Sandoz/Par/Watson[b]
104	Lamivudine/ Zidovudine	Combination for HIV	2	Teva/Lupin/Aurobindo/Camber
105	Latanoprost	Glaucoma and ocular hypertension	3	Sandoz/Greenstone/Pfizer/ Valeant
106	Leflunomide	Moderate to severe rheumatoid arthritis and psoriatic arthritis	1	Heritage/Apotex/Teva
107	Levothyroxine	Hypothyroidism	2	Mylan/Sandoz/Lannett
108	Lidocaine	Arrhythmia and pain reliever	3	Sandoz/Taro
109	Loperamide	Diarrhea	2	Teva/Mylan
110	Medroxyprogesterone	Abnormal menstruation and uterine bleeding	2	Teva/Greenstone/Pfizer
111	Meprobamate	Short-term anxiety, tension, and insomnia	1	Heritage/Dr. Reddy's

Table 7.2. (cont.)

	Drugs	Complaint[a]	Use	Firms
112	Methazolamide	3	Glaucoma	Sandoz/Perrigo
113	Methotrexate	2	Cancer	Teva/Mylan
114	Methylphenidate HCL	3	ADHD	Sandoz/Actavis/Sun/ Mallinckrodt
115	Metronidazole	3	Vaginal infections and rosacea	Sandoz/Taro/G&W/ Actavis
116	Moexipril HCL	2	High blood pressure	Teva/Glenmark
117	Mometasone Furoate	3	Skin conditions, hay fever, and asthma	G&W/Glenmark
118	Nabumetone	2	NSAID for arthritis	Teva/Glenmark/Sandoz/ Actavis
119	Nadolol	2	High blood pressure	Teva/Mylan/Sandoz
120	Nafcillin Sodium	3	Bacterial infection	Sandoz/Aurobindo
121	Niacin/Niacin ER	2	Cholesterol	Teva/Lupin/Zydus
122	Nimodipine	1	Bleeding in brain	Heritage/Sun/Ascend
123	Nitrofurantoin MAC Capsules	2	Urinary tract infection	Teva/Mylan/Alvogen
124	Norethindrone Acetate	2	Endometriosis	Teva/Amneal/Glenmark
125	Norethindrone and Ethinyl Estradiol	2	Combination for contraception	Teva/Lupin
126	Nortriptyline HCL	2	Depression	Teva/Taro/Actavis
127	Nystatin	1, 3	Fungal infections	Teva/Heritage/Sun; Sandoz/ Perrigo/ Actavis

128	Nystatin	Fungal skin infection	3	Sandoz/Taro
	Triamcinolone			
129	Omega-3-Acid Ethyl Esters	Lipid regulator	2	Teva/Par
130	Oxacillin Sodium	Bacterial infection	3	Sandoz/Aurobindo
131	Oxaprozin	NSAID for arthritis	2	Teva/Dr. Reddy's/Pfizer
132	Oxybutynin Chloride	Bladder and urinary conditions	2	Teva/Upsher-Smith
133	Paricalcitol	Parathyroid hormone in long-term kidney disease	2	Teva/Zydus/Dr. Reddy's
134	Paromomycin	Intestine amoeba infection and liver disease	1	Heritage/Sun
135	Penicillin V Potassium	Moderate bacterial infections	2	Teva/Sandoz/ Aurobindo/Pfizer
136	Pentoxifylline	Poor blood circulation	2	Teva/Apotex/Mylan
137	Phenytoin Sodium ER	Seizures	3	Taro/Mylan/Sun/Amneal
138	Pioglitazone HCL	High blood sugar	3	Sandoz/Aurobindo/Mylan
	Metformin HCL			
139	Piroxicam	NSAID for arthritis	2	Teva/Greenstone/Pfizer
140	Portia and Jolessa	Combination for contraception	2	Teva/Sandoz
141	Pravastatin	High cholesterol	2	Teva/Glenmark/Lupin/Apotex/Zydus
142	Prazosin HCL	High blood pressure	2	Teva/Mylan
143	Prochlorperazine	Nausea, vomiting, anxiety, and schizophrenia	2	Teva/Mylan/Sandoz

Table 7.2. (cont.)

	Drugs	Complaint[a]	Use	Firms
144	Prochlorperazine Maleate	3	Severe nausea and vomiting	Perrigo/G&W
145	Promethazine HCL	3	Allergies and motion sickness	Perrigo/G&W/Actavis
146	Propranolol HCL	2	High blood pressure, irregular heartbeats, and shaking (tremors)	Teva/Actavis/Mylan
147	Raloxifene	2	Osteoporosis	Teva/Camber
148	Ranitidine	2	Heartburn and stomach ulcers	Teva/Glenmark/Sandoz/Amneal
149	Sotalol Hydrochloride	2	Heart arrhythmia	Teva/Mylan
150	Tacrolimus	3	Rejection of organ transplant	Sandoz/Perrigo
151	Tamoxifen Citrate	2	Breast cancer	Teva/Actavis/Mylan
152	Temozolomide	2	Some brain cancers	Teva/Sandoz
153	Terconazole	3	Fungal and yeast infection	Sandoz/Taro/Actavis
154	Theophylline ER	1	Asthma, chronic bronchitis, and emphysema	Heritage/Teva
155	Tizanidine	2	Muscle relaxer	Dr. Reddy's/Sandoz/Mylan
156	Tobramycin	2	Eye drop for bacterial infections	Teva/Sandoz
157	Tolmetin Sodium	2	Rheumatoid arthritis and osteoarthritis	Mylan
158	Tolterodine ER	2	Overactive bladder	Teva/Mylan

159	Tolterodine Tartrate	2	Overactive bladder	Teva/Greenstone/Pfizer
160	Topiramate Sprinkle Capsules	2	Seizures and migraines	Teva/Zydus/Actavis
161	Triamcinolone Acetonide	3	Eczema, dermatitis, allergies, and rash	Sandoz/Taro/Perrigo
162	Trifluoperazine HCL	2	Psychotic disorder and anxiety	Mylan/Sandoz
163	Valsartan	2	High blood pressure and heart failure	Mylan/Sandoz
164	Verapamil	1	Hypertension, angina, and heart rhythm disorder	Heritage/Mylan/Actavis
165	Warfarin Sodium	2	Blood clots	Teva/Taro/Zydus
166	Zoledronic Acid	1	High blood calcium levels	Heritage/Dr. Reddy's

[a] Complaint 1 refers to *In re Generic Pharmaceuticals Pricing Antitrust Litigation*, No. 16-AG-27240 (D.C.E. Penn. 2017), Complaint. Complaint 2 refers to *State of Connecticut v. Teva Pharmaceuticals* (D.C. Conn. 2019), Complaint. Complaint 3 refers to *State of Connecticut v. Sandoz Inc.* (D.C. Conn. 2020), Complaint.

[b] Watson acquired Actavis in 2013 and went by that name.

REFERENCES

Benner, Katie. (2020). Generic Drug Maker Admits to Fixing Prices for Cholesterol Medication. *New York Times*. www.nytimes.com/2020/05/07/us/politics/just ice-department-antitrust-drugs.html.

Berndt, Ernst R., and Murray L. Aiken. (2011). Brand Loyalty, Generic Entry and Price Competition in Pharmaceuticals in the Quarter Century after the 1984 Waxman-Hatch Legislation. *International Journal of the Economics of Business* 18: 177–201.

Centers for Medicare & Medicaid Services. (2021). NHE Fact Sheet. www.cms.gov/ Research-Statistics-Data-and-Systems/Statistics-Trends-and-Reports/National HealthExpendData/NHE-Fact-Sheet.

Clincalc. (2021). *Pravastatin Sodium: Drug Usage Statistics, United States, 2008–2018*. ClinCalc. https://clincalc.com/DrugStats/Drugs/PravastatinSodium.

Conrad, Ryan, and Randall Lutter. (2019). *Generic Competition and Drug Prices: New Evidence Linking Greater Generic Competition and Lower Generic Drug Prices*. US Food and Drug Administration. www.fda.gov/about-fda/center-drug-evalu ation-and-research-cder/generic-competition-and-drug-prices.

Dave, Chintan V., Abraham Hartzema, and Aaron S. Kesselheim. (2017). Prices of Generic Drugs Associated with Numbers of Manufacturers. *New England Journal of Medicine* 377: 2597–2598.

Department of Justice. (2019a). Pharmaceutical Company Admits to Price Fixing in Violation of Antitrust Law, Resolves Related False Claims Act Violations. www .justice.gov/opa/pr/pharmaceutical-company-admits-price-fixing-violation-anti trust-law-resolves-related-false.

Department of Justice. (2019b). Second Pharmaceutical Company Admits to Price Fixing, Resolves Related False Claims Act Violations. www.justice.gov/opa/pr/ second-pharmaceutical-company-admits-price-fixing-resolves-related-false-claims-act.

Department of Justice. (2020). Generic Drugs – Update 2020. www.justice.gov/atr/ division-operations/antitrust-division-update-2020/generic-drugs.

Department of Justice. (2021). Generic Drugs Investigation Targets Anticompetitive Schemes – Division Update Spring 2021. www.justice.gov/ atr/division-operations/division-update-spring-2021/generic-drugs-investiga tion-targets-anticompetitive-schemes.

Frakt, Austin. (2017). When a Drug Coupon Helps You but Hurts Fellow Citizens. *New York Times*. www.nytimes.com/2017/09/25/upshot/when-a-drug-coupon-helps-you-but-hurts-fellow-citizens.html.

Lande, Robert H. (1993). Are Antitrust "Treble" Damages Really Single Damages? *Ohio State Law Journal* 54: 115–174.

Mikulic, Matej. (2020). *Savings through Generic Drug Usage in the US, 2008–2019.* Statista. www.statista.com/statistics/277492/savings-through-generic-drug-usage-us/.

Poitras, Colin. (2019). *Price-Fixing, Fraud and Collusion, CT Attorney General Offers Sobering View of Generic Drug Market.* Yale School of Medicine. https://medicine.yale.edu/news-article/price-fixing-fraud-and-collusion-ct-attorney-general-offers-sobering-view-of-generic-drug-market/.

8 The Hatch-Waxman Act, Patent Infringement Suits, and Reverse Payments

8.1 INTRODUCTION

It is often the case that the road to hell is paved with good intentions. This also seems to be the case with the Hatch-Waxman Act of 1984. The Act has two goals: (1) extend the patent life of a pioneer drug to compensate for delays in the FDA approval process and (2) accelerate the entry of generic drugs to combat rising pharmaceutical prices. Extending the patent life would increase the incentive of a pioneer firm to invest in the search for new cures to alleviate human suffering. Expedited entry of generic substitutes for popular branded drugs would be welcomed by consumers, insurance companies, and government, as it could reduce expenditures by billions of dollars.

The Act has been quite successful in increasing the number of generic drugs on the market. Unfortunately, the Act has serious flaws that encourage both generic producers and pioneer firms to game the system. In the pursuit of economic profit, some producers of generic drugs use the Hatch-Waxman Act to challenge the valid patents of pioneer drugs. This conduct undermines the value of the patent awarded to the pioneer firm by the US Patent and Trademark Office (PTO). At the same time, pioneer firms can stall generic competition by filing perhaps baseless patent infringement suits. After 30 months, the pioneer firm and the would-be entrant often strike deals that result in payments by the pioneer firm to the generic producer for delaying its entry into the market, which protects the pioneer firm's monopoly profits. This conduct has aroused antitrust concerns that are the subject of this chapter.

In Section 8.2, we examine the successes and failures of the Hatch-Waxman Act and introduce the concept of reverse payments.

We discuss patent infringement suits in Section 8.3 and describe the settlements of such suits in Section 8.4. We also examine two appellate court decisions that required Supreme Court resolution. The resulting opinion in *Federal Trade Commission* v. *Actavis*[1] provided limited antitrust guidance. In Section 8.5, we discuss the aftermath of the landmark *Actavis* case as well as the future of reverse payment settlements. With this in mind, we introduce some antitrust remedies in Section 8.6. In Section 8.7, we elaborate on private damages, and in Section 8.8 we provide concluding remarks.

8.2 THE HATCH-WAXMAN ACT

In the Hatch-Waxman Act,[2] Congress conferred some benefits on producers of pioneer brands in the form of extended patent life under certain conditions. But the Act also created a mechanism for accelerating the entry of generic substitutes that would reduce the profits of the pioneer brand.[3]

Benefits to Pioneer Firms

Patents have a 20-year life that begins when the pioneer firm submits its patent application to the PTO. It takes some time for the patent office to review the application and, if appropriate, award a patent. Following the patent's approval, the pioneer firm must begin the testing required by the Food and Drug Administration (FDA) to ensure both safety and efficacy. Generally, the pharmaceutical company will have conducted research on how the drug affects animals or certain living tissues before obtaining a patent. Once this preclinical research is done, the pioneer firm must complete Phase I, Phase II, and Phase III clinical trials that include humans to establish the drug's safety and efficacy.

---

[1] 570 US 136 (2013).

[2] Drug Price Competition and Patent Term Restoration Act of 1984, 35 USC 156, Public Law 98-417 Title II (1984). We refer to this act as the Hatch-Waxman Act in the rest of the chapter.

[3] See Grabowski and Vernon (1986) for an analysis of the trade-offs.

In Phase I trials, the drug is administered to a small group of people to determine whether it is safe. Generally, doses are incrementally increased to monitor side effects and determine safe dosage levels. In this way, researchers can study how the drug works and can determine effective dosage. Then, a Phase II trial is implemented in a larger group of participants. Participants are placed either into a control group, which receives a placebo or similar drug, or a treatment group, which receives the new drug. The groups are compared, and the drug's effects are analyzed over a greater period of time in order to evaluate safety and efficacy. Finally, in Phase III trials, thousands of participants – who vary on age, gender, race, ethnicity, geographic location, and other determinants of health – test the drug. The trial focuses on the efficacy of the drug and also tests the effects of combining the drug with other medications. Once the drug passes these three trials, the FDA will review the application and, if appropriate, grant the pioneer firm approval to sell the drug. After entry, the FDA continues to monitor the effects of the drug in Phase IV trials.[4]

In some cases, delays at the patent office and the FDA can reduce the patent life substantially. Congress sought to alleviate this problem by extending the patent life on a pioneer brand under the following three conditions: (1) the drug's patent must not have expired at the time of the application, and the patent term must not have been extended previously; (2) the application must be submitted by the owner of the patent or his or her agent; and (3) the drug must have gone through a regulatory review process, such as clinical trials required by the FDA, which would not allow the drug to be marketed before their completion. If successful, the patent could be extended for up to five years to account for delays during clinical testing.[5] No doubt, this provision of the Hatch-Waxman Act was most welcome

---

[4] After Phase III trials, the FDA must approve drug labeling and also inspect the facilities where the drug will be produced. More detailed information is available from the US Food and Drug Administration.

[5] Hatch-Waxman Act, 35 USC 156, Public Law 98-417 1598-1599,1602 Title II (1984).

to the pharmaceutical firms that produce pioneer drugs. But there was something in the Act for producers of generics as well.

Accelerating Generic Entry

Prior to the Hatch-Waxman Act, generic entry was delayed well past the expiration of the pioneer brand's patent. The generic entrant would have to go through the same expensive FDA testing and approval process as the pioneer firm. Under the Hatch-Waxman Act, the would-be entrant could instead file an Abbreviated New Drug Application (ANDA), which allows the generic producer to rely on the pioneer firm's testing that established the safety and efficacy of the drug. The generic producer simply has to prove that its drug is therapeutically equivalent to the pioneer brand. In effect, the generic version has to be identical in all material respects: strength, absorption rate, and delivery form, such as a capsule or a tablet. If the FDA is satisfied that the generic is therapeutically equivalent to the pioneer brand, it will permit the generic drug to enter the market. The Hatch-Waxman Act also grants the first generic filer a 180-day period of exclusivity, which gives generic producers a powerful incentive to file quickly. In many cases, the first generic filer makes most of its profits during this six-month exclusivity period.

In addition to establishing therapeutic equivalence, the generic producer must certify that the generic drug does not infringe any valid patent in one of four ways. The generic producer can certify (1) there was never a valid patent on the original drug; (2) the patent expired; (3) the patent is about to expire; or (4) the patent is invalid or is irrelevant to the drug being contested. Using the last point to establish the validity of the generic drug, denoted a *paragraph IV certification*, often leads to a patent infringement suit and a perplexing number of reverse payments, which occur when a plaintiff pays a defendant to settle a lawsuit.

When the FDA is prepared to authorize generic entry, it is required to inform the pioneer firm that holds the patent for the branded drug. The pioneer firm then has 45 days to file a patent infringement suit against the generic firm if it believes the generic firm has infringed its patent. Under the terms of the Hatch-Waxman Act, the patent infringement suit stays FDA approval of the generic for 30 months or the final resolution of the litigation, whichever comes first. During those 30 months, the pioneer firm continues to enjoy monopoly profits, which far exceed the profits – if any – that it will earn once generic entry is permitted. Given the glacial pace of patent litigation, the 30 months usually arrives first.[6] At that point, the FDA may authorize entry by the generic firm. It is difficult to say just what might happen at this juncture. The issue of patent infringement is still in play. If the generic producer enters and loses the patent infringement suit, it will be vulnerable to damage claims by the pioneer firm, which could be substantial.

The pioneer and generic firms often settle the litigation, but on somewhat peculiar terms. The pioneer firm pays the would-be entrant to settle the suit. Since the pioneer firm is the plaintiff, these cases are often called *reverse payments* or *pay-for-delay settlements*. In the next section, we discuss these reverse payment settlements and the incentives for both parties to use them to game the system.

8.3   REVERSE PAYMENT SETTLEMENTS

When a plaintiff has suffered an injury allegedly due to the wrong-doing of the defendant, the case is likely to settle before trial. Typically, the defendant pays the plaintiff to drop its case. This scenario is consistent with our intuition: The plaintiff has suffered

---

[6] There is an incentive for the pioneer firm to stall the litigation for the full 30 months to ensure that it maintains its monopoly profits during that time. For example, Pfizer claimed that the generic versions of its blockbuster cancer treatment drug, Ibrance, infringed its patents. Ibrance had US sales of $3.25 billion in 2019. Although it is not clear whether the patent infringement suit is valid, Pfizer could presumably earn more than $6 billion in profits if it forestalled generic competition by 30 months (Yasiejko 2020). Additionally, in *AbbVie Inc.* v. *FTC*, US, No. 20-1293, the FTC alleged that AbbVie knowingly filed sham patent litigation against Teva Pharmaceuticals in order to stall generic entry in the AndroGel market. Teva's formulation of AndroGel used different materials than AbbVie, implying that the patent would not be infringed.

an injury, and the wrongdoer compensates him or her for that injury. The payment certainly seems to flow in the right direction.[7]

Patent infringement suits filed pursuant to provisions of the Hatch-Waxman Act also primarily settle before trial. Interestingly, these settlements involve a *plaintiff* paying the *defendant* a settlement fee. This scenario is rarely found outside of disputes in the pharmaceutical industry.

In patent infringement suits under the Hatch-Waxman Act, there has been no injury at the time of the suit. The purpose of the suit is to forestall the entry of an allegedly infringing generic substitute and thereby prevent injury to the pioneer firm. When the parties settle, the generic producer generally agrees to refrain from entering. Since the pioneer firm pays the generic firm to settle, the pioneer firm is paying the generic firm to not inflict injury in the form of lost profits on the pioneer firm. This agreement seems a bit odd. Moreover, such settlements raise competitive concerns.

Without generic entry, the pioneer firm enjoys patent protection and charges the monopoly price, which maximizes its profits. If generic firms do not enter, it will continue to earn monopoly profits for the duration of the patent's life. These profits will decrease substantially if there is generic entry. Since the reverse payment settlement involves a commitment to refrain from entering in exchange for a substantial sum, it has the appearance of an agreement not to compete.

These reverse payments can take the form of a lump sum fee, yearly fees, percentages of revenue, or a number of non-fee settlement terms such as payment for backup production, marketing, or generic exclusivity.[8] Generic firms, meanwhile, agree not to enter the market

---

[7] See the Appendix to this chapter for the economic rationale behind settlements.

[8] The terms of the reverse payment will vary from one dispute to another and can involve compensation, preferential licensing agreements, and fair value for services, among other terms. Sometimes, the pioneer firm may offer generic exclusivity if the generic firm agrees to delay entry. That is, the pioneer firm will not introduce its own authorized generic when the generic firm enters the market.

with their generic drug. On its face, this agreement certainly appears to be anticompetitive because consumers appear to be denied the benefits of generic competition. There is, however, a wrinkle. At the time of the settlement, no one knows for sure whether the patent infringement claim is valid.

In general, the courts presume any patent issued by the PTO is valid. In many reverse payment cases, however, the generic firm argues that its drug does not infringe on a patent because the drug does not include elements covered by the patent. If the patent is valid and the generic drug infringes it, the pioneer firm is entitled to its monopoly profits. Any competition provided by the infringing generic drug is unlawful. Consumers are not entitled to the benefits of illegitimate competition.[9] In contrast, if the drug does not infringe the patent, then the generic producer is entitled to entry and the profits from selling its generic version of the drug. Potentially, the foregone profits due to the patent litigation delay could be considered antitrust damages. The problem is that no one knows whether the patent was valid at the time of settlement. The troublesome policy question is this: Under what conditions is a reverse payment settlement an antitrust violation? As we will see in the rest of the section, the answer is not obvious.

A reverse payment should be legal if it can be assumed that the generic firm would not enter after 30 months of litigation. Due to the powerful incentive of the 180-day exclusivity period that the Hatch-Waxman Act grants the first generic filer, generic firms may gamble with their drugs and file inappropriate ANDAs on the off chance that their application is granted. Some pioneer brands enjoy sales in the hundreds of millions of dollars. Producers of generics understandably want to tap into such pots of gold.[10] Additionally, the prevalence of reverse payments would minimize the risk of filing since the generic

---

[9] In fact, those who consumed the infringing generic drug are also liable for patent infringement damages. See Blair and Cotter (2002) for an analysis.

[10] Grabowski et al. (2011).

could expect to at least break even if the pioneer firm pays for its litigation fees in the settlement. In this case, generic firms do not want to risk entering the market after 30 months of patent litigation. They know that they will be required to pay patent infringement damages that could bankrupt them. Even generic firms with a reasonable prospect of winning the case may elect to stay out of the market if they are risk averse or the expected profits of entering are negative.

The following example shows why it may be unprofitable for a generic to enter the market after the 30 months of litigation. Suppose a pioneer firm had a patent for a drug with a perfectly inelastic demand. The pioneer firm sold 1 million doses per month at $100, each of which cost $10 per dose to produce. The pioneer firm would earn $90 million per month in profit.

Now suppose Generic Firm 1 enters the market. Since it is the first generic firm to enter, it receives a 180-day period of market exclusivity and is the sole manufacturer of the drug besides the pioneer firm.[11] They split the market.[11] The pioneer firm charges $100 each for 500,000 doses and receives profits of $45 million per month. Generic Firm 1 charges $80 each for the remaining 500,000 doses and receives profits of $35 million per month.[12]

After the first six months, suppose Generic Firm 2 enters the market. The pioneer firm sells only 250,000 doses at $100 each, reducing its profits to $22.5 million per month. The two generic firms split the market equally for the remaining 750,000 doses. They each charge a price of $60 per dose and receive combined profits of $37.5 million per month.

The total loss of profits to the plaintiff is $270 million for the first six months and $405 million for the second six months, for a

---

[11] Due to state substitution laws, generic drugs generally capture a much higher percentage of the market.

[12] In this example, we assume that the generic drug is considered inferior to the branded drug by doctors or consumers. Thus, even though the price is lower, some consumers do not want to buy the generic drug. In fact, there are often brand-loyal consumers who will purchase brand-name drugs even when they are more expensive.

grand total loss of $675 million. Generic Firm 1 gains $210 million in profits for the first six months and $112.5 million in the second six months, for a total of $322.5 million. Generic Firm 2, which only operated during the second six months, gains profits of $112.5 million. Since the total profits earned by the generic producers add up to only $435 million, while the pioneer firm has a loss of $675 million in profits, the generic firms could not repay the damage if they wrongly entered the market.

A reverse payment in this case makes both parties happy and ends costly litigation. The generic firm loses nothing since its costs are covered by the pioneer firm – and the pioneer firm protects its patent. FTC reports of reverse payments offer some evidence for this claim. Many of the settlements that they analyzed in 2016 resulted in delayed generic entry, but compensation to generic firms was generally not much higher than the litigation costs. It may be that the generic firms were not planning to enter the market after 30 months of litigation due to the risks involved with paying infringement damages. Allowing the pioneer firms to pay their litigation fees allowed the generic firms to break even.

But the reverse payment will be illegal if the patent is invalid. In this case, the pioneer and generic firms are gaming the system by using the settlement as a means of dividing the market. Such market division schemes are per se violations of Section 1 of the Sherman Act. The pioneer firm's profits will be greater than those of the generic firm, which makes it profitable for the pioneer firm to pay off the generic firm to delay entry while harming consumers in the process. Payments would have to be less than the monopoly profits of the manufacturer, but greater than the expected profits that the generic firm would have received for the duration of the delay tempered by its probability of winning the patent infringement suit. In other words, the deal needs to be profitable for both the pioneer and generic firms. The pioneer firm will pay more if it believes that its patent is likely to be found invalid and that the generic firm will win the suit. Thus, a large payment may be a sign of an invalid patent. In the next section, we discuss how the courts have dealt with the question of reverse payments.

8.4   THE *ACTAVIS* DECISION

The disputes arising from pay-for-delay settlements expose the tension between antitrust law and patent law. Antitrust policy is aimed at protecting the competitive process in order to protect and promote consumer welfare. It does this by prohibiting collusion among ostensible competitors[13] and prohibiting monopolizing conduct by individual firms.[14] The Patent Act seeks to promote consumer welfare by encouraging innovation. A patent permits an innovator to monopolize the production, use, and sale of the patented item for a limited period of time.[15] There is a certain amount of tension between those two approaches to promoting consumer welfare. This conflict led to a split between the Courts of Appeals for the Sixth and Eleventh Circuits on the legality of reverse payments, which the Supreme Court attempted to remedy in *FTC* v. *Actavis*.[16]

Cardizem CD Antitrust Litigation

Hoechst Marian Rousell (HMR) sold a branded version of diltiazem hydrochloride under the brand name Cardizem CD.[17] The patent on the basic molecule had expired in November 1992, but other patents on the formulation and delivery mechanism had not expired. Andrx Pharmaceutical Inc., a generic pharmaceutical manufacturer,

---

[13] Section 1 of the Sherman Act forbids "contracts, combinations . . . or conspiracies in restraint of trade or commerce" (15 USC §1).

[14] Under Section 2 of the Sherman Act, any person who monopolizes or attempts to monopolize any part of trade or commerce is guilty of a felony (15 USC §2).

[15] This exclusivity provides the patentee with an incentive to devote resources to innovation, which is fraught with uncertainty. Any benefits that consumers might enjoy from the illicit competition of patent infringers may be too small to offset the costs of decreased innovation. Thus, public policy favors forgoing such consumer benefits in favor of protecting the incentive to invent.

[16] 570 US 136 (2013).

[17] Cardizem CD is prescribed for the treatment of angina and hypertension to prevent heart attacks and strokes.

produced a generic version of Cardizem CD that it proposed to market under the name Cartia XT. Andrx satisfied the FDA requirements that Cartia XT was therapeutically equivalent to Cardizem CD. As required by the Hatch-Waxman Act, Andrx provided a paragraph IV certification that Cartia XT did not infringe any valid patent covering Cardizem CD. Pursuant to the Hatch-Waxman Act's provisions, HMR filed a patent infringement suit against Andrx.[18] In response, Andrx filed an antitrust counterclaim against HMR alleging a violation of Section 2 of the Sherman Act. Under the terms of the Hatch-Waxman Act, HMR's suit stayed FDA approval of Cartia XT for 30 months. At the end of the 30-month period, HMR's patent infringement suit was unresolved, but the FDA was prepared to authorize the entry of Cartia XT into the market in competition with Cardizem CD.

When the FDA approved Andrx's entry, neither the patent infringement suit nor the antitrust counterclaim had been resolved. Although Andrx informed the FDA that it would enter the market as soon as it received permission, this was no sure thing. If Andrx had entered the market, it would have faced the risk of patent infringement damages. Consequently, Andrx may not have entered because potential damages would have exceeded Andrx's profits on the sales of Cartia XT. At the same time, HMR faced the prospect of paying treble damages to Andrx on the antitrust counterclaim.[19] These opposing risks made a settlement attractive.

As soon as the FDA authorized Andrx to begin supplying Cartia XT, HMR and Andrx entered into an agreement that settled both the patent infringement suit and the antitrust counterclaim. The terms of the agreement delayed the entry of Cartia XT. HMR agreed to pay $10 million per quarter to Andrx to refrain from entering the market. "Andrx also agreed to dismiss its antitrust and unfair competition counterclaims, to diligently prosecute its ANDA, and to not

[18] *In re Cardizem CD Antitrust Litigation*, No. 00-2483 218 F.R.D. 508 (E.D. Mich. 2003).
[19] If Andrx prevailed, its antitrust damages would seem to be limited to the forgone interest on the profits that it would have earned had it entered earlier.

'relinquish or otherwise compromise any right accruing thereunder or pertaining thereto' including its 180-day period of exclusivity."[20] Additionally, HMR pledged to pay $100 million per year minus the previous payments if the patent were deemed to be not infringed in a "final and unappealable determination." Andrx, as promised, stayed out of the market and began to receive payments from HMR. Less than a year later, Andrx reformulated its drug and sought FDA approval. When the FDA approved Andrx's reformulation, the HMR–Andrx agreement was terminated. HMR paid Andrx a final $50.7 million under the terms of the original settlement, and Andrx began to sell its reformulated product.

In the aftermath of their settlement, a class of Cardizem CD buyers sued HMR and Andrx. The class alleged that the HMR–Andrx settlement violated the antitrust laws and that the class paid higher prices for Cardizem CD than it would have paid for Cartia XT and thereby suffered antitrust injury. In the course of the litigation, the plaintiffs filed a partial summary judgment motion asking the district court to find the HMR–Andrx agreement unlawful per se under Section 1 of the Sherman Act. When the district court granted the plaintiff's motion, the defendants appealed to the Sixth Circuit Court of Appeals, which affirmed the district court's ruling.

The Sixth Circuit court focused on the fact that Andrx was paid $10 million per quarter to refrain from introducing Cartia XT into the US market. This payment led the court to find that the HMR–Andrx settlement agreement amounted to a horizontal market allocation scheme in violation of Section 1 of the Sherman Act.[21] The Sixth Circuit was not persuaded that Andrx would have stayed out of the market due to the fear of patent infringement damages. The court pointed to the $89.83 million that HMR had paid to Andrx as evidence that Andrx would not have been deterred. The court's economic logic, however, is unclear.

---

[20] *In re Cardizem CD Antitrust Litigation*, No. 00-2483 218 F.R.D. 508 (E.D. Mich. 2003).
[21] 332 F.3d 896 (6th Cir. 2003).

Presumably, the $89.83 million was more than Andrx's expected profit and less than HMR's expected loss. Consequently, patent infringement damages would have exceeded Andrx's profits.

In the Sixth Circuit, antitrust law trumped patent protection. Ordinarily, a patentee has the right to bar competition from any entity that would wrongly infringe its patent. In *Cardizem CD*, HMR alleged that entry by Andrx's Cartia XT would infringe its patents. HMR paid Andrx to refrain from infringing its patent rather than suffer the disruption in the market due to ongoing litigation. In effect, the Sixth Circuit ruled that a patentee cannot protect its intellectual property rights in this way. A patentee must continue to litigate or be found guilty of market division, which is per se unlawful under Section 1 of the Sherman Act.[22]

The AndroGel Litigation

Solvay Pharmaceuticals held a patent license on AndroGel, which is a synthetic testosterone supplement in gel form. Although the patent on the synthetic testosterone had expired, the gel formulation patent had not expired. Solvay began marketing AndroGel in 2001 following FDA approval. The product was quite successful, with sales of $1.8 billion during the 2001–2007 period.

On the heels of Solvay's successful entry, Watson Pharmaceuticals filed an ANDA with its generic substitute. At nearly the same time, Paddock Laboratories filed an ANDA of its own. Both generic manufacturers submitted paragraph IV certifications asserting that their products did not infringe any patent covering AndroGel. Pursuant to the provisions of the Hatch-Waxman Act, Solvay filed a patent infringement suit against both Watson and Paddock.[23] To reduce its exposure to the financial burdens of defending the patent infringement suit, Paddock partnered with Par Pharmaceuticals.

---

[22] *Palmer* v. *BRG of Georgia, Inc.*, 498 US 46 (1990) found a market division scheme to be a per se violation of Section 1 of the Sherman Act.
[23] 677 F.3d 1298 (11th Cir. 2012), *Cert.* granted 122 S. Ct. 787 (2012).

As usual, the patent litigation was unresolved at the end of 30 months in December 2005. Pursuant to the Hatch-Waxman Act, the FDA then authorized generic entry by Watson Pharmaceuticals. At that point, the parties settled the patent litigation on terms that involved reverse payments. Solvay, the plaintiff, agreed to pay $10 million per year for six years to Par/Paddock. In addition, it agreed to pay another $2 million per year to Par for its agreement to provide backup production support to Solvay. Watson received a profit-sharing agreement from Solvay that was expected to generate $19–30 million per year.

In exchange for its largesse, Solvay received commitments from the generic manufacturers. Par Pharmaceuticals agreed to provide backup production capability for Solvay, which reduced Solvay's business risk. Watson agreed to market AndroGel to urologists, whereas Paddock agreed to market AndroGel to primary care physicians. Although those costly marketing services were valueable to Solvay, the most important term of the settlement involved delayed entry. Both Watson and Par/Paddock agreed to stay out of the US market until August 31, 2015.

To put these settlement terms into perspective, recall that Solvay's revenues for 2000–2007 exceeded $1.8 billion, for an annual average of $225 million. Watson forecasted its price to be 25 percent of the AndroGel price, which would have caused Solvay's sales to fall by 90 percent, thereby costing Solvay $125 million per year in profits.[24]

Paying for delayed entry would appear to be a sound business decision. Solvay agreed to pay $31–42 million per year to avoid a $125 million loss in profits. In addition, Solvay avoided the risk of having its patent deemed invalid. Finally, Solvay received marketing services from Par and Watson as an added bonus.

In 2009, the Federal Trade Commission filed suit against Solvay, Par, Paddock, and Watson, alleging that the reverse payment

[24] *Federal Trade Commission* v. *Watson Pharmaceuticals, Inc.*, No. 10-12729 (11th Cir. 2012).

settlement was a violation of Section 1 of the Sherman Act and a violation of Section 5 of the FTC Act. The Eleventh Circuit rejected the FTC's claims largely because the settlement did not extend beyond the scope of Solvay's patent. The exclusionary terms of the agreement ended in 2015 while Solvay's patent extended until August 2020.

In the Eleventh Circuit, a reverse payment settlement was immune from antitrust challenge as long as its anticompetitive potential fell within the exclusionary potential of the patent. The FTC argued that Solvay was not likely to prevail with its patent infringement claim. In the event that Solvay lost, it would not have had the right to exclude competitors from the market.

The Eleventh Circuit found the FTC's argument to be unpersuasive. Even if a favorable outcome for Solvay was unlikely, that did not mean that the probability was zero. Thus, the FTC was asking the court to speculate, and it was not prepared to do so. But the Eleventh Circuit decision gave pioneer firms the opportunity to protect invalid patents by using reverse payment settlements to pay competitors to stay out of the market.

The Supreme Court Weighs In

In *Actavis*,[25] the Supreme Court found that neither the Sixth Circuit nor the Eleventh Circuit had correctly addressed reverse payments. Reverse payment settlements were neither per se unlawful as the Sixth Circuit held nor per se lawful as the Eleventh Circuit held.[26] Instead, reverse payment settlements must be evaluated under the rule of reason, which involves a three-step process that shifts the burden of proof from the plaintiff to the defendant and then back to

---

[25] *Federal Trade Commission* v. *Actavis*, 570 US 136 (2013).

[26] The case was remanded to the district court, and the parties came to an agreement in February 2019. AbbVie, the new owner of Solvay, agreed that it would not enter into any reverse payment agreements with producers of generic drugs (Federal Trade Commission 2019).

the plaintiff. First, the plaintiff's burden is to establish that the conduct in question is demonstrably anticompetitive. Second, if the plaintiff is successful in making its case, the defendant must refute the plaintiff's claims in one of two ways. The defendant could argue that the plaintiff's allegations are simply incorrect; that is, there is no factual foundation for the claims. Alternatively, the defendant could offer a procompetitive justification for its conduct. Third, the burden of proof shifts back to the plaintiff to offer a less restrictive means of accomplishing the same ends for the defendant. The outcome of the legal dispute depends on which party is most successful in meeting its burden of proof.

In patent infringement suits under the Hatch-Waxman Act, the patent's validity is at the center of the dispute. If a patent is found to be invalid, then the patentee has no basis for preventing competition from producers of generic equivalents. Any agreement to preclude or curtail competition would be proscribed by Section 1 of the Sherman Act.

In this context, the antitrust challenge arises because the patent dispute has not been settled. The patentee holds a patent that presumably is valid since it was issued by the PTO. But, because the suit was settled before the patent's validity was determined in court, we simply do not know whether the patent is valid.

The Supreme Court recognized the obvious conflict between antitrust law and intellectual property law in its *Actavis* decision. It found that antitrust challenges to reverse payment settlements should be resolved through a rule of reason analysis and thereby took the middle ground. The Court indicated that reverse payments could be anticompetitive, and further analysis must be conducted to determine the competitive impact. Since the legality of any specific reverse payment settlement had to be determined through a rule of reason analysis, it was left to the lower courts to develop the law.

The Supreme Court offered five considerations in rendering its decision. First, the Court found that reverse payments can have serious anticompetitive effects that would harm consumers.[27] If the litigation had continued and the patent had been deemed invalid, the settlement would then have been nothing more than a platform for monopoly profit sharing. This eliminates the presumption that a reverse payment is always legal. Second, reverse payments can be justified based on "traditional settlement considerations, such as avoided litigation costs or fair value for services" actually rendered.[28] Therefore, the Court concluded that reverse payments are also not per se unlawful. Third, where a reverse payment threatens to cause unjustified anticompetitive harm, the patentee likely possesses the power to actually bring about that harm. Fourth, evaluating a reverse payment is more feasible than first thought by the Eleventh Circuit. The Court suggested using the size of the settlement as an indication of the patent's weakness. If the patent is more likely to be invalid, the pioneer firm will pay a premium to keep the generic out of the market. Therefore, unjustified large payments could signal patent invalidity. Fifth, reverse payments are not the only way to settle patent litigation issues. If firms prefer reverse payments over other methods solely because of monopoly profit sharing, then they should be considered anticompetitive. One common method of settlement that does not involve a reverse payment is a licensing agreement. The patentee agrees to license its patent to the generic firm, which enters the market once the litigation has settled.

These considerations, however, leave many unanswered questions for the lower courts, which have led to confusion and inconsistency in rulings.[29] At issue is the lack of guidance on the threshold for

---

[27] Interestingly, the majority and the dissenting justices reemphasized their commitment to consumer welfare in the *Actavis* case. The courts would not look favorably on an agreement that raised total and producer welfare at the cost of consumer welfare.

[28] *Federal Trade Commission* v. *Actavis*, 570 US 136 (2013).

[29] In the years since the *Actavis* case, reverse payments in the traditional sense have declined. Pharmaceutical firms, however, have found other ways to settle litigation that may be anticompetitive while flying under the radar of the Supreme Court's test (Karas, Anderson, and Feldman 2019).

large and unjustified payments. A reasonable assessment of "large" must consider the cost of litigation. The median litigation costs in 2013, according to an American Intellectual Property Law Association survey, were between $2.65 and $6 million, depending on the damages at stake. Another study suggested that patent litigation cost generic firms an average of $10 million. Thus, a $5 or $10 million upper threshold may be justified.[30] In its view, the FTC generally uses a $7 million threshold.[31] Arguably, payments below this threshold would not cause anticompetitive harm. By accepting such a settlement, the generic firm would be signaling that it does not have a strong case, which would support an inference of patent validity. Anything above this threshold would require further justification.

Litigation costs incurred, however, are not the whole story. For example, if a plaintiff had a claim with an expected recovery of $100,000, the plaintiff would not settle for, say, $15,000, which would be the avoided litigation costs. In the context of patent infringement suits under the Hatch-Waxman Act, the issues are more complex because the suit seeks to prevent infringement rather than seek compensation after the fact.

Another possible justification of a large payment is compensation for the fair value of services rendered, such as backup production or marketing. This justification, however, requires the lower courts to decide the "fair value" of a service, which can lead to more confusion and inconsistency in court rulings. Without this evaluation, however, pioneer firms could disguise anticompetitive reverse payments as payment for services. For example, in the reverse payment settlement of *Actavis*, the FTC alleged that Solvay entered into unprofitable deals with the generic firms for backup production and marketing.[32] Such deals between drug manufacturers are quite

---

[30] Carrier (2014).   [31] Towey and Albert (2019).

[32] In its complaint, the FTC alleged that Solvay's payment for services was far above value. Before the litigation, Solvay did not include co-promotion in its business plan due to evidence showing its ineffectiveness. Yet, in its settlement, Solvay not only entered into co-promotion deals but also vastly overpaid. The firm would have paid

uncommon outside the context of litigation, which further supports the inference that a payoff may have occurred. Thus, courts must analyze these deals closely even though they may not have good information or sufficient expertise to determine fair value. A fair value for services justification could soon become an administrative nightmare.

Finally, the Supreme Court dismissed the notion that a pioneer firm with a valid patent may pay off the generic firm to reduce its risk of an erroneous finding on patent invalidity. This seems to be a serious mistake. Suppose a pioneer firm earns $200 million per year on its patented drug and that the patent has five years left. Further, suppose that the probability of an erroneous finding of invalidity is 0.10. The patentee's expected loss from an erroneous verdict is $20 million per year or $100 million over the next five years. If the pioneer firm can settle the patent litigation for, say, $50 million, it will avoid the expected loss of $100 million and avoid litigation costs of perhaps $10 million. Although the settlement may seem disproportionate to the avoided litigation costs, it stems from a relatively small probability of error. Lower courts may consider this settlement to be large and unjustified even though it is efficient. The increase in standards for reverse payment settlements may decrease the number of these settlements, including some that would have been justified. Insofar as the courts encourage settlement over trial, this ruling may be inefficient.

8.5   THE POST-*ACTAVIS* EXPERIENCE[33]

The Supreme Court's *Actavis* opinion did not provide much guidance to the lower courts. The opinion mandated rule of reason treatment, but it did not spell out the balancing – if any – that the lower courts would have to conduct in determining whether a particular reverse

about $300 per sales call when the industry average was only about $45. Similarly, before litigation, Solvay had no intention of organizing backup production. Yet, it entered into an agreement with a generic firm to provide backup production during the settlement (Carrier 2014).

[33] For an excellent survey, see Areeda and Hovenkamp (2021) at ¶2046f.

payment settlement was anticompetitive. A superficial reading of *Actavis* suggests that reverse payments can be found competitively unreasonable only if they involve cash payments. As an economic matter, this makes no sense since in-kind payments can serve much the same purpose as cash payments. It appears that this loophole has been closed by subsequent lower court rulings. Yet, drug companies are finding other ways of restricting generic entry without ringing alarm bells.

Nonmonetary Settlements

Pioneer firms have learned that reverse payments involving cash will be subject to increased scrutiny by the Federal Trade Commission. Thus, they have turned to other nonmonetary settlements as compensation for delayed entry. Pioneer firms may enter into agreements with generic firms to provide backup production or marketing, as was the case with Solvay. Additionally, the pioneer firm may offer a license to the generic firm to sell a generic version of its branded drug. The pioneer firm may even offer the generic firm a license to sell a different drug. For example, AbbVie agreed to license a different drug to Teva as a reward for Teva's delayed entry into the generic AndroGel market.[34]

The Threat of Authorized Generics

Some pioneer firms have introduced an "authorized," or "branded," generic version of their pioneer drug. Thus, the pioneer firm sells precisely the same product under a different label at a different price. The presence of an authorized generic provides immediate competition for the drug introduced by a generic firm, since it is not subject to the 180-day period of exclusivity. Consequently, the entry of a branded generic will substantially reduce the profit that the generic producer could earn during its 180-day exclusivity period. A study

---

[34] *Federal Trade Commission* v. *AbbVie, Inc., et al.*, No. 2621 (3rd Cir. 2014).

showed that generic prices would be 16 percent lower on average when an authorized generic was present.[35]

In some cases, the pioneer firm has settled its patent infringement case by agreeing not to introduce an authorized generic during the 180-day exclusivity period in exchange for a delayed entry of the generic drug. Although this is obviously not a cash payment, this promise certainly has value. This seemingly clever settlement does not seem to be anticompetitive, but it does delay the entry of competing generics to the market. If the original patent is invalid, the prices will be higher, the quantities sold will be lower, and consumers will be harmed. We offer several examples of antitrust litigation involving branded generics.[36]

A recent example of this agreement occurred with Lamictal. A class of direct purchasers of Lamictal, which treats epilepsy, sued GlaxoSmithKline PLC (GSK) and Teva Pharmaceutical Industries Ltd. (Teva) for suppressing generic competition through a pay-for-delay agreement.[37] As part of the agreement, GSK, the original manufacturer of Lamictal, agreed to "pay" Teva to delay the entry of its generic by six months by assuring Teva that they would not introduce their own authorized generic during Teva's period of exclusivity. The Third Circuit concluded that the "no-authorized-generic" agreement would be considered the same as a cash payment.[38]

Another case involving the drug Intuniv, which treats attention-deficit hyperactivity disorder (ADHD), provides some guidance.

[35] *In re Effexor XR Antitrust Litigation*, No. 11-5479 (D. N.J. 2014).

[36] Hikma Pharmaceuticals entered into an agreement with Jazz Pharmaceuticals (Jazz), such that Jazz would delay entry of its narcolepsy drug Xyrem for six months in exchange for the license to sell an "authorized" version of Xyrem and thereby share in the monopoly profits. If any other pharmaceutical firm were to enter the market before the end of the six months, the terms of the contract would allow Jazz to enter (Leonard 2021).

[37] *King Drug Co. of Florence, Inc.* v. *SmithKline Beecham Corporation*, 791 F.3d 388 (3rd Cir. 2015). For a more recent class action suit, see *In re Lamictal Direct Purchaser Antitrust Litigation*, No. 19-1655, (3rd Cir. 2019).

[38] *King Drug of Florence, Inc.* v. *SmithKline Beecham Corporation*, 791 F.3d 388 (3rd Cir. 2015).

As part of the settlement agreement, Shire, LLC, the original manufacturer of Intuniv, agreed to delay entry of its authorized generic during Actavis's 180-day period of exclusivity in return for delayed generic entry. The District of Massachusetts, which tried the case, reasoned that "if a brand company agrees to sacrifice some of its profits and transfer them to a generic as part of a settlement agreement, the Court may infer that the unexplained payment was given in exchange for the generic delaying entry."[39] Thus, the court concluded that using the threat of an authorized generic to delay entry was not necessarily free from antitrust scrutiny. The plaintiffs (direct and indirect purchasers) settled with Actavis for $1.1 million and with Shire for $1.85 million.

Other Loopholes

Amgen and Teva faced a lawsuit for a rather clever reverse payment.[40] Amgen patented and sold its blockbuster drug, Sensipar, which reduces calcium in the blood for those with chronic kidney disease. Annual sales of the drug have netted Amgen more than $1 billion since 2015. When the FDA gave final approval for Watson Pharmaceuticals' non-infringing patent for generic Sensipar, Teva, which owned the rights, immediately launched its own generic. Launching the generic was risky since Amgen had appealed the patent infringement decision. After a week on the market in which Teva earned a profit of $393 million, Teva and Amgen reached a settlement. Teva exited the market and agreed to delay the entry of its generic. Additionally, Teva paid Amgen $40 million in damages due to its weeklong entry. Although not an explicit reverse payment, the plaintiffs alleged that the settlement was a net reverse payment since the damages Teva paid to Amgen were only a fraction of the profits it made by launching its generic for a week.

---

[39] *In re Intuniv Antitrust Litigation*, No. 1:16-cv-12653-ADB (D. Mass. 2020). Revised Memorandum and Order on Motions for Summary Judgement.
[40] *In re Sensipar (Cincalcet Hydrochloride Tablets) Antitrust Litigation*, No. 19-md-2895 (D. Del. 2020).

In some cases, the drug companies may come to agreements on the court steps. Bausch Health Companies Inc. and Assertio Therapeutics, Inc., secretly conspired with Lupin Pharmaceuticals to keep Lupin's generic version of Glumetza, which treats diabetes, off the market for six months. The settlement involved a no-authorized-generic agreement.[41]

Although traditional reverse payment settlements are on the decline, drug companies are devising clever ways to get around the rules.[42] The *Actavis* decision has contributed considerably to the decline in the number of traditional reverse payment settlements, as seen in Table 8.1. The Federal Trade Commission's latest report of reverse payments from 2017 indicates that no reverse payment included an unjustified payment above $7 million, which is their threshold for litigation costs.[43] Additionally, there were no agreements that included the threat of authorized generic entry. The threat of legal action has played a substantial role in this decline.[44]

Surprisingly, however, even though the number of seemingly anticompetitive agreements has dropped significantly, the number of settlements has increased. For example, from 2015 to 2016, the number of settlements between pharmaceutical companies rose from 170 to 232, as seen in Table 8.1. As long as these settlements are truly procompetitive, social welfare is optimized. It is reasonable to say,

---

[41] Bausch Health Companies Inc. has agreed to pay $300 million to settle the antitrust lawsuit (Pierson 2021). Assertio Therapeutics, Inc., also settled for an undisclosed amount (Barker 2020). Lupin Pharmaceuticals agreed to settle for $150 million (Brittain 2021).

[42] *Impax Laboratories, Inc.* v. *Federal Trade Commission*, No. 19-60394 (5th Cir. 2019) is an example of a recent reverse payment case. There is also ongoing private litigation: *In re Opana ER Antitrust Litigation*, No. 14-cv-10150 (N.D. Ill. 2021).

[43] Federal Trade Commission (2020).

[44] After 2000, when the FTC declared that it would begin prosecuting reverse payment settlements, the number of settlements declined. The numbers jumped back up after a 2005 circuit court decision that was sympathetic to reverse payments. See *Schering-Plough Corporation* v. *Federal Trade Commission*, No. 04-10688 (11th Cir. 2005).

Table 8.1. *Reverse payment agreements, 2004-2017*[a]

Year	Resolved patent litigation	Restricted generic entry	Payment and restriction	Payment above litigation fees (>$7 million)	Notes
2004	14	5	0	0	
2005	11	4	3	3	
2006	28	20	14	13	*Schering-Plough v. FTC*[b]
2007	33	25	14	14	
2008	66	46	16	15	
2009	68	57	19	11	
2010	113	97	31	17	
2011	156	128	28	25	
2012	140	121	40	33	
2013	145	104	29	15	*Actavis*
2014	160	140	21	11	
2015	170	150	14	5	
2016	232	195	30	1	
2017	226	197	20	3	

[a] The data were obtained from FTC reports available at www.ftc.gov/system/files/documents/reports/reports/agreements-filed-federal-trade-commission-under-medicare-prescription-drug-improvement-modernization/mma_report_fy2017.pdf.
[b] In this decision, the Eleventh Circuit ruled that a reverse payment that restricted generic entry and offered the generic firm compensation was not a violation of the Federal Trade Commission Act.

however, that some of these reverse settlements may have included patents that were invalid and should have been overturned. Delayed generic entry harms consumers; thus, a better method of evaluating these settlements could improve consumer welfare. In the next section, we discuss some possible remedies.

8.6 LEGISLATIVE REMEDIES

Both state and federal legislators are concerned about the high prices of pharmaceutical products. When patent infringement litigation results in deferred entry of generic substitutes, there is an understandable frustration. In spite of the Supreme Court's decision in *Actavis*, legislators appear to be impatient and have proposed legislation that is aimed at curtailing reverse payments and the corresponding losses of generic competition.

State Legislation

The State of California has taken dead aim at reverse payment settlements with the Preserving Access to Affordable Drugs Act, which went into effect in January 2020. In California, there is a presumption of illegality. Any reverse payment settlement that includes (1) a generic firm receiving "anything of value" from the branded firm and (2) delayed entry by the generic substitute would be deemed anticompetitive. The firms would then have to prove that the agreement was justified and procompetitive by establishing that the payment amounted to no more than the litigation costs that were avoided plus the true value of any services provided by the generic producer.

The sanctions for violating the statute could reach $20 million or three times the value of the settlement payment to the generic firm. In essence, the California statute bans reverse payments that pay for delay. There does not appear to be any wiggle room for reverse payments that share the monopoly profits. Interestingly, the law would be applicable to any reverse settlement agreement that involved a drug sold in California, which could extend the law's influence to the rest of the United States.[45] This law may be overly restrictive since it likely would also criminalize payments in cases where a patent would be valid, that is, where a reverse payment would be procompetitive. If this is the case, the law may decrease incentives to innovate.

Federal Legislative Proposals

There are a number of congressional proposals that would reduce, or even eliminate, anticompetitive reverse payments. For example, the Strengthening Health Care and Lowering Prescription Drug Costs Act, which passed the House in 2019,[46] includes a section that makes unjustified reverse payments illegal. "[I]t shall be unlawful for a ... [New Drug Application] or [Biologics License Application] holder and subsequent filer ... to enter into, or carry out, an agreement resolving or settling a covered patent infringement claim on a final or interim basis" if the generic firm receives anything of value or the subsequent filer limits or forgoes research, development, manufacturing, marketing, or sales. The bill does allow these agreements if it can be shown that they result from fair compensation for other services. This legislation is quite similar to that of California and would reduce unlawful reverse settlements.

The Competitive DRUGS Act of 2019[47] takes a different approach to reverse payments. First, it emphasizes that the FTC has the power to challenge reverse payment settlements in court. Second, the Act would impose other penalties on the pioneer and generic firms for engaging in reverse payment settlements. These manufacturers could lose research and development tax benefits, and they may need to pay a tax of half of the value of the settlement payment. By

---

[45] California was only able to create this law because of its passage of the Cartwright Act, which does not apply to other states (Ford, Spaeth, and Luo 2020).

[46] Strengthening Health Care and Lowering Prescription Drug Costs Act, H.R. 987, 116th Congress (2019). This bill was passed by the House but has not been passed by the Senate.

[47] Competitive DRUGS Act of 2019, H.R. 1344, 116th Congress (2019). The bill did not receive a vote and died in Congress.

imposing these penalties, the Act would make it riskier for the drug manufacturers to agree to a reverse payment settlement.

Amending the Hatch-Waxman Act

The antitrust approach to reverse settlements focuses on patent litigation. But amending the Hatch-Waxman Act may be another avenue to pursue. The Hatch-Waxman Act tried to balance the need for innovation while encouraging generic entry that would lead to affordable prices. The incentives, however, are not well balanced. Specifically, the introduction of the 30-month stay on generic entry during patent litigation gives pioneer firms unjustified monopoly profits, and the 180-day exclusivity period may encourage sham paragraph IV certifications.

First, during the 30-month period of patent litigation where generic entry is prevented, the pioneer firm will earn monopoly profits that may be unjustified. In many circumstances, when a pioneer firm receives notice that a generic producer has filed a paragraph IV certification, it has an incentive to file a patent infringement suit even if it knows, or suspects, that its patent will be deemed invalid. Consider Solvay's situation. It was earning about $225 million in annual revenues. If its return on sales had been 80 percent, then its annual profit would have been $180 million. Even if Solvay planned to abandon the suit at the end of the 30-month stay, its profits (undiscounted) would have amounted to $450 million! Even after deducting the cost of maintaining the litigation and the profit that it would have earned with generic competition, there would remain a substantial profit.

To some extent, the 30-month stay is justified because the initial stages of the patent litigation could give both parties a sense of the strength of each other's claims. That sense would inform the generic firm on whether it should enter the market after the 30-month period. At the same time, the decision to enter with a looming patent infringement suit is not much different whether it occurs at the beginning of the patent infringement suit or after 30 months.

The 30-month stay, then, provides an unnecessary incentive for pioneer firms to initiate patent infringement suits, even if their claim is weak. In some cases, it delays the entry of rightful generics that would reduce costs for consumers. Additionally, if the first generic firm to file settles with the pioneer firm, a new generic firm must wait another 30 months before it can get its drug approved for market, which could delay generic entry until the end of the patent's life.

Second, the 180-day exclusivity period provides a strong incentive for generics to file ANDAs, even if their claims are weak. If the market is lucrative enough, the reward of duopoly profits may make it worthwhile to attempt to enter even if the risk of winning a patent infringement suit is low. In these cases, the pioneer firm would likely initiate a patent infringement suit that it should win. Thus, resources are wasted on litigation. Additionally, the small but positive chance of a generic firm winning such a suit would reduce incentives to innovate. The 180-day exclusivity requirement could be revised such that generic firms would only be allowed to gain 180-day exclusivity if they successfully defeated the pioneer brand in court – only the first successful challenger would get the reward. This would also eliminate the loophole that allows the first generic firm to file an ANDA to hold its 180-day exclusivity period until it enters.[48] The problem with this proposal lies in the fact that patent infringement litigation is extremely slow. Few – if any – patent challenges are resolved in 30 months. After the final court verdict, the loser can appeal. The pioneer firm could continue to delay generic entry by extending patent litigation with appeals and other tactics. This would further delay generic entry and could be more profitable than a reverse payment settlement.

Europe takes a different approach to approving generic entry that may mitigate some of the concerns noted above. In Europe,

---

[48] A provision in the Hatch-Waxman Act would force the generic producer to forfeit its 180-day exclusivity after 75 days of non-use. Unfortunately, this forfeiture clause only works if the generic producer knew whether the patent was valid. Since most reverse settlements do not specify validity, generic firms can maintain their 180-day exclusivity.

generics are approved without consideration of existing patents.[49] Thus, a generic drug could be approved for any drug product whether on patent or not. Once approved, the generic firm has the option of entering the market immediately, but it must weigh the consideration that its patent may infringe on the pioneer firm's patent if it enters. This method eliminates the 30-month delay in generic entry and the possibility of the pioneer firm earning unjustified monopoly profits. Additionally, although there is no period of exclusivity that functions as a direct incentive to be the first to file, profits from being one of the first generic firms to enter may be substantial.[50]

Review by the Patent and Trademark Office

Once the PTO issues a patent, subsequent challenges to its validity are resolved in court. But is this process sensible? Courts lack the expertise to resolve this question. It may make more sense to have the PTO review its initial decision.

The courts could delegate the determination of patent validity to the PTO. Much of the ambiguity surrounding the legality of reverse payments concerns the validity of the patent. If the patent is invalid, any settlement that delays generic entry would seem to be a per se violation of Section 1 of the Sherman Act. If the patent is valid, then the patentee is entitled to prevent entry even if it has to bribe the generic producer to refrain from entering.[51] Determining patent validity, however, is not an antitrust matter and requires experience and knowledge that most courts do not possess. The PTO does have this expertise and knowledge.

---

[49] Gallasch (2016).

[50] Note that entering a market first does indeed bring an advantage even without a period of exclusivity. For the time that the firm is exclusive, it can make huge profits. Take, for example, Teva, which earned $393 million in the first week of selling generic cinacalcet hydrochloride tablets. *In re Sensipar (Cinacalcet Hydrochloride Tablets) Antitrust Litigation*, No. 19-md-2895 (D. Del. 2020).

[51] The pioneer firm has the right to exclude anyone from the market. Payments for delay, then, are irrelevant. Recognizing this, the pioneer firm would not offer a settlement with a payment larger than its nuisance cost.

A reverse settlement with a certain threshold payment in a patent infringement suit could trigger a second look by the PTO's Patent Trial and Appeal Board in an *inter partes* review. Then, a patent can be challenged only for novelty or obviousness issues. Once challenged, the patent undergoes an administrative trial that includes the parties and judges with the relevant technical and patent litigation knowledge. This review proffers results within one year and is more efficient than traditional court litigation.[52] Additionally, patents can be reviewed parallel to district court cases. This policy would serve two purposes. First, invalid patents would be overturned, and strong patents would receive a seal of approval that would diminish the risk of future paragraph IV certifications. Second, a determination from the PTO would remove the need for a reverse settlement.[53]

Rather than settling disputes through the PTO, the parties in the patent infringement suits could hire expert witnesses who could discuss the validity of the patent. For example, in *In re Zetia (Ezetimibe) Antitrust Litigation*,[54] the plaintiffs introduced a patent lawyer who gave an expert opinion concerning the plaintiff's likelihood of prevailing in the case. But this method has been criticized as being too speculative.

The threat of litigation by the Agencies and private parties has been quite effective at reducing the number of anticompetitive reverse payment agreements. Legislative proposals, revisions of the Hatch-Waxman Act, and *inter partes* analysis would refine the process to further winnow the wheat from the chaff.

8.7 PRIVATE DAMAGE ACTIONS

Settlements of patent infringement suits involving the delayed entry of a generic substitute for a pioneer drug have spawned private

---

[52] The *inter partes* review can be extended for six months if there is good reason to do so.

[53] For more details about a possible role of the PTO, see Areeda and Hovenkamp (2021, ¶2046).

[54] *In re Zetia (Ezetimibe) Antitrust Litigation*, No. 2:18-md-02836 (D. E. Vir. 2018).

antitrust damage suits. An unlawful settlement is a contract that restrains trade. To the extent that the pioneer firm and the generic producer agree not to compete, health care consumers and their insurers are denied the benefits of competition – they have paid more and consumed less. Instead of paying lower prices for generic substitutes, they must pay the pioneer firm's monopoly prices. The plaintiff, therefore, alleges that it would have paid less for a therapeutically equivalent generic substitute than it actually paid for the pioneer brand. In other words, the plaintiff alleges that it has been overcharged.

While the legal issues surrounding the question of liability seem to be quite complicated, the focus of the damage inquiry is straightforward. This is not to say, however, that measuring the damages will be easy. The antitrust damages would be

$$\Delta = \left(P_a - P_{bf}\right)Q_a,$$

where P_a is the price actually paid for the pioneer brand, P_{bf} is the price that would have been charged but for the illicit settlement terms, and Q_a is the quantity actually purchased. Most of the antitrust damage claims are class actions that span several years. Consequently, obtaining accurate data on P_a and Q_a may require a monumental accounting effort. Adjustments for discounts, rebates, coupons, returns, and any other variable affecting the actual price and/or the actual quantity must be included. For example, an uninsured patient may be charged the list price of, say, $100 but have a $25 coupon from the producer. The net price of $75 is the correct value of P_a for that patient. In some cases, the pioneer brand may reduce its price in response to generic entry.[55] In other cases, the pioneer firm may introduce an authorized generic of its own. It does not take much imagination to see that there may well be many different values for P_a.

The more troublesome problem is finding a suitable value for the but-for price, P_{bf}. The values of the but-for price do not reside

---

[55] Often, the pioneer brand raises its price after generic entry so that it can extract a higher margin on its brand-loyal consumers.

in any accounting records. These values must be estimated, and this may prove to be extremely difficult. First, no before-and-after methodology can be employed. Since the allegedly infringing generic has never been sold and will not be sold due to the delay, there is no "before" or "after" period. This leaves the yardstick methodology, which relies on experience in another market as a surrogate for the market in question. In other words, the plaintiff might identify another pioneer brand that faced generic entry and track the generic prices in that market. The pattern of declining prices of the generic substitute would then be applied to the market under review. For the yardstick damage methodology to provide reliable estimates, the yardstick market must be comparable to the plaintiff's market in all important respects.[56] Therefore, finding a suitable yardstick can prove quite difficult.

The question then becomes whether this effort provides a reliable inference or speculation. If this methodology and its application are found to be reliable, the damage estimation problem will be solved. If a judge deems the estimates speculative, however, they will be inadmissible – the jury will never see them. Fortunately, most of these cases settle before a final decision is reached, and no reliable damage calculation must be estimated.

In the aftermath of the *Actavis* decision, there has been a flood of private antitrust damage suits. These suits have included a case against Celgene for keeping generic substitutes of its drugs Thalomid and Revlimid off the market, which resulted in a $55 million settlement;[57] a California case against Teva, Cephalon, and Barr Laboratories for a reverse payment settlement agreement concerning the wakefulness drug Provigil, which resulted in a $69 million settlement;[58] the case against Allergen for reverse payments that delayed

---

[56] See Areeda and Hovenkamp (2021, ¶392) for further discussion.
[57] Lichtenberg (2019).
[58] Bauman (2020). Note that this settlement was made with the State of California. Other class actions concerning Provigil have yielded other settlements.

generic Namenda for six years, which settled for $750 million;[59] and a case involving Takeda and Endo's agreement to delay entry of generic Amitiza, which allegedly led to hundreds of millions of dollars in overcharges.[60]

8.8 CONCLUDING REMARKS

Reverse payments are found in pharmaceutical patent infringement cases due to the provisions of the Hatch-Waxman Act that delay generic entry for 30 months while patent litigation is ongoing. As long as this provision remains, every paragraph IV certification that is filed by a generic firm may be met with a patent infringement suit, even if the patent is invalid or not infringed. This could cause considerable harm to consumers in the form of higher drug costs. On the other hand, it is important to recognize that the patent may be valid and a reverse payment settlement is a means to end costly litigation, which would be efficient. Since reverse payment settlements are neither invariably anticompetitive nor invariably procompetitive or competitively neutral, rule of reason treatment seems appropriate. Even so, the lack of concrete instruction has led to some confusion in the lower courts. Currently, Congress is attempting to resolve this discrepancy by passing definitive laws that should make it easier to isolate anticompetitive reverse payments.

APPENDIX: THE ECONOMICS OF SETTLEMENTS

Consider an example of litigation involving two parties, Jones and Miller. Jones alleges that she was injured by Miller and sues him for an amount S. In the vast majority of cases, this dispute will be settled before trial. Here, we explain why.

Jones recognizes that litigation is risky and assigns a probability of p to winning and a probability of $(1 - p)$ to losing the case. Whether she wins or loses,

---

[59] Sullivan (2019).

[60] *KPH Healthcare Services, Inc.* v. *Takeda Pharmaceutical Co.* No. 1:21-cv-11255 (D. Mass. 2021).

she incurs costs of litigation equal to C_J. Consequently, the expected value of the litigation to Jones is

$$E[L]_J = pS + (1 - p)(0) - C_J = pS - C_J.$$

For Miller, there is no upside. If he wins, he pays nothing but incurs his costs of litigation, C_M. If he loses, he pays S and still incurs costs of C_M. For Miller, the expected cost of the litigation is

$$E[L]_M = qS + (1 - q)(0) + C_M = qS + C_M,$$

where q is Miller's assessment of the probability that he will lose.

If Miller's expected loss exceeds Jones's expected gain, the litigation is more valuable to Miller and he will buy it from Jones by settling. If $E[L]_M > E[L]_J$, then $qS + C_M > pS - C_J$. This settlement condition will be satisfied whenever p and q are the same. The important point to remember is that the defendant pays the plaintiff – not the other way around. This is why settlements under the Hatch-Waxman Act are an anomaly – the plaintiff pays the defendant.

REFERENCES

Areeda, Phillip, and Herbert Hovenkamp. (2021). *Antitrust Law*, Vol. XII. 5th ed. New York: Wolters Kluwer.

Areeda, Phillip E., Herbert Hovenkamp, Roger D. Blair, and Christine Piette Durrance. (2021). *Antitrust Law*, Vol. IIA, 5th ed. New York: Wolters Kluwer.

Barker, Holly. (2020). *Glumetza Class Certified in Lawsuit Alleging $2.3 Billion Injury*. Bloomberg Law. https://news.bloomberglaw.com/mergers-and-anti trust/gulemtza-class-certified-in-lawsuit-alleging-2-3-billion-injury.

Bauman, Valerie. (2020). *Pharma Pay-for-Delay Deals Called "Cost of Doing Business."* Bloomberg Law. https://news.bloomberglaw.com/pharma-and-life-sciences/pharma-pay-for-delay-settlements-cost-of-doing-business.

Blair, Roger D., and Thomas F. Cotter. (2002). Are Settlements of Patent Disputes Illegal Per Se? *Antitrust Bulletin* 47: 491–539.

Brittain, Blake. (2021). *Lupin Agrees to Pay $150 Mln to settle Glumetza Antitrust Claims*. Reuters. www.reuters.com/legal/litigation/lupin-agrees-pay-150-mln-settle-glumetza-antitrust-claims-2021-09-21/.

Carrier, Michael A. (2014). *Payment After Actavis. Iowa Law Review* 100: 7–49.

Federal Trade Commission. (2019). Last Remaining Defendant Settles FTC Suit That Led to Landmark Supreme Court Ruling on Drug Company "Reverse Payments." www.ftc.gov/news-events/press-releases/2019/02/last-remaining-defendant-settles-ftc-suit-led-landmark-supreme.

Federal Trade Commission. (2020). Agreements Filed with the Federal Trade Commission under the Medicare Prescription Drug, Improvement, and Modernization Act of 2003: Overview of Agreements Filed in FY 2017. www.ftc.gov/system/files/documents/reports/agreements-filed-federal-trade-com mission-under-medicare-prescription-drug-improvement-modernization/mma_ report_fy2017.pdf.

Ford, Mark A., Peter A. Spaeth, and Christina Luo. (2020). *Unprecedented State Law on Pharmaceutical "Reverse Payments" Goes into Effect*. www .wilmerhale.com/en/insights/client-alerts/20200108-unprecedented-state-law-on-pharmaceutical-reverse-payments-goes-into-effect.

Gallasch, Sven. (2016). Activating *Actavis* in Europe: The Proposal of a "Structure Effects-Based" Analysis for Pay-for-Delay Settlements. *Legal Studies* 36: 683–705.

Grabowski, Henry, Margaret Kyle, Richard Mortimer, Genia Long, and Noam Kirson. (2011). Evolving Brand-Name and Generic Drug Competition May Warrant a Revision of the Hatch-Waxman Act. *Health Affairs* 30: 2157–2166.

Grabowski, Henry, and John Vernon. (1986). Longer Patents for Lower Imitation Barriers: The 1984 Drug Act. *American Economic Review* 76: 195–198.

Karas, Laura, Gerard F. Anderson, and Robin Feldman. (2019). Pharmaceutical 'Pay-for-Delay' Reexamined: A Dwindling Practice or a Persistent Problem? *Hastings Law Journal* 71: 959–974.

Leonard, Mike. (2021). *Jazz Pharma, Hikma, Others Ordered to Face Xyrem Antitrust Case*. Bloomberg Law. https://news.bloomberglaw.com/us-law-week/jazz-pharma-hikma-others-ordered-to-face-xyrem-antitrust-case.

Lichtenberg, Nick. (2019). *Celgene Settles Class Action Antitrust Case for $55M: Law Firm*. Bloomberg Law. https://news.bloomberglaw.com/pharma-and-life-sciences/celgene-settles-class-action-antitrust-case-for-55m-law-firm.

Pierson, Brendan. (2021). *Bausch to Pay $300 Mln in Antitrust Suit over Diabetes Drug*. Reuters. www.reuters.com/business/healthcare-pharmaceut icals/bausch-pay-300-mln-antitrust-suit-over-diabetes-drug-2021-09-09/.

Sullivan, Thomas. (2019). *Allergan Subsidiary Forest Settles for $750 Million in Namenda Class Action Pay for Delay Suit*. Policymed. www.policymed .com/2019/11/allergan-subsidiary-forest-settles-for-750-million-in-namenda-class-action-pay-for-delay-suit.html.

Towey, Jamie, and Brad Albert. (2019). Then, Now, and Down the Road: Trends in Pharmaceutical Patent Aettlements after *FTC* v. *Actavis*. www.ftc .gov/news-events/blogs/competition-matters/2019/05/then-now-down-road-trends-pharmaceutical-patent.

US Food and Drug Administration. (2021). Drug Approval Process. www.fda.gov/media/82381/download.

Yasiejko, Christopher. (2020). *Pfizer Files More Patent-Infringement Suits on Ibrance Capsules*. Bloomberg Law. https://news.bloomberglaw.com/ip-law/pfizer-files-more-patent-infringement-suits-on-ibrance-capsules.

9　The Alleged Insulin Conspiracy

More than 10 percent of the US population suffers from diabetes. For many of those diabetics, insulin stands between them and ill health or death. This makes the demand for insulin extremely inelastic. For many low-income diabetics, the cost of insulin accounts for a large fraction of their disposable income, which makes it difficult for them to pay rent, maintain a healthy diet, and provide for the needs of their children and aging parents. As a result, it is important for policymakers and the antitrust Agencies to preserve and promote competition in the insulin market. But the price of insulin continues to rise, which indicates that the insulin market may not be competitive. We review two possible explanations for rising prices. First, there have been allegations that pharmacy benefit managers (PBMs), whose primary role is to negotiate lower pharmaceutical prices, may be encouraging higher insulin prices to increase rebates, which would increase their profits. Second, there have been allegations that the three major producers of insulin – Eli Lilly, Novo Nordisk, and Sanofi – have been cooperating rather than competing. This chapter addresses these allegations and the antitrust response.

In Section 9.2, we provide a brief history of insulin production and development and lay the foundation for Section 9.3, which examines the market structure for insulin and its distribution and pricing. Section 9.4 introduces PBMs, who negotiate pharmaceutical drug prices on behalf of health insurers. We discuss the perverse incentives inherent in their compensation scheme that may have encouraged rising insulin prices. In Section 9.5, we examine models of oligopoly pricing and tacit collusion and review the possible antitrust responses to such activities. We provide concluding observations in Section 9.6.

9.2 INSULIN: A BRIEF HISTORY

Before the synthesis and distribution of insulin in 1923, 60 percent of diabetics died within one year of diagnosis. Early treatments ranged from opium to dietary intervention, which lengthened a patient's life span by a minimal amount. In 1921, Frederick Banting, an orthopedic surgeon with little formal training in medicine, and Charles Best, a graduate student, began experiments at the University of Toronto that eventually culminated in the discovery of insulin as an effective treatment for diabetes. With the aid of John James R. Macleod, who offered lab space and advice, as well as James Bertram Collip, a biochemist who purified the insulin solution, the first diabetes patient was treated in 1922.[1] The team went on to receive the Nobel Prize in 1923 for their work.

Shortly after treating their first patient, Banting, Best, and Collip filed a patent for insulin in order to keep it out of the hands of disreputable pharmaceutical companies. They sold the patent for $3 to the University of Toronto, which they hoped could produce and distribute insulin cheaply for diabetes patients. The University of Toronto, however, proved incapable of producing insulin on a substantial scale. As a result, the university joined forces with Eli Lilly in 1923, which played a crucial role in designing large-scale processes that allowed it to expand production. Eli Lilly's patent license covered the United States, while licenses were issued to other pharmaceutical producers for production and sales outside the United States.[2] After visiting the University of Toronto and the insulin researchers,

---

[1] There is a great deal of controversy surrounding who deserves credit for the discovery of insulin. See Rosenfeld (2002) for a comprehensive analysis of the history.

[2] Although the University of Toronto had a patent on the substance, Eli Lilly patented its production techniques and purification process, which improved the purity of the insulin by 10–100 times. A lab at Washington University in St. Louis had also discovered the same purification process at about the same time. Washington University in St. Louis threatened to oppose the patent on the University of Toronto's behalf. This threat allowed the University of Toronto to impose better license terms with Eli Lilly that included a nonexclusive contract, which allowed it to license insulin to other manufacturers.

one such license was granted to Scandinavian professor August Krogh. Krogh and Hans Christian Hagedorn founded Nordisk Insulinlaboratorium in 1923 as a nonprofit organization to produce insulin for the European market. Novo Terapeutisk Laboratorium was founded two years later by brothers Harold and Thorvald Pederson, who had previously worked at Nordisk.[3] These firms later merged in 1989 and became Novo Nordisk, which is the second biggest player in the US insulin market. Additionally, Hoechst AG produced insulin for the German market in 1923. Hoechst AG was later integrated into what is now Sanofi – the third major player in the US insulin market.[4]

Due to mergers and new patents, Eli Lilly, Novo Nordisk, and Sanofi are the major insulin producers in the United States and global markets. In 2016, the companies controlled nearly 87 percent of the world's insulin production. A number of smaller firms produce insulin in other countries.[5] Specifically, Southeast Asian and Latin American insulin markets are comprised of a number of small-scale manufacturers.[6]

Insulin has existed for nearly 100 years, but the insulin of the 1920s is not the insulin of today. There have been vast improvements in terms of convenience and efficacy. In the 1920s, insulin was extracted from the pancreases of slaughtered cows and pigs.[7] Patients needed to inject insulin three to four times per day because its effects were not long-lasting. Researchers in the 1930s added zinc and protamine to the insulin, which prolonged its therapeutic effectiveness to 24–36 hours.

Diabetes patients continued to use animal-derived insulin until the early 1980s, when it was replaced by recombinant DNA insulin, which is a much better derivation of human insulin.[8] The 1990s saw

---

[3] Diabetesmuseum München (2020).   [4] Vecchio et al. (2018).
[5] For example, Berlin-Chemie, which was acquired by the Menarini Group, produces insulin for 30 countries in Europe and the steppes of Asia.
[6] Envision Intelligence (2018).
[7] In total, 7.5 million pancreases were required to produce 100 kilograms of insulin.
[8] Recombinant insulin is created by changing the genetic code of bacteria to enable them to produce the insulin. By using this strategy, animals were no longer needed to produce insulin.

the rise of analog insulin, which used recombinant DNA with minor modifications so that the insulin administered acted more like human insulin. Insulin innovation, such as an artificial pancreas, marches steadily forward, making the insulin of today much different from the one discovered at the University of Toronto in 1921. Since then, benefits from innovation have provided diminishing rates of return over time while allowing pharmaceutical firms to maintain patent monopolies. Now prices are rising at such a dramatic pace that many diabetes patients struggle to afford the medication that they need. The original producers of insulin wanted to avoid precisely this scenario. In the next section, we discuss the current state of the insulin market.

9.3 THE US INSULIN MARKET

The Centers for Disease Control and Prevention (CDC) estimated that about 34.2 million Americans, or about 10.5 percent of the population, suffered from diabetes in 2018.[9] This number is expected to rise to more than 54.9 million by 2030 due to an aging population and falling morbidity rates for those with the disease.[10] This increase in diabetic patients has fueled the rise of a valuable insulin market, which was worth around $10.42 billion in 2018.[11] Although diabetes management and treatment continue to benefit from innovation, the price of managing diabetes can be overwhelming for some patients. In this section, we discuss the market structure of insulin, product distribution, and recent pricing patterns and trends.

Market Structure of Insulin

The most common types of insulin on the market are those of the analog variety, which were developed in the 1990s. Table 9.1 shows that analog insulin is divided into rapid-acting, short-acting, intermediate-acting, long-acting, and premixed. Eli Lilly, Novo

---

[9] CDC (2020).   [10] Rowley et al. (2017).   [11] Fortune Business Insights (2018).

Table 9.1. *Common types of insulin with prices*

Type	Drug	Manufacturer	Average retail price[a]	Generic available?
Rapid-acting	Aspart (NovoLog)	Novo Nordisk	$348.94	Yes
	Aspart (Fiasp)	Novo Nordisk	$339.45	No
	Aspart (generic)	Novo Nordisk	$180.29	
	Lispro (Humalog)	Eli Lilly	$325.70	Yes
	Lispro (Admelog)	Sanofi	$273.08	No
	Lispro (generic)	Eli Lilly	$167.61	No
	Glulisine (Apidra)	Sanofi	$217.94	No
Short-acting	Regular (Novolin R)	Novo Nordisk	$160.65	No
	Regular (Humulin R)	Eli Lilly	$182.08	No
Intermediate-acting	NPH (Humulin N)	Eli Lilly	$181.79	No
	NPH (Novolin N)	Novo Nordisk	$160.23	No
Long-acting	Glargine (Basaglar)[b]	Eli Lilly	$397.47	No
	Glargine (Lantus)[c]	Sanofi	$283.56	No
	Detemier (Levemir)	Novo Nordisk	$399.32	No
Premixed	Humulin 70/30	Eli Lilly	$180.82	No
	Aspart 70/30 (Novolog 70/30)	Novo Nordisk	$365.63	Yes
	Aspart 70/30 (generic)	Novo Nordisk	$184.32	

[a] Pricing information was collected from Goodrx.com on May 26, 2021. The price represents one 10 mL vial with 100 units of insulin.

[b] Pricing was based on cartons of pens rather than vials.

[c] Pricing data came from Sanofi (2019).

Nordisk, and Sanofi produce these drugs in the United States.[12] A careful review of 2021 financial documents yielded the following sales revenue on insulin in the US market: Eli Lilly had over $2.74 billion,[13] Novo Nordisk had over $2.29 billion, and Sanofi had over $4.16 billion.[14] These figures indicate that the three firms have similar US market shares. Consequently, the insulin market in the United States is considered a three-firm oligopoly.

In the absence of significant barriers to entry, we would expect new firms to enter lucrative markets. Not surprisingly, there are a number of barriers to entry in the insulin market. The most notable barrier is patent protection. Using strategies such as product hopping (Chapter 4), along with litigation strategies (Chapter 8), these firms have extended the patent protection for their top-selling insulin drugs. Although the patents covering the compounds for the analog drugs that were developed in the 1990s have recently expired, Sanofi and Novo Nordisk have extended their patents on certain insulin products beyond 2030. At the same time, all three companies are working to research new and better insulin products or diabetes treatments for patients. This innovation, which is beneficial to diabetic patients, will result in patents that create barriers to entry for firms that hope to sell generic insulin. At this time, a few generics are beginning to enter the market due to the expiration of analog insulin patents. Eli Lilly introduced a generic for its Humalog insulin, while Mylan and Biocon jointly introduced Semglee, a generic for Sanofi's Lantus.[15]

---

[12] Mylan and Biocon received FDA approval for a generic version of Lantus in June 2020. Additionally, Pfizer has shown interest in developing diabetes treatments and generic insulin for the market. Currently, however, Eli Lilly, Novo Nordisk, and Sanofi control the US market (Mylan N.V. 2020).

[13] Eli Lilly sells a variety of noninsulin medications for diabetes, such as Trulicity, which yielded $4.9 billion in sales revenue in 2021. Noninsulin revenue is not included in the above calculations.

[14] Revenues for Sanofi and Novo Nordisk were presented in euros and Danish Kroner, respectively – 3,658 million euros and 14,944 million DKK. These numbers were converted to US dollars based on the December 31, 2021 foreign exchange rate.

[15] Mylan and Biocon received FDA approval for Semglee in June 2020. In 2021, the FDA said that Semglee was equivalent to its branded counterpart. This allows

Another barrier to entry is the fact that patients generally need prescriptions to purchase insulin. As discussed in Chapter 3, this requirement can lead to undesirable effects for insulin consumers. When prescriptions are required, patients must rely on doctors, who are not as price sensitive, to choose their insulin for them. Doctors will generally choose higher-quality insulins even if they are more expensive, so they may prescribe newer, patented insulins even if the quality increase does not justify the cost increase that patients would have to bear. This preference by doctors makes it challenging for generic firms to enter the market with older versions of the drug. Currently, both Eli Lilly and Novo Nordisk sell relatively inexpensive versions of insulin based on their 1980s formula that consumers can buy "behind the counter" without a prescription.[16] The insulin is relatively inexpensive, but due to its older formulation, the drug is not as effective as those being produced with newer formulations. Additionally, without doctor supervision, which patients may not be able to afford, self-managing a dosage and timing schedule can be dangerous and lead to emergency department visits or even death.[17] This nonprescription insulin is not a close substitute for newer insulins, but it may be utilized by low-income individuals and the uninsured.

Product Distribution

The distribution of insulin is fairly systematic. As shown in Figure 9.1, producers sell their output to wholesale distributors, which resell the insulin to pharmacies. The retail pharmacies sell the insulin to

pharmacies to automatically substitute generic Semglee for Sanofi's Lantus, which should increase its popularity (Walker 2021).

[16] The drug is held behind the counter rather than out on the shelf, so the pharmacist can control the distribution to some extent.

[17] It can be dangerous for diabetics to self-manage their disease, especially if they switch to a new type of insulin. Dosage and timing schedules can depend on a variety of factors, such as type of insulin, gender, diet, exercise, stress levels, emotions, and even the weather. It can be particularly difficult to adjust dosages to the optimal level initially, which often leads to over- or underdosing (Tribble 2015).

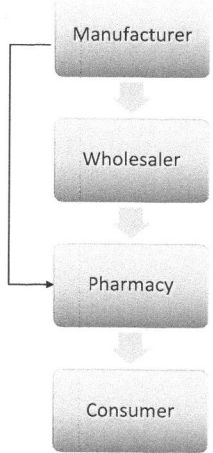

FIGURE 9.1 Pharmaceutical distribution chain

diabetic patients. Thus, the distribution of the physical product is linear and largely uncomplicated. The payment flow, however, is a complicated web of negotiated payments and rebates among patients, drug companies, wholesalers, retailers, pharmacy benefit managers, and insurers, depending on whether patients have insurance.

Determining Net Payments

Identifying the net payments for insulin by patients and their insurers is quite complicated. Determining how much the insulin producer receives for its sale of insulin after adjusting for coupons and rebates is also quite confusing. We will illustrate these observations by comparing the price an uninsured patient pays and the price an insured patient pays for Lantus, a long-acting insulin drug produced by Sanofi.

The uninsured patient receives a prescription for Lantus. According to Sanofi, one 10 mL vial had a list price of $284 in 2019.[18] Generally, patients will pay much less than $284 for a vial. Uninsured patients may shop around and pay a discounted price for

[18] Sanofi (2019). Most patients use two to four vials a month.

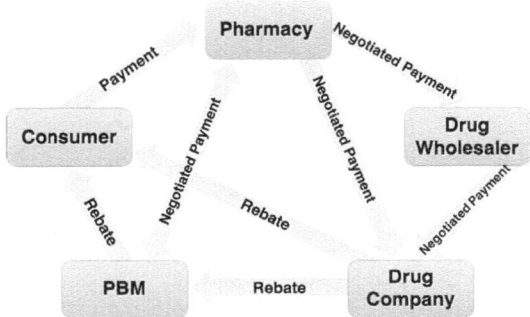

FIGURE 9.2 Flow of payments for an uninsured patient

Lantus at a pharmacy. They may also qualify for a rebate from Express Scripts, a PBM that negotiates insulin prices with Sanofi, which further reduces the price. Additionally, uninsured patients of little means may enroll in Sanofi's rebate program, the Patient Assistance Connection program, and receive a 90-day supply of Lantus for free or at a reduced cost.

The supply side of the dollar flow is a veritable web of negotiations and rebates (see Figure 9.2). Drug companies set high list prices in large part because they know they must offer discounts to sell their products. Drug companies, therefore, negotiate payments with wholesalers and pharmacies. Additionally, they can use a PBM that acts as a middleman between the drug company and other sellers on the marketplace. Finally, pharmacies and drug wholesalers negotiate prices and payments between themselves.

Now, suppose an insured patient receives a prescription for Lantus. If Lantus is covered under the patient's insurance plan, she pays a copayment at the pharmacy, which might be about $40 if she were on Medicare.[19] Depending on the patient's income, she may have the option to apply for copay assistance from Sanofi. If Lantus is not covered under the patient's insurance plan, she faces options

---

[19] Cubanski et al. (2020). Some Medicare copayments were lower, and others ranged up to $106.

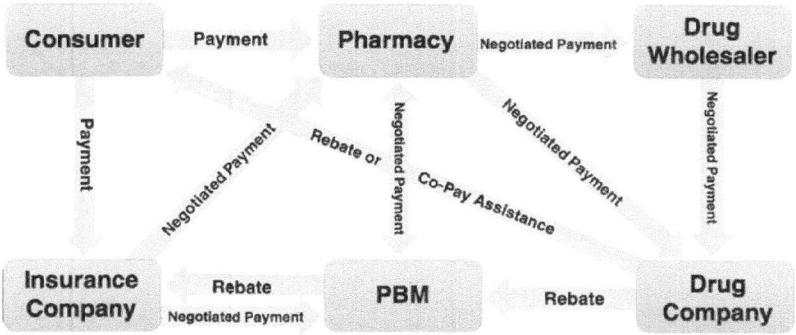

FIGURE 9.3 Flow of payments for an insured patient

similar to those of the uninsured patient. She may be able to pay a discounted price by applying for a rebate from Sanofi or may use a rebate from Express Scripts.

Supply-side payment negotiations for the insured patient are similar in format to those for uninsured patients (see Figure 9.3). The only difference is that insurance companies enter the picture. Patients pay for insurance and insurers cover part of the patients' prescription drug costs. Additionally, since insurers have greater bargaining power, they can often negotiate lower payments for insulin with the pharmacy and the PBM on behalf of their policyholders. The PBM may offer a rebate to the insurance company, which reduces the price. Similar to the case of uninsured patients, pharmacies negotiate with drug companies, wholesalers, and PBMs, and drug wholesalers negotiate directly with the drug company.

Pricing Patterns

Over the past two decades, the price of insulin has risen dramatically. From 2002 to 2013, the prices of insulin nearly tripled; from 2012 to 2016, the prices doubled. In 2002, a diabetic patient may have paid about $43 per 10 mL vial on average.[20] In 2021, these patients faced

---

[20] Hua et al. (2016).

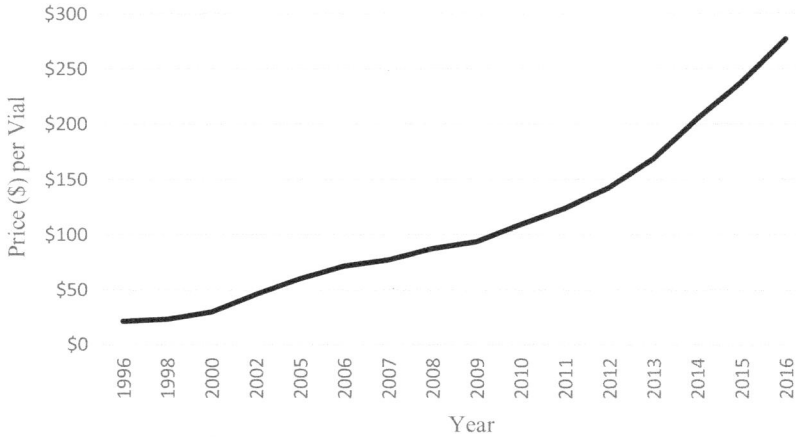

FIGURE 9.4 Humalog insulin price per vial by year
Source: Stark and Wood (2020).

prices of up to $300 per vial, depending on which insulin they were prescribed. In Figure 9.4, we display the dramatic price increases of the common insulin drug Humalog, which is produced by Eli Lilly. Other insulin drugs had similar pricing trends. These high prices foreclose many patients from lifesaving medicine, causing some to ration their insulin, a practice that can land them in the emergency department or even kill them. Although each of the three firms has some form of rebate program that assists patients who cannot afford the high price of insulin,[21] many still suffer under the high prices. In 2020, the Trump administration put forward an executive order that would lower the cost of insulin for patients, but in 2021, the order was first put on hold and later rescinded by the Biden administration.[22] Other policy proposals have been considered that

[21] There are various rebate programs. For example, Sanofi has the Patient Assistance Connection program, which gives Sanofi drugs at no cost to the uninsured with income below 400 percent of the US poverty guideline. Additionally, Sanofi has the Valyou Savings Program, which allows eligible patients to pay $99 for up to 10 vials of insulin. For more information, visit www.sanofipatientconnection.com.

[22] US White House (2020), Sullivan (2021).

would limit out-of-pocket spending for insulin and/or treat insulin as a preventive medicine with no patient cost sharing.[23]

In this chapter, however, we offer two potential explanations identifying possible factors that drove the increase in prices. First, as mentioned previously, insulin manufacturers compete not for patients but for prescriptions from doctors. These firms, therefore, focus on promoting their products to prescribing physicians. One important avenue for promoting insulin sales is the prominent placement on formularies, which are managed by pharmaceutical benefit managers. PBMs prefer higher list prices because it ensures that they can get larger rebates when negotiating with other players in the market. This preference leads to the unsettling conclusion that the three insulin manufacturers may be competing to increase their list prices to incentivize PBMs to grant their drugs a prominent placement on formularies. Second, there may be collusion among the three manufacturers. Since the insulin market can be considered a three-firm oligopoly, one might expect noncompetitive prices well above the competitive level. Given the market structure, there may be tacit collusion, which could result in monopoly prices.

9.4   PHARMACY BENEFIT MANAGERS

Overview of Pharmacy Benefit Managers

There is no doubt that pharmacy benefit managers (PBMs) have an imposing presence in the prescription drug market. The top three PBMs – CVS Health, Express Scripts, and OptumRx – report combined annual revenue of over $200 billion.[24] Together, these three firms control about 85 percent of the prescription drug market and negotiate pharmaceutical pricing for more than 266 million insured Americans. But the PBMs are secretive – their transactions and negotiated rebates are not transparent. Consequently, whether PBMs promote or hinder competition is an open public policy question.

---

[23] Hayes, Barnhorst, and Farmer (2020).

[24] *Boss* v. *CVS Health Corp.*, No. 17-cv-01823 (D. N.J. 2017), at 5.

PBMs emerged in the 1960s to administer health insurance company prescription drug benefits by processing claims.[25] PBMs effectively consolidate the demand for myriad prescription drugs, increasing the buying power of the PBM and reducing the prices health insurers must pay for those drugs. Originally, independent PBMs generated revenue through administrative fees, similar to how group purchasing organizations operate (Chapter 13). In the 1990s, PBMs were acquired by drug manufacturers, but were later forced to divest by the antitrust Agencies, which raised concerns over conflicts of interest where drug manufacturers would have an improved ability to coordinate prices through the PBM.[26] In recent years, there have been more consolidations involving PBMs. In 2007, CVS bought the PBM Caremark (and was renamed CVS Health), Express Scripts merged with Medco Health in 2012, and OptumRx merged with Catamaran in 2015. There were also consolidations with health insurance companies – Cigna and Express Scripts, CVS and Aetna. Additionally, OptumRx is owned by United Healthcare. Now, PBMs have taken on additional roles: PBMs serve as intermediaries in the prescription drug supply chain, negotiating with pharmaceutical manufacturers, health insurers, and pharmacies; creating the prescription drug formulary; and maintaining a network of pharmacies.

PBMs act as middlemen in negotiating drug prices with pharmaceutical manufacturers and control which drugs earn preferred positions on formularies for health insurers. Formularies tier pharmaceutical drugs that are reimbursed by health insurers based on the expense to patients.[27] The drugs in higher tiers are more expensive drugs that demand higher copays and, as such, command a higher consumer price. In addition, health insurers will not

---

[25] *Boss* v. *CVS Health Corp.*, No. 17-cv-01823 (D. N.J. 2017), at 38, 45.

[26] *Boss* v. *CVS Health Corp.*, No. 17-cv-01823 (D. N.J. 2017), at 45.

[27] The formulary is typically divided into three or four tiers, where the lowest tier is composed of generic drugs and higher tiers incrementally include drugs that are higher cost, higher copay for the consumer, more brand-name drugs, and/or specialty drugs.

reimburse their policyholders for drugs that are not placed on a formulary. Drug manufacturers are therefore incentivized to offer rebates for preferential formulary placement, as this directly impacts its access to consumers. In this way, the formulary, and therefore the PBM, has considerable power in driving consumer purchasing behavior based on what is covered and at what copayment. Given rising prices of prescription drugs, and insulin in particular, there are open policy questions and considerable finger-pointing as to the responsibility for these rising prices. There is also a good deal of confusion surrounding the negotiations between PBMs and pharmaceutical manufacturers, as well as the economic effects of PBMs.

PBMs tout their ability to lower drug prices by using formularies and generic substitution, obtaining volume discounts or rebates, and negotiating with pharmacies for lower reimbursement rates. Revenue sources for PBMs include percentages on the rebates the PBMs negotiate (i.e., negotiated price reductions on the list price) in addition to administrative fees. The former revenue source may provide the PBM with a perverse incentive to encourage higher list prices in order to raise potential rebates.

In recent years, PBMs have come under scrutiny because of their rebate negotiations with pharmaceutical manufacturers. Critics of PBMs are concerned that these intermediary functions could lead to higher prices through the collection of fees and/or the failure of PBMs to pass on sufficient portions of the negotiated rebates.[28] Policymakers have questioned to what extent PBMs pass on the negotiated rebate to the health insurer and, as such, whether PBMs are effectively reducing pharmaceutical drug pricing to health insurers and ultimately consumers. Neither PBMs nor health insurers share information about the price that the PBM negotiates for the pharmaceutical drug. Some critics worry that manufacturer list prices could actually increase if drug makers build in the expected rebate to

---

[28] Bergin (2019).

the PBM, leading to higher prices for health care consumers since copayments and PBM fees are ultimately based on the drug's list price.[29]

In addition to concerns about negotiations with the drug manufacturers and associated rebates, PBMs have also received criticism for their reimbursement policies for pharmacies. PBMs set the maximum allowable cost, which determines the rate pharmacies are reimbursed for a particular drug. With concerns about disadvantaging independent pharmacies and reimbursement rates that were below pharmacy acquisition cost, Arkansas Act 900 required PBMs to reimburse pharmacies at or above their acquisition costs. In December 2020, the Supreme Court upheld the Arkansas law (i.e., Act 900).[30] This ruling had impacts beyond Arkansas, as at least 36 other states have similar PBM regulations.[31] With respect to concerns over rebate negotiations, PBMs and pharmaceutical drug manufacturers have faced antitrust scrutiny in private damage actions. For example, Mylan (manufacturer of EpiPen injectors) and PBMs (e.g., CVS Caremark, Express Scripts, and OptumRx) were alleged to have engaged in a conspiracy where Mylan paid inflated rebates (i.e., bribes) to PBMs. PBMs, in turn, agreed to ignore price increases in the market for EpiPen injectors, which increased substantially in 2016.[32] Moreover, in 2019, the US House passed two bills (H.R. 2115[33] and H.R. 1781[34]) to improve PBM transparency by requiring them to disclose and publish rebates. PBMs and drug manufacturers have also faced legal challenges in the market for insulin.

---

[29] Bergin (2019).

[30] *Rutledge* v. *Pharmaceutical Care Management Association*, No. 18-540, 592 US ___ (2020). The Supreme Court upheld an Arkansas law that requires PBMs to reimburse pharmacies at no less than their acquisition costs.

[31] Wheeler (2020).

[32] Leonard (2021). See *In re EpiPen Direct Purchaser Litigation*, No. 20-cv-827 (D. Minn. 2021).

[33] Public Disclosure of Drug Discounts and Real-Time Beneficiary Drug Cost Act, H.R. 2115, 116th Congress (2019).

[34] Payment Commission Data Act of 2019, H.R. 1781, 116th Congress (2019).

Pharmacy Benefit Managers and the Insulin Market

There has been a great deal of public and private attention devoted to rising insulin prices, and in response, much litigation aimed at both drug manufacturers and PBMs.[35] In this section, we focus on a class action lawsuit filed in 2017 against insulin manufacturers, including Sanofi (Lantus, Apidra), Novo Nordisk (Levemir, Novolog), and Eli Lilly (Humalog), and against PBMs (CVS Health, Express Scripts, and OptumRx). The lawsuit alleged an "insulin pricing scheme" among the drug manufacturers and PBMs that increased prices of insulin drugs above the competitive level.[36] This litigation, in combination with other suits, was consolidated into *In re Insulin Pricing Litigation*.[37]

The plaintiffs alleged that PBMs failed to disclose negotiated net prices, rebates obtained from drug manufacturers, and what percentage of the rebates the PBMs retained. The list prices are defined as the starting point for purchase negotiations while the net price is the price the manufacturer receives after all rebates are applied.[38] If list prices rise while net prices fall, this creates problems with affordability for health care consumers because payments at the pharmacy (i.e., out-of-pocket spending or copayments) are based on higher list prices – not lower net prices.[39]

In addition to the insulin litigation, the Senate Finance Committee also investigated the rising prices of insulin over a two-year period and issued their findings in a 2021 report.[40] The conclusions of the committee suggest that PBMs have (1) obtained

---

[35] There have been numerous suits filed in this space (Balto 2017).

[36] *Boss* v. *CVS Health* is a class action suit on behalf of named plaintiffs who are health care consumers of insulin and Type 1 Diabetes Defense Foundation, a nonprofit organization. *Boss* v. *CVS Health Corporation*, No. 17-cv-01823 (D. N.J. 2017).

[37] *In re Insulin Pricing Litigation*, No. 17-00699 (D. N.J. 2017).

[38] *Boss* v. *CVS Health Corporation*, No. 17-cv-01823 (D. N.J. 2017), at 10.

[39] A 2020 move by CVS Caremark would decrease out-of-pocket spending for insulin consumers through a program called RxZERO, which would achieve zero cost-sharing by leveraging generic and preferred brand-name insulin products. See, for example, Campbell (2020).

[40] US Senate Finance Committee (2021).

substantially higher rebates since 2013 and (2) instituted contracting practices that would not reduce list prices for insulin products. For example, some have alleged that PBMs include the most expensive drugs in their formularies so that they can extract the highest rebates from the drug manufacturers. Given the lack of transparency in who benefits from the negotiated rebates, this practice could have led to a "race to the top," where the three insulin manufacturers competed for the best formulary placement by increasing their list prices for insulin products so that they could offer higher rebates to the PBMs.

In 2019, under the Trump administration, a proposal entitled "Pharmacy Benefit Manager Rebate Rule" would have taken direct action against PBM rebate practices, requiring disclosure of negotiated rebates from list prices.[41] Although this proposal was not pushed forward, other possible reforms have called for requirements to pass on all or most of the negotiated rebates to payers, substantially reducing that source of revenue for PBMs.[42]

There appear to be both public policy and private concerns about the contracting behavior of PBMs, which may play some role in the increasing list prices and out-of-pocket costs of insulin. In the next section, we consider whether collusion among the three manufacturers could have contributed to rising insulin prices.

9.5 COLLUSION IN THE INSULIN MARKET

In the insulin market, three manufacturers – Eli Lilly, Novo Nordisk, and Sanofi – comprise a three-firm oligopoly. Given this market structure, each firm recognizes its ability to affect price by adjusting quantity, although this ability is mitigated to some extent by the influence of the other firms in the market. We can, therefore, require non-collusive pricing from a competition policy perspective, but we cannot necessarily expect competitive prices.

For a three-firm Cournot oligopoly, price and output will be both non-collusive and noncompetitive. If demand is given by

---

[41] US Health and Human Services (2019).   [42] Seeley and Kesselheim (2019).

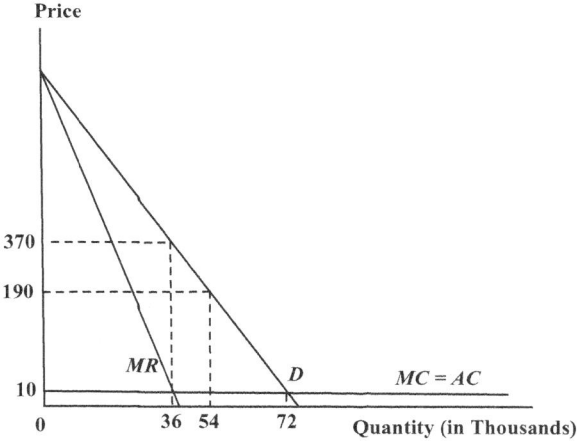

FIGURE 9.5 Competition, monopoly, and Cournot oligopoly

$$P = 730 - 0.01Q,$$

where P and Q are price and output, and the constant marginal (and average) production cost is 10, the competitive price will be $10 and the corresponding output will be 72,000 units. See Figure 9.5 for a graphical depiction of the following example.

We can show that the Cournot equilibrium output is equal to $n/(n+1)$ times the competitive output, where n is the number of firms in the market. For a three-firm Cournot oligopoly, $n = 3$ and

$$Q = \frac{n}{n+1}(72{,}000) = 54{,}000,$$

which yields a decidedly noncompetitive price of $190. Each firm produces one-third of the output, or 18,000 units. This outcome yields economic profit for each firm, but it does not involve any collusion since each firm acts unilaterally. Each firm earns the following economic profit:

$$\Pi = (190 - 10)(18{,}000) = \$3{,}240{,}000.$$

As Cournot oligopolists, the firms have done nothing illegal. The price and output are clearly noncompetitive, but since they are not the product of collusion, there is no antitrust violation. There is, however, a social welfare loss:

$$\frac{1}{2}(Q_1 - Q_2)(P_2 - MC) = \frac{1}{2}(72{,}000 - 54{,}000)(190 - 10) = \$1{,}620{,}000.$$

Given the market structure, there appears to be no antitrust remedy. Section 1 of the Sherman Act, which forbids agreements among competitors that restrain trade,[43] is not violated in the absence of an agreement. And the Cournot oligopoly model assumes that each firm acts independently to maximize profit without any consideration of the effect on any other firm's profits.

But the three firms can improve their profits if they choose to collude. The firms can achieve the highest profits by agreeing to produce the monopoly output and charge the monopoly price. In that event, the industry output will be one-half of the competitive output, $Q = 36{,}000$, and the corresponding price will be \$370 rather than \$190. With collusion, each identical firm would produce 12,000 units and firm profit would rise to

$$\Pi = (370 - 10)(12{,}000) = \$4{,}320{,}000.$$

Moving from Cournot oligopoly to the monopoly solution is good for the firms but harmful for everyone else. When the quantity falls and the price rises due to collusion, the social welfare loss increases from \$1.62 million to \$6.48 million. Consumer surplus falls from \$14.58 million to \$6.48 million, as wealth is redistributed from patients to pharmaceutical firms.[44] The reduction in sales volume means that some patients are either rationing their medication, which will adversely affect their health, or not taking their medicine at all, which will eventually kill them.

There are two things to notice about this example. First, even when price is well above the marginal cost of production, we cannot

---

[43] Chapter 6 discusses the requirements necessary to prove a conspiracy under Section 1 of the Sherman Act.

[44] Consumer surplus is calculated by the equation $CS = \frac{1}{2}(Q_a)(730 - P_a)$, where Q_a and P_a represent actual quantity and actual price, respectively.

infer collusion. The Cournot solution yields noncompetitive, yet non-collusive, prices. Second, the monopoly price and output can be the product of either overt collusion, which is unlawful, or tacit collusion, which is not unlawful. In the absence of convincing evidence of overt collusion, the antitrust Authorities cannot challenge the price increase. Section 1 of the Sherman Act can only be used if there is evidence – direct or circumstantial – of collusion. In the absence of such proof, Section 1 will be ineffective. Put differently, if the market structure leads to noncompetitive outcomes without collusion, there appears to be no antitrust remedy. Generally, antitrust challenges depend on direct or circumstantial evidence of collusion.

One significant problem with circumstantial evidence is that it is often ambiguous on the question of collusion. For example, suppose that the three insulin producers all deal with the same PBMs, each offers coupons to help low-income patients, none advertises on network television, and each relies on sales representatives to market its products to physicians. The firms are all doing the same thing – but it is not clear whether this is due to competition or collusion. As a policy matter, if conduct is equally consistent with competition and collusion, a plaintiff is not entitled to an inference of collusion.

Collusion: Overt or Tacit

Section 1 of the Sherman Act forbids agreements among competitors that restrain trade. As a legal matter, there must therefore be evidence of an actual (or overt) agreement for a violation of Section 1 of the Sherman Act. The evidence may be direct; that is, there may be confessions of participants, wiretaps, email correspondence, and internal documents. The evidence may be circumstantial; that is, there may be observed conduct or patterns of behavior that seem to require an overt collusive agreement.[45] But whether the evidence of

---

[45] Proof of parallel pricing is not proof of collusion. Although parallel pricing is consistent with collusion, it is also consistent with unilateral conduct based on conscious parallelism, which is not in and of itself unlawful. In addition to proof of parallel pricing, the plaintiff must offer some so-called "plus factors" that tip the

an agreement is direct or circumstantial, it must exist if a plaintiff is going to prove a Section 1 violation. If the evidence does exist, the Department of Justice can file an antitrust suit against the firms and private parties can sue for antitrust damages.

The so-called folk theorem of modern game theory holds that under suitable circumstances, the monopoly price and output quantity may emerge without any overt collusion. Tacit collusion, which can be traced to Edward Chamberlin (1933), gets the rival to the same economic outcome but does not involve an overt agreement and, therefore, does not amount to a Section 1 violation. According to Chamberlin and modern game theorists, well-informed business decision makers recognize that cooperation is more profitable than competition. Without overt agreement, the decision makers play their parts and arrive at a cooperative outcome that is more profitable than the Cournot solution. One such superior outcome is the monopoly solution, which will maximize industry profit.[46]

Tacit collusion is an obvious contradiction in terms since it requires reaching an agreement without any communication. But it has come to have meaning in terms of oligopolistic interaction. The idea is that intelligent business executives understand what must be done to maximize industry profit, and each knows what its firm's role should be. If each firm plays its part, industry profit is maximized and the firms share that profit, which will be greater than the profit that any other course of action would generate. In principle, this makes sense from an economic perspective.

Chamberlin introduced the concept of tacit collusion in a critique of the Cournot duopoly model. Faced with entry by an equally efficient firm, an incumbent monopolist would accommodate the entrant by

scales in favor of collusion rather than the latter conduct. Parallel pricing may result from price leadership. In a three-firm oligopoly, one firm may announce its price in advance of the others. If the other two firms follow the leader with matching price changes, that conduct will be lawful – if not economically regrettable – as long as all firms behave unilaterally. Without an agreement, there is no collusion.

[46] There are incentives for each individual firm to cheat to maximize its own profits.

reducing its output to one-half of the monopoly output. An intelligent entrant would also produce one-half of the monopoly output. Profit would remain at the monopoly level and each firm would earn one-half of the profit, which is more than one-half of any other profit.

This all sounds clear in the bare-bones model that Chamberlin employed, but things are rarely so simple. The two firms in a real market would have to agree without communication on a wide array of important variables of interest to the consumer, such as quality, location, delivery terms, credit terms, warranties, return policies, damage allowances, advertising, promotions, and technical support. Any significant product differentiation would complicate matters further.

George Stigler (1964) provided additional reasons for being skeptical of tacit collusion. In most markets, customers come and go in a predictable but somewhat random fashion. If a tacit colluder finds unexpected movement, it might infer cheating when, in fact, none had occurred. There are several sources of possible confusion. First, a seller always loses some customers and will come to expect constant turnover. Second, a seller will usually acquire new customers who are leaving one of its rivals and comes to expect it. Third, a seller expects to get its fair share of new customers entering the market. These changes are probabilistic to some extent. Consequently, the realized results may deviate from the expected value by chance, but they may arouse suspicion of cheating, which can undermine tacit collusion. If one firm believes the other is cheating, it will most likely retaliate to punish the suspected cheater. If the suspected firm was not cheating, the unwarranted retaliation will destabilize the cartel agreement.[47]

9.6 CONCLUDING REMARKS

Insulin is essential to the health of millions of diabetics in the United States. Over the last two decades, the prices of insulin drugs have

---

[47] For more information on how cartels punish each other for cheating, see Ayres (1987). See Pepall, Richards, and Norman (2014) for a discussion of the tit-for-tat strategy.

surged and many patients face a dilemma: Buy insulin or meet other family needs. If the soaring prices are non-collusive, there is no antitrust remedy. But if they result from overt, albeit clandestine, agreement, the Department of Justice can file criminal antitrust charges and private parties can sue for damages. If the rising prices flow from tacit collusion, there is no antitrust remedy. Section 1 of the Sherman Act requires an agreement – a contract, combination, or conspiracy. This rules out tacit collusion.

PBMs play a role in the market for prescription drugs broadly and insulin specifically, as they affect the list prices for branded insulin. Because of the nature of the negotiations between drug manufacturers and PBMs, there is a lack of transparency in pricing and rebates and clear evidence of rising list prices. Ongoing litigation in this area as well as public policy toward PBM negotiating tactics may affect this process in the future. As the United States grapples with reducing prescription drug expenditures for health insurers and consumers, further scrutiny of the practices of PBMs is likely.

For many diabetics, hope is on the way. A number of generics are beginning to enter the insulin market now that patents on the active ingredients of analog insulin are expiring. For example, Mylan and Biocon launched a generic of Lantus, which received FDA approval in June 2020. Other pharmaceutical firms have also expressed interest in entering the generic market for insulin, and branded generics have already entered the market. Eli Lilly, for example, has introduced a generic of Humalog at 50 percent of the price of branded Humalog. Generic entrants will increase competition in the insulin market and therefore make insulin more affordable for patients.

REFERENCES

Ayres, Ian. (1987). How Cartels Punish: A Structural Theory of Self-Enforcing Collusion. *Columbia Law Review* 87: 295–325.
Balto, David. (2017). *Federal and State Litigation Regarding Pharmacy Benefit Managers*. PBM Watch. www.pbmwatch.com/pbm-litigation-overview.html.

Bergin, Jessica M. (2019). A Primer on Pharmacy Benefit Managers. *Antitrust Health Care Chronicle* 33: 7–15.

Campbell, Todd. (2020). *CVS Announces Plan to Eliminate Co-Pays for Diabetes Drugs.* Fool. www.fool.com/investing/2020/01/29/cvs-announces-plan-to-eliminate-diabetes-co-pays.aspx.

Centers for Disease Control and Prevention. (2020). National Diabetes Statistics Report: Estimates of Diabetes and Its Burden in the United States. www.cdc.gov/diabetes/pdfs/data/statistics/national-diabetes-statistics-report.pdf.

Chamberlin, Edward. (1933). *The Theory of Monopolistic Competition.* Cambridge, MA: Harvard University Press.

Cubanski, Juliette, Tricia Neuman, Sarah True, and Anthony Damico. (2020). *Insulin Costs and Coverage in Medicare Part D.* Kaiser Family Foundation. www.kff.org/medicare/issue-brief/insulin-costs-and-coverage-in-medicare-part-d/.

Diabetesmuseum München. (2020). Insulin: 2020 – Thanks for 99 Years of Insulin. https://diabetesmuseum.de/insulin.

Envision Intelligence. (2018). Globally, Top 10 Insulin Manufacturers Are Dominated by Europe and North America. www.envisioninteligence.com/blog/globally-top-10-insulin-manufacturers/.

Fortune Business Insights. (2018). Human Insulin Market Size, Share & Industry Analysis, by Type (Analogue Insulin, Traditional Human Insulin), by Diabetes Type (Type 1, Type 2), by Distribution Channel (Retail Pharmacy, Hospital Pharmacy, Online Pharmacy), and Regional Forecast, 2019–2026. www.fortunebusinessinsights.com/industry-reports/human-insulin-market-100395.

Hayes, Tara O'Neill, Margaret Barnhorst, and Josee Farmer. (2020). *Federal and State Actions to Address Insulin Costs.* American Action Forum. www.americanactionforum.org/insight/federal-and-state-actions-to-address-insulin-costs/.

Hua, Xinyang, Natalie Carvalho, Michelle Tew, Elbert S. Huang, William H. Herman, and Philip Clarke. (2016). Expenditures and Prices of Antihyperglycemic Medications in the United States: 2002–2013. *Journal of the American Medical Association* 315: 1400–1402.

Leonard, Mike. (2021). *EpiPen Gouging Suit Advances against Mylan, CVS, Express Scripts.* Bloomberg Law. https://news.bloomberglaw.com/antitrust/epipen-gouging-suit-advances-against-mylan-cvs-express-scripts.

Mylan N.V. (2020). *Mylan and Biocon Announce US FDA Approval of Semglee.* Cision PR Newswire. www.prnewswire.com/news-releases/mylan-and-biocon-announce-us-fda-approval-of-semglee-insulin-glargine-injection-301074847.html.

Pepall, Lynne, Dan Richards, and George Norman. (2014). *Industrial Organization: Contemporary Theory and Empirical Applications.* 5th ed. Hoboken, NJ: Wiley.

Rosenfeld, Louis. (2002). Insulin: Discovery and Controversy. *Clinical Chemistry* 48: 2270–2288.

Rowley, William R., Clement Bezold, Yasemin Arikan, Erin Byrne, and Shannon Krohe. (2017). Diabetes 2030: Insights from Yesterday, Today, and Future Trends. *Population Health Management* 20: 6–12.

Sanofi. (2019). How Much Should I Expect to Pay for Lantus? www.lantus.com/-/media/EMS/Conditions/Diabetes/Brands/lantus-final/Header/Lantus-Pricing.pdf.

Seeley, Elizabeth, and Aaron S. Kesselheim. (2019). *Pharmacy Benefit Managers: Practices, Controversies, and What Lies Ahead.* The Commonwealth Fund. www.commonwealthfund.org/publications/issue-briefs/2019/mar/pharmacy-benefit-managers-practices-controversies-what-lies-ahead.

Stark, S., and J. Wood. (2020). Humalog Insulin: Investigating the Potential Implications of Insulin Price Hikes on Company Financial Data. https://insulin.substack.com/p/humalog-insulin-investigating-the?s=r.

Stigler, George J. (1964). A Theory of Oligopoly. *Journal of Political Economy* 72: 44–61.

Sullivan, Thomas. (2021). *Biden Administration Rescinds Trump Administration Insulin Pricing Rule.* Policymed. www.policymed.com/2021/10/biden-administration-rescinds-trump-administration-insulin-pricing-rule.html.

Tribble, Sarah Jane. (2015). *You Can Buy Insulin without a Prescription, but Should You?* KHN. https://khn.org/news/you-can-buy-insulin-without-a-prescription-but-should-you/.

US Health and Human Services. (2019). Trump Administration Proposes to Lower Drug Costs by Targeting Backdoor Rebates and Encouraging Direct Discounts to Patients. www.hhs.gov/sites/default/files/20190131-fact-sheet.pdf.

US Senate Finance Committee. (2021). Insulin: Examining the Factors Driving the Rising Cost of a Century Old Drug. www.finance.senate.gov/imo/media/doc/Grassley-Wyden%20Insulin%20Report%20(FINAL%201).pdf.

US White House. (2020). Executive Order on Access to Affordable Life-Saving Medications. www.whitehouse.gov/presidential-actions/executive-order-access-affordable-life-saving-medications/.

Vecchio, Ignazio, Cristina Tornali, Nicola Luigi Bragazzi, and Mariano Martini. (2018). *The Discovery of Insulin: An Important Milestone in the History of Medicine.* Frontiers in Endocrinology. www.frontiersin.org/articles/10.3389/fendo.2018.00613/full.

Walker, Joseph. (2021). FDA Lets Pharmacies Substitute Branded Insulin with Knockoff Product, in First for a Biologic Drug. *Wall Street Journal.* www.wsj

.com/articles/fda-lets-pharmacies-substitute-branded-insulin-with-knockoff-product-in-first-for-a-biologic-drug-11627589200.

Wheeler, Lydia. (2020). *High Court Upholds State Law Reining in Pharmacy Drug Middlemen*. Bloomberg Law. https://news.bloomberglaw.com/us-law-week/high-court-upholds-state-law-reining-in-pharmacy-drug-middlemen.

10 Licensing of Health Care Professionals

10.1 INTRODUCTION

The premise of the antitrust laws is that society is best served when competitive market forces direct economic activity.[1] In the absence of market failure, this premise is well-founded. As a result, antitrust laws ordinarily forbid interference with the competitive process. But market failure, which can arise due to market power, externalities, public goods, or asymmetric information, undermines our confidence in a well-functioning market. Market failure due to asymmetric information is common in health care markets. Consequently, state legislatures have displaced competition in some health care markets in favor of regulation under the state action doctrine.

When a state identifies an area of the economy in which it wants to displace competitive market forces with regulation, it may do so through specific legislation. Participants in that regulated industry are protected from antitrust scrutiny if the state (1) has clearly articulated its desire to displace competition as a disciplining force and (2) actively supervises the regulatory activity.[2] The need for active state supervision is especially acute when members of a profession participate in the regulatory activity, since the economic self-interest of the regulatory board members may take precedence over the promotion of public health, safety, and welfare.

Most health care professions are regulated by state licensing boards. In the United States, approximately 25 percent of workers require a license to work; for health care professionals, closer to

---

[1] This chapter relies heavily upon Blair and Durrance (2015a, 2015b).
[2] Areeda and Hovenkamp (2021, ¶¶221–231).

70 percent require licensure.[3] State licensing boards are charged with promoting public health, safety, and welfare by preventing charlatans, incompetents, and quacks from practicing. Typically, these boards are populated by members of the regulated profession since they have the requisite expertise to police the profession. Over half a century ago, however, Milton Friedman warned us that an inevitable conflict of interest would result from such self-regulation.[4] Recently, the Federal Trade Commission characterized it as putting the proverbial fox in the henhouse.[5] Professionals with the power to grant licenses may have a financial incentive to use that power to reduce competition and exclude other medical professionals. Concerned about this conflict of interest, the Supreme Court agreed that the state should supervise such boards. In *North Carolina Dental*, the issue before the Court was whether the State of North Carolina actively supervised the dental licensing board that was dominated by those whom it regulated. The Court found an absence of active supervision and, therefore, held that the board did not have antitrust immunity.[6] In the wake of this decision, many antitrust suits have been filed against medical boards. At the same time, a number of states have introduced legislation to proactively deter possible competitive abuses by regulatory boards.

When the discipline of competitive market forces is replaced by regulation, there are benefits and costs. On the benefit side, licensing boards protect consumers and should thereby improve the quality of care. On the cost side, however, reduced competition leads to higher prices and reduced access to health care. In this chapter, we explore the competitive concerns economists and the antitrust Agencies have regarding professional licensure regulations. We identify two general antitrust concerns: (1) the exclusion of some competitors through

---

[3] National Conference of State Legislatures (2017).   [4] Friedman (1962).
[5] Federal Trade Commission (2014b).
[6] *North Carolina Board of Dental Examiners* v. *Federal Trade Commission*, 574 US 494 (2015).

entry limitations or practice restrictions and (2) supervision requirements that make the employment of competitors less attractive.

In Section 10.2, we summarize the economic concerns with
licensing of health care professionals. We review the state action
doctrine along with relevant Supreme Court precedent, including
North Carolina Dental, in Section 10.3. In Section 10.4, we present
a simple economic model of exclusion, which reveals the benefits to
non-excluded medical professionals and the costs to excluded medical
professionals as well as to health care consumers. In Section 10.5, we
examine the economic consequences of supervision requirements for
the supervisor, the supervised, and the public. In Section 10.6, we
summarize the empirical evidence on the economic consequences of
professional licensing. There is ample empirical evidence of increased
prices and reduced access – but little evidence of improved quality.
These results should alarm state legislators if they are truly concerned
with public welfare. We offer concluding remarks in Section 10.7.

10.2   ECONOMIC CONCERNS WITH
PROFESSIONAL LICENSING

Ordinarily, price, quantity, quality, and other relevant product characteristics should be determined by unrestricted competition in the
market. There are times, however, when policymakers conclude that
competition will not yield the socially optimal results. In these cases,
regulation or some other deviation from unfettered competition
seems warranted, which creates the need for an exemption from the
proscriptions of the Sherman Act. If certain requirements are met, the
state action doctrine permits the state legislature to enact policies
that restrict competition in ways that courts would otherwise consider antitrust violations.

In *Parker* v. *Brown*,[7] the Supreme Court allowed a state statute
that substituted state regulation for competitive market forces. The

---

[7] *Parker* v. *Brown*, 317 US 341 (1943). The case involved the California Raisin
Proration Program, which stabilized the price of raisins in 1941 during the time of an

Parker requirements were restated in *California Retail Liquor Dealers Association* v. *Midcal Aluminum, Inc.*, where the Supreme Court adopted a two-pronged standard for satisfying the state action doctrine: (1) "the challenged restraint must be 'clearly articulated and affirmatively expressed as state policy'" and (2) "the policy must be 'actively supervised' by the State."[8]

The resulting state action doctrine extends to occupational licensing generally and health care profession licensing specifically. It has become clear that professional licensure enjoys a good deal of protection from antitrust scrutiny afforded by the state action doctrine. Competitive concerns continue to fester, however, and occasionally result in challenges in court.[9] *North Carolina Dental*, which we discuss in Section 10.3, is the latest challenge to reach the Supreme Court, although there has been a flurry of lower court decisions on its heels.

Over half a century ago, Milton Friedman warned us about the economic consequences of professional regulation.[10] Ostensibly, the regulatory statutes emerge from the need to protect the public from charlatans and incompetents.[11] The presumption is that the public is incapable of selecting a competent professional and therefore must be protected from its own ignorance. But Friedman pointed out that, in general, demands for occupational licensing stem from professionals in that occupation rather than people who have been abused by those professionals.

"The arrangements made for licensures almost invariably involve control by members of the occupation which is to be

---

economic crisis. Brown, a short seller of raisins, sued to enjoin the program. The Supreme Court unanimously decided that the program was not subject to the Sherman Act since it was a "state action" rather than an effort by private parties.

[8] *California Retail Liquor Dealers Association* v. *Midcal Aluminum, Inc.*, 445 US 97, 105 (1980).

[9] The results of these challenges are summarized in Areeda and Hovenkamp (2021, ¶¶ 221–231).

[10] Friedman (1962).

[11] Friedman (1962) argued that protecting the public from medical incompetents was unnecessary in the absence of externalities since the usual malpractice risk does not justify licensing; that risk is a private assessment.

licensed."[12] He went on to observe that there is an inevitable conflict of interest that arises when professions are regulated by members of the regulated profession. This follows because professionals can abuse their licensure powers "to obtain a monopoly position at the expense of the rest of the public."[13] In order to protect this monopoly position, it is necessary to control entry and curtail competition from outsiders. Since the practice of medicine, for example, is limited to those who have the appropriate training, it is necessary to define "the practice of medicine," and that is typically left to the profession. Because the enabling legislation allows the profession to restrict the practice of medicine to its members, the profession is able to control entry and competition.

Entry into the medical profession is restricted both in terms of who can enter the medical profession through medical school and who ultimately passes the threshold to receive a license to practice. But the profession is further insulated by defining the practice of medicine broadly through the physician's scope of practice. Friedman argues that technicians and other skilled people can often provide good substitute services that are currently restricted to licensed professionals. Such restrictions require consumers to purchase services (at higher cost) from licensed providers, leaving them with no substitute choices.

Licensing restrictions affect a number of parties. First, licensing reduces the opportunities available to those who want to enter the profession. Second, those who are able to enter the profession benefit from entry restrictions in the form of higher compensation. Third, consumers pay higher prices to obtain services from those who entered the profession.

Moreover, by insisting on licensing restrictions to offer consumers quality, first-rate care, some patients may be priced out of the market and get no care at all. The professions argue that licensing restrictions will increase the quality of medical care by protecting

[12] Friedman (1962, 140).   [13] Friedman (1962, 148).

consumers from inferior care. Friedman argues that it is not enough to simply look at the average quality of care actually received. An appropriate analysis must also include the effect of some consumers receiving no care at all due to the higher prices.

The Federal Trade Commission (FTC) shares some of Friedman's concerns with professional self-regulation:

> [O]ccupational regulation can be especially problematic when regulatory authority is delegated to a nominally "independent" board comprised of members of the very occupation it regulates. When the proverbial fox is put in charge of the henhouse, board members' financial incentives may lead the board to make regulatory choices that favor incumbents at the expense of competition and the public. This conflict of interest may lead to the adoption and application of licensure restrictions that discourage new entrants, deter potential competition from professionals in related occupations, and suppress innovative forms of service delivery that could challenge the status quo. Such entry and innovation can have substantial consumer benefits.[14]

Although the FTC recognized that professional licensure may have some benefits, their central message was that licensure can be anticompetitive.[15] The FTC argued that not all professional licensure is necessary. Moreover, the benefits of the restrictions may not offset the harms to competition. The FTC pointed out that it had observed "many examples of licensure restrictions that likely impede competition and hamper entry into professional markets, yet offer few, if any, significant consumer benefits."[16] Consequently, regulation may lead to higher prices, lower quantities of services and products offered, lower quality, and less convenience, which not only harms consumers

[14] Federal Trade Commission (2014b).

[15] The Obama White House (2015) also expressed concerns about occupational licensing, acknowledging that licensing should protect consumers without placing unnecessary restrictions on employment or competition.

[16] Federal Trade Commission (2014b).

but can also "cause lasting damage to competition and the competitive process by rendering markets less responsive to consumer demand."[17]

Additionally, the FTC pointed out that licensure does not necessarily increase quality. But licensing may prevent consumers who need access to such services from receiving those services due to higher prices. In addition, the FTC has questioned other restrictions such as mandated supervision requirements or collaborative practice agreements. These restrictions, which we discuss in more detail later in this chapter, give the supervisor the ability to restrict access to the market. In many cases, the FTC warns that these restrictions may do more harm than good.

10.3   *NORTH CAROLINA DENTAL* AND THE STATE ACTION DOCTRINE

Although there has been a flurry of licensing-related litigation, the most recent Supreme Court guidance in this area comes from *North Carolina Dental (NC Dental)*.[18] Beginning in the 1990s, dentists began to offer teeth-whitening services; in 2003, non-dentists entered the market for teeth-whitening services and charged lower prices.[19] In response, the North Carolina Dental Board, which is comprised of dentists who compete with non-dentist teeth whiteners, sent

---

[17] Federal Trade Commission (2014b).

[18] Legal challenges of this kind have not been limited to health care. The courts have seen challenges in legal services (e.g., *LegalZoom.com* v. *N.C. State Bar*, N.C. Super. Ct., Wake Cnty, No. 11 CVS 1511 (N.C.B.C. 2012)) and the liquor market (e.g., *Spec's Family Partners Ltd.* v. *Texas Alcoholic Beverage Commission*, No. 19-20661 (5th Cir. 2020)).

[19] A number of challenges have been filed against dental boards for restricting non-dentists from selling teeth-whitening services. A similar case was filed against the Georgia Dental Board for taking action against non-dentist teeth whiteners Enlightened Expressions LLC. The court held that plaintiffs could pursue antitrust claims (*Colindres* v. *Battle*, No. 1:15-cv-2843-SCJ (N.D. Ga., 2016)). In another dental board dispute, the US Court of Appeals for the Second Circuit held that the Connecticut Dental Board was protecting patients from possible harm by restricting the practice of teeth whitening (with an LED light) to dentists. The Supreme Court declined to review this case (*Sensational Smiles, LLC* v. *Mullen*, No. 14-1381 (2nd Cir. 2015)).

"cease-and-desist letters to … non-dentist teeth whiten[ers]," indicating that the non-dentists were practicing illegally and should stop offering these services.[20] Many providers complied. The Federal Trade Commission, however, learned of the restrictions and filed suit against the dental board.

The central issue in *NC Dental* involved the state action doctrine. When state legislatures decide to regulate professions through licensing, they insulate the group from competition and Sherman Act scrutiny. But to do so, the legislatures must satisfy the requirements of the state action doctrine, which requires the following: (1) the state must clearly articulate its intention to displace the discipline of competitive markets with regulation, and (2) the state must actively supervise the professional group.

The first requirement for state action immunity is the presence of a "clear state purpose" to displace the antitrust laws.[21] In other words, the enabling legislation must clearly articulate the state's intention to exempt the members of a profession from the Sherman Act's mandate to engage in free and open competition. The Federal Trade Commission encourages policymakers to carefully consider the restrictions imposed by licensure requirements and their likely effect on competition and consumers, including whether less restrictive options could achieve the same goal.[22] Although the FTC has not specifically challenged the establishment of general licensing requirements (e.g., entry qualifications for a profession), it is more concerned with additional restrictions on licensing of particular professionals (e.g., supervisory relationships between advanced practice registered nurses [APRNs] and physicians).

The second requirement of the state action doctrine is active state supervision. It is not enough for a state to authorize otherwise

---

[20] *North Carolina Board of Dental Examiners* v. *Federal Trade Commission*, 574 US 494 (2015).

[21] For a detailed overview of the state action doctrine, see Areeda and Hovenkamp (2021).

[22] Federal Trade Commission (2014b).

unlawful restraints of trade. For antitrust immunity under the state action doctrine, the state must supervise the conduct to ensure that abuses are minimal. Specifically, state supervision is not adequate if the members of the profession make decisions for themselves. Adequate supervision requires decision making on the part of public officials. Absent sufficient public control, antitrust immunity will not be granted. If the supervising government body is solely made up of the interested producers, there is inadequate state supervision since that body will have a conflict of interest. This conflict of interest, however, is common for medical, legal, and other professional associations.

In most states, licensing boards are comprised of active members of the occupation being regulated. For example, physicians regulate physicians and dentists regulate dentists. This practice makes sense since physicians, for example, are best positioned to regulate the practice of medicine due to their specific expertise. Of course, there are a multitude of reasons why this supervision could be compromised. First, the board member physicians are also market participants with a financial interest in the regulation of the practice of medicine. This can create a problematic conflict of interest. The FTC noted that a state regulatory board may avoid antitrust scrutiny if the board serves only in an advisory capacity or if the board is staffed by individuals who do not benefit financially from the regulation of the occupation in question. Second, board member physicians may be more sympathetic to other practicing physicians and choose disciplinary actions that may be more generous to a fellow physician.[23]

The FTC challenges behavior when the actions of a board appear to go beyond the scope of its stated purpose as a regulatory agency, by

---

[23] Medical boards do not always ensure quality among physicians. As has become evident in the opioid crisis in the United States, many physicians have been involved in overprescribing opioids and other controlled substances (some knowingly, some unknowingly). Rebecca Haw Allensworth (2020) attended medical board meetings in the State of Tennessee, where myriad physicians regained prescribing privileges after losing them for reasons related to inappropriate overprescribing.

furthering the interests of its own members to the potential detriment of consumers. Such was the case in *NC Dental*.

In *NC Dental*, the FTC challenged the North Carolina Board's conduct, alleging that its actions led to higher prices for teeth whitening, reduced consumer choice, and suppressed competition.[24] The board pointed to the state action doctrine and argued that it was immune from antitrust liability since it acted like a regulatory body.[25] In contrast, the FTC argued that the board could not have antitrust immunity because it was composed of dentists who stood to benefit from the exclusion of non-dentist providers, and because it had no active state supervision. The board's counterargument was that it did not require state supervision since it was a state entity. The Court of Appeals sided with the FTC, finding that a board run by market participants was a private actor. The Supreme Court agreed.[26] Following *NC Dental*, the FTC issued guidance on active state supervision.[27]

In the wake of the *NC Dental* decision, a plethora of other licensing litigation was filed in the health care sector.[28,29] Because

---

[24] See *North Carolina Board of Dental Examiners* v. *Federal Trade Commission*, 574 US 494 (2015). Even more recently, the FTC has challenged actions by the National Association of Teachers of Singing. See *In re National Associationn of Teachers of Singing, Inc.*, No. C-4491, WL 5298209 (F.T.C. 2014), Complaint, 1. The association's code of ethics restricted members from soliciting other members' students, that is, no poaching. We cover no-poaching restrictions in Chapter 16.

[25] NC State Board of Dental Examiners v. *Federal Trade Commission*, 717 F.3d 359 (4th Cir. 2013), 366.

[26] Edlin and Allensworth (2014) argued that the state action doctrine should not prevent legitimate competitive concerns from being challenged under the antitrust laws.

[27] Federal Trade Commission (2015b).

[28] Opternative, Inc. challenged the South Carolina Board of Medical Examiners because the board's rules prohibit an ophthalmologist from using an automated eye test when writing a prescription (*Opternative, Inc.* v. *South Carolina Board of Medical Examiners*, No. 2016CP4006276 (S.C. Ct. Com. Pl 2016)).

[29] A chiropractor filed an antitrust suit against the Virginia Board of Medicine after she was suspended and fined for allegedly offering services (laser fat removal, treatment for thyroid conditions, treatment for diabetes) outside her scope of practice. The Supreme Court declined to hear this case, but the US Court of Appeals for the Fourth Circuit found that the chiropractor had not provided evidence that other chiropractors in Virginia were foreclosed from offering similar services nor that

most boards are primarily comprised of current licensed professionals, it follows that many boards will face the same questions of inadequate state supervision that were at issue in *NC Dental*.[30] For example, in *Teladoc, Inc. v. Texas Medical Board*,[31] the Texas Medical Board (TMB) instituted rules that required physicians to conduct in-person examinations of a patient before prescribing medications. When Teledoc entered the market and began providing telemedicine services to patients, it filed an antitrust suit in 2015, alleging that the TMB had overstepped its bounds as a regulatory agency. Similar to *NC Dental*, the TMB argued that it held antitrust immunity because its members were practicing physicians who were supervised by the state. Eventually, Texas made legislative changes to telemedicine, instituting changes permitting the kind of telemedicine that Teledoc provided; in response, Teledoc dropped its antitrust suit.

Other challenges have emerged in additional dental settings. SmileDirectClub, through its SmileShops, provides teledentristy services that are used for teeth straightening. A non-dentist takes digital photographs of patients' teeth and gums, which can be used by an offsite dentist to create teeth aligners for patients without ever having to visit a dentist office. SmileDirectClub argued that their innovative business model decreases prices for teeth alignment treatment. Dental boards in California,[32] Georgia,[33] and

---

there was competitive harm (*Petrie* v. *Virginia Board of Medicine*, No. 15-1007 (4th Cir. 2016)).

[30] Allensworth (2017) conducted a review of all licensing boards (not just health professions) in the United States and found that approximately 85 percent of those boards required most members to be current, licensed professionals.

[31] *Teladoc, Inc.* v. *Texas Medical Board*, No. 1:15-cv-00343 (W.D. Tex. 2015).

[32] *Sulitzer* v. *Tippins*, No. 19-cv-8902 (C.D. Cal. 2019). In July 2020, a California judge dismissed SmileDirectClub's suit against the California dental board. The case was appealed to the Court of Appeals for the Ninth Circuit. The US Department of Justice filed a motion on SmileDirectClub's behalf in 2021. *Sulitzer* v. *Tippins*, No. 20-55735 (9th Cir. 2020).

[33] *SmileDirectClub, LLC* v. *Battle*, No. 19-12227 (11th Cir. 2019). The 11th Circuit ruled that the Georgia dental board did not qualify for antitrust immunity because it is not actively supervised by the state. In February 2021, the Georgia dental board submitted an appeal to the US Court of Appeals for the Eleventh Circuit to reverse the ruling of denial of state action immunity.

Alabama[34] attempted to prevent SmileDirectClub from continuing to provide these services, alleging that the services were unauthorized because they were performed without a supervising dentist. As a result, SmileDirectClub filed antitrust suits against the dental boards. There has been a flurry of court decisions in this set of antitrust litigations. In California, the court found that the actions of the dental board were within its regulatory purview. SmileDirectClub has taken its challenge to the Court of Appeals for the Ninth Circuit and has been supported by the Department of Justice, which has submitted an amicus brief on its behalf. The Ninth Circuit reversed the ruling (Grzinic 2022) in favor of SmileDirectClub. In Georgia, the Court of Appeals for the Eleventh Circuit rejected the dental board's position that it held antitrust immunity with active state supervision. In Alabama, the parties reached an undisclosed settlement in August 2021.[35]

While the *NC Dental* Court found inadequate state supervision, state governments have reacted to the decision in several ways. The Supreme Court in *NC Dental* did not specify what constitutes active state supervision. Rather, the Court indicated that the state's supervisory role is variable and dependent on the facts of the specific case. Reacting to the Supreme Court ruling, states have begun to reconsider occupational licensing. Between 2017 and 2019, over 2,000 pieces of legislation involving occupational licensing were introduced across all 50 states.[36]

---

[34] *Leeds* v. *Board of Dental Examiners of Alabama*, No. 2:18-cv-1679 BL 11643 (N.D. Ala., 2018); *Leeds* v. *Jackson*, No. 19-11502 (11th Cir. 2019). In Alabama, the dental board sent SmileDirectClub a cease-and-desist letter. The Alabama dental board reacted to the FTC investigation and its support for SmileDirectClub by filing suit against the FTC. The Board alleged, as did the dental board in *NC Dental*, that it had state action antitrust immunity (*Board of Dental Examiners of Alabama* v. *Federal Trade Commission*, No. 20-cv-1310 (N.D. Ala. 2020)). In February 2021, the Alabama dental board's lawsuit against the FTC was dismissed because the judge ruled that an agency cannot refuse to respond to an FTC investigation by claiming immunity. In October 2021, the FTC and the Board of Dental Examiners of Alabama reached a proposed settlement agreement where the board agreed to remove the requirement of a supervising dentist for teeth alignment treatment (Bulusu (2021).

[35] *SmileDirectClub, LLC* v. *Board of Dental Examiners of Alabama*, No. 2:18-cv-1679 (N.D. Ala. 2018).

[36] National Conference of State Legislatures (2020).

Some states have proactively reorganized professional board membership compositions to be responsive to the Court's concerns. Other states have made formal legal pathways for antitrust challenges to problematic board behavior. Still other states have investigated whether new or existing regulations are required within occupational licensing. Most recently, President Joe Biden issued an executive order instructing the FTC to issue new rules limiting unnecessary and cumbersome licensing requirements issued by state licensing boards.[37]

Many scholars have written on the topic of occupational licensing. Kleiner (2015), for example, offered some specific thoughts on how governments should approach professional licensing. First, he suggested that governments should employ cost-benefit analysis (CBA) to determine whether licensing makes sense – if the gains to consumers from licensing professions outweigh the costs from restricted competition. Second, governments should provide guidance on best practices for licensing occupations. Third, to ease unnecessary restrictions in the labor market, governments should lower cross-state labor market restrictions and enhance reciprocity. Finally, governments should identify the least restrictive licensed environment and convert existing licensing arrangements to certification or no regulation where warranted. Allensworth (2017) identifies two changes states could enact to respond to occupational licensing concerns and the *NC Dental* ruling. First, she suggests that states should better supervise professional boards, perhaps with a new regulatory body responsible for supervision. Second, board membership should be reconsidered so that both active, currently practicing professionals and nonpracticing professionals make decisions.

10.4   LICENSING TO EXCLUDE COMPETITION

We use the case of *NC Dental* to examine the economic effects of excluding competitors.[38] In most local markets for teeth-whitening

---

[37] Bulusu, Hao, and Mulvaney (2021).

[38] Exclusion has also occurred in the case of vision services. Before the 2004 Fairness to Contact Lens Consumers Act, some optometrists forced patients to purchase eyewear from them by refusing to release the customer's prescription. Norris and

services, there is ample competition. In Chapel Hill, for example, there are approximately 150 dental offices in a community of 60,000 people. While there is no clear demarcation between competitive and non-competitive markets, there are a sufficient number of dentists for competition to prevail. Practice restrictions in the case of *NC Dental* take the form of restrictions on which kind of providers can perform teeth-whitening services. In this setting, practice restrictions are equivalent to the exclusion of one group of suppliers (i.e., non-dentist teeth whiteners). In spite of the competitive structure of the dental services market, the exclusion of a source of supply confers economic benefits on those who are not excluded. These economic benefits come at the expense of patients and those who are excluded. As we will show in this section, the exclusion of a group of providers will only be socially beneficial if the benefits associated with increased quality (if any exist) outweigh the welfare losses associated with the exclusion.

In Figure 10.1, *D* represents the demand for teeth-whitening services in a local market and *S* represents the supply of teeth-whitening services from all sources. The market for these services will be in equilibrium when supply (*S*) and demand (*D*) are equal. In this example, the quantity demanded and quantity supplied will be equal at Q_1 while the price paid and received will be P_1. Consumer surplus, which is a measure of consumer welfare, is equal to the area under the demand curve and above the price, that is, area abP_1 in Figure 10.1. Producer surplus, which is profit to the suppliers, is the area above the supply curve and below the price, that is, area P_1bc in Figure 10.1. Social welfare, or total welfare, is the sum of consumer and producer surplus, which is represented by the triangular area *abc*. Competition in this market maximizes social welfare; that is, no other price and output will generate as much total surplus as the competitive price and output. This is the reason competition is considered optimal.

Timmons (2020) found that when the Act came into effect and forced optometrists to release prescription records, optometrist wages were reduced by 13 percent.

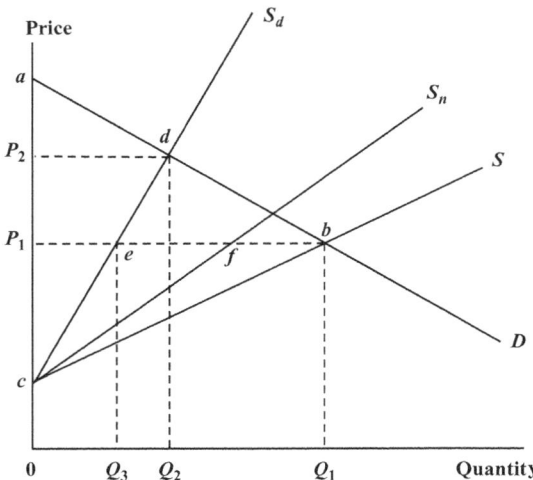

FIGURE 10.1 The economic effects of excluding non-dentist teeth whiteners

The demand and supply model illustrates the consequences of excluding a source of supply. Figure 10.1 includes a disaggregation of supply into two sources: S_d, which is the supply of teeth-whitening services by dentists, and S_n, which is the supply of teeth-whitening services by non-dentists. The horizontal sum of S_d and S_n is S.

If the non-dentists are excluded from the market for teeth-whitening services, the supply becomes S_d. The price rises from P_1 to P_2 and the quantity falls from Q_1 to Q_2. The dentists actually sell more teeth-whitening services than they previously sold and do so at a higher price. Before the exclusion of the non-dentists, the price was equal to P_1 and the dentists supplied Q_3. After the exclusion of the non-dentists, the price rises, and the quantity supplied by the dentists expands to Q_2. As a consequence, the dentists earn higher profits. Their profits are equal to area cdP_2, with an increase of area P_1P_2de in Figure 10.1. It is clear from this example that the dentists have a profound economic incentive to exclude non-dentists from supplying teeth-whitening services. There are, however, costs for other market participants.

First, the non-dentists had enjoyed producer surplus of P_1fc but now earn no profits since they are precluded from offering teeth-whitening services. The non-dentists are, therefore, worse off as a result of their exclusion. Consumers are also worse off. With competition, consumer surplus had been equal to area abP_1; after exclusion, it falls to adP_2. The reduction in social welfare is captured by area cbd. Gains to the dentists are outweighed by losses to others. On Kaldor–Hicks grounds, therefore, the exclusion unambiguously reduces social welfare.[39] Without more evidence that non-dentists are offering harmful services, the state legislature should not displace competition in this market.

Summary

The effects of removing a source of supply from a market are (1) higher market prices, (2) lower market output, (3) higher profits for the dentists, (4) lower profits for the non-dentists and (5) reduced consumer welfare. In the market for health care, fewer health care services received may be even less desirable than may be first apparent. If the costs of preventive health services increase, for example, and fewer of those services are consumed, individuals may be worse off if they delay receiving care. Such delay can lead to increased costs in the future if consumers require more complex or emergency care. Without licensing, the cost of those preventive services may be lower and more of those services may have been consumed. Although the quality of services offered may be lower, this may be a better option for those consumers who would otherwise be priced out of the market.

10.5 ECONOMIC EFFECTS OF MANDATED SUPERVISION

As Friedman predicted, entry restrictions into a profession often result in the rise of alternatives.[40] Those alternative sources of professional

---

[39] A good discussion of the Kaldor–Hicks compensation principle can be found in Just, Hueth, and Schmitz (2004). For the seminal articles, see Kaldor (1939) and Hicks (1939).

[40] Friedman (1962) pointed to the emergence of osteopathy and chiropractic as alternatives to traditional medical practice.

services provide competition with attendant lower prices and greater quantities of services consumed. Traditional practitioners experience lower revenues, which is a decidedly undesirable outcome for them. In some instances, however, the profession can mitigate the effects of substitution and thereby protect their incomes through the imposition of supervision requirements.

Dental hygienists are supervised by dentists, nurse anesthetists are supervised by anesthesiologists, and nurse practitioners and physician's assistants are supervised by physicians. This supervision promotes the interests of the supervisor at the expense of the supervised and, of course, the patients. We illustrate and analyze these results in the context of a specific example.

In 2003, the FTC challenged the South Carolina Board of Dentistry, alleging that the board had illegally restricted the provision of dental services.[41] Dental hygienists often perform dental cleanings on children at schools, which reduces transaction costs for parents and specifically helps low-income children. In South Carolina, however, dental hygienists could not provide teeth-cleaning services without being supervised by a dentist, which increased the cost of the service. In 2000, the state legislature removed the requirement that a dentist must examine a child before a hygienist could perform preventive services in schools, which made dental services more accessible for low-income children. But in 2001, the board reimposed the dental examination requirement. As a result, the FTC filed a complaint against the dental board, alleging that the action unnecessarily restrained competition.

In Figure 10.2, D represents the demand for dental hygiene services and S_1 represents the competitive supply of such services from this program. The competitive equilibrium quantity is Q_1, and the fee for those services is P_1. This fee and quantity maximize the sum of consumer surplus, represented by the area abP_1, and producer

---

[41] *In re South Carolina State Board of Dentistry*, No. 9311 WL 22168993 (FTC 2003), Complaint, 1.

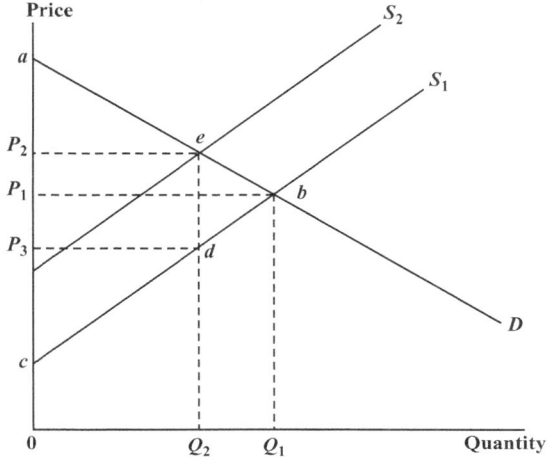

FIGURE 10.2 The economic effects of mandated supervision

surplus, represented by P_1bc. This sum is a measure of social welfare, which is maximized in competitive markets.[42]

The fee for supervision by a dentist acts like a per-unit tax on dental hygiene services. In Figure 10.2, S_2 represents the supply of dental hygiene services plus the mandated supervision. The vertical distance between S_1 and S_2 is equal to the fee for the supervision. The new equilibrium occurs at a quantity of Q_2 and a combined fee for services and supervision of P_2. There are winners and losers. The dentists are the clear winners since they collect fees for supervision. In Figure 10.2, these fees amount to the difference between P_2 and P_3 times the quantity of services performed by the dental hygienists: $(P_2 - P_3)Q_2$. The dental hygienists are the losers since they perform fewer services – Q_2 as opposed to Q_1 – and receive a lower fee – P_3 as opposed to P_1. Compared to the competitive equilibrium, producer

[42] In this analysis, we assume that the supervision confers no benefit. At least implicitly, this is the view of the Directors of Policy Planning, the Bureau of Economics, and the Bureau of Competition at the FTC. See their joint letter from January 17, 2014, to Representative Kay Khan of the Massachusetts House of Representatives (Federal Trade Commission 2014a).

surplus is reduced from P_1bc to P_3dc. The dental hygienists are clearly worse off.

The patients are also worse off due to the mandated supervision. The fee they must pay rises from P_1 to P_2, and the quantity of dental hygiene services consumed falls from Q_1 to Q_2. Compared to the competitive equilibrium, consumer surplus falls from abP_1 to the area aeP_2. Consumers are clearly worse off.

In sum, the deadweight social welfare loss is captured by the triangular area ebd. From a social welfare perspective, however, this implicitly assumes that the supervision services are worth the total cost of $(P_2 - P_3)Q_2$.

It is also important to observe that those who are priced out of the market because of the dental supervision rule are injured. Dental hygienists provide preventive services and can spot problems that require dental services before they become acute. Low-income children who do not receive the dental hygienists' services may experience future problems that could have been avoided.

The FTC supports reducing unnecessary supervision requirements wherever possible. For example, the FTC advised the state legislature in Massachusetts that removing unnecessary supervision requirements for nurse anesthetists and nurse practitioners would increase competition, reduce health care costs, and improve access to health care. Specifically, the legislature was considering a bill to no longer require a supervisory relationship with a Massachusetts physician to "(1) order tests and therapeutics, (2) issue written prescriptions, and (3) administer and dispense certain controlled substances."[43]

A number of states have proposed legislation targeting supervision requirements for non-physician medical professions such as advanced practice registered nurses (APRNs) and nurse practitioners (NPs). Additionally, the FTC has issued letters of support for bills that expand scope of practice or relax mandatory supervision

---

[43] Federal Trade Commission (2014a).

requirements, while enhancing competition in the marketplace, reducing prices, increasing access, and protecting patient safety. In Kansas, for example, HB 2412 proposed eliminating the requirement that APRNs have a collaborative agreement with a physician in order to prescribe medications.[44] In Massachusetts, HB 2009 proposed removal of supervisory requirements for both APRNs and NPs.[45] Similarly, in Ohio, HB 177 proposed the removal of the supervisory requirement for all APRNs.[46] In South Carolina, two opposing bills were proposed. HB 3508 would increase supervisory requirements for APRNs, whereas HB 3078 would remove the supervisory collaborative agreement with a physician to expand the APRNs' scope of practice.[47] Although APRNs and NPs do not have the same rigorous training as doctors, their education and training equips them to deal with ordinary cases. Allowing them to practice medicine and prescribe medication increases the supply of such services, especially in rural areas, and mitigates the negative effects of the doctor shortage.

10.6 THE EMPIRICAL EVIDENCE

Several hypotheses flow from the economics of professional licensing. First, licensing limits entry and reduces competition within the profession. This should lead to higher income for those who are licensed to practice. Second, the increased professional fees that licensing engenders reduce the quantity of professional services consumed. Third, higher fees improve the likelihood that alternatives will emerge and pose a competitive threat that the profession may want to curtail. For example, due to the high cost of physician services, APRNs and NAs have emerged. Practice restrictions imposed on these substitutes reduce the incentives to turn to them for professional services and may insulate the wages and employment of those in the protected profession. Fourth, licensing should result in higher quality of care.

---

[44] Federal Trade Commission (2020).   [45] Federal Trade Commission (2014a).
[46] Federal Trade Commission (2020).   [47] Federal Trade Commission (2015a).

The literature is full of research that addresses the economic effects of occupational licensing across myriad occupations. Other work has reviewed this literature in detail.[48] Researchers have employed a variety of data sets and advanced econometric methodology to investigate the markets for physicians and nurses, optometrists and ophthalmologists, midwives, dentists and dental hygienists, chiropractors, physical therapists, radiologic technicians, and massage therapists. In short, the literature is replete with findings that support Milton Friedman's concerns: More restrictive occupational licensing is associated with increased wages, reduced output within the profession, and higher prices of health care services for consumers. Moreover, the literature generally supports findings that relaxing occupational licensing restrictions or expanding nonphysician scope of practice leads to improved economic outcomes for those non-physician professions and increased utilization of non-physician services. Importantly, there is little (if any) evidence that expansions in scope of practice lead to reductions in health care quality.

10.7 CONCLUDING REMARKS

The fundamental premise of the Sherman Act is that competition will yield socially optimal results. As such, deviations from competition result in suboptimal outcomes. But the competitive model presumes that all market participants have full information, which is generally not the case when it comes to professional health care services. The presence of asymmetric information provides a rationale for systematically deviating from unfettered competition. Such deviations are permitted under the state action doctrine, provided that the state clearly articulates its intention to replace competition with some form of regulation and actively supervises that regulatory process to ensure that the benefits of abandoning competition are realized.

---

[48] Blair and Durrance (2015b).

Professional licensing falls under the state action doctrine. In many cases, licensing boards have restricted entry, excluded rival groups, and imposed supervisory requirements in ways that impair competition. We have presented two simple economic models that illustrate the gains to the protected profession and the losses to the patients and foreclosed rivals. The net loss from reduced competition can only be justified if the benefits of enhanced quality swamp those losses. In the absence of persuasive evidence that quality is greatly improved, state legislatures should pause and reflect before displacing market discipline in favor of licensing regulation. The empirical research on the effects of occupational licensing is expansive. The effects on price and quantity are both ubiquitous and consistent with economic theory – prices rise and quantities shrink – which means that some patients do not receive the care they need due to the licensing. Those results are inconsistent with antitrust's goal of promoting consumer welfare. On the other hand, occupational licensing arguably serves the public interest by protecting consumers from charlatans and incompetents. And so, we should expect licensing to improve quality. The empirical evidence on this issue is fairly limited, but the evidence that does exist fails to support a claim of substantially improved quality. Consequently, occupational licensing appears to impose costs without conferring many benefits.

REFERENCES

Allensworth, Rebecca Haw. (2017). Foxes at the Henhouse: Occupational Licensing Boards Up Close. *California Law Review* 105: 1567–1610.

Allensworth, Rebecca Haw. (2020). Licensed to Pill. *The New York Review*. www.nybooks.com/daily/2020/07/21/licensed-to-pill/.

Areeda, Philip, and Herbert Hovenkamp. (2021). *Antitrust Law*. 5th ed., Vol. II. New York: Wolters Kluwer.

Blair, Roger D., and Christine Piette Durrance. (2015a). Economic Effects of Licensing Health Care Professions. *Antitrust Health Care Chronicle* 28: 29–34.

Blair, Roger D., and Christine Piette Durrance. (2015b). Licensing Health Care Professionals, State Action, and Antitrust Policy. *University of Iowa Law Review* 100: 1943–1967.

Bulusu, Siri. (2021). *FTC Settles with Alabama Dental Board over Teledentistry Rules*. Bloomberg Law. https://news.bloomberglaw.com/health-law-and-busi ness/ftc-settles-with-alabama-dental-board-over-teledentistry-rules.

Bulusu, Siri, Claire Hao, and Erin Mulvaney. (2021). *Worker License Rules Emerge as FTC Competition Oversight Priority*. Bloomberg Law. https://news .bloomberglaw.com/antitrust/worker-license-rules-emerge-as-ftc-competition-oversight-priority.

Edlin, Aaron S., and Rebecca Haw Allensworth. (2014). Cartels by Another Name: Should Licensed Occupations Face Antitrust Scrutiny? *University of Pennsylvania Law Review* 162: 1093–1164.

Federal Trade Commission. (2014a). FTC Letter to Massachusetts House of Representatives. www.ftc.gov/sites/default/files/documents/advocacy_docu ments/ftc-staff-comment-massachusetts-house-representatives-regarding-house-bill-6-h.2009-concerning-supervisory-requirements-nurse-practitioners-nurse-anesthetists/140123massachusettnursesletter.pdf.

Federal Trade Commission. (2014b). Prepared Statement of the Federal Trade Commission: Competition and the Potential Costs and Benefits of Professional Licensure. www.ftc.gov/system/files/documents/public_state ments/568171/140716professionallicensurehouse.pdf.

Federal Trade Commission. (2015a). FTC Letter to South Carolina House of Representatives. www.ftc.gov/system/files/documents/advocacy_documents/ ftc-staff-comment-south-carolina-representative-jenny.horne-regarding-house-bill-3508-3078-advanced-practice-registered-nurse-regulations/151103scaprn.pdf.

Federal Trade Commission. (2015b). FTC Staff Guidance on Active Supervision of State Regulatory Boards Controlled by Market Participants. www.ftc.gov/ system/files/attachments/competition-policy-guidance/active_supervision_of_ state_boards.pdf.

Federal Trade Commission. (2020). FTC Letter to Kansas House of Representatives. www.ftc.gov/system/files/documents/advocacy_documents/ftc-staff-comment-kansas-house-representatives-concerning-kansas-house-bill-2412/v200006kan sashb2412aprnscomment.pdf.

Friedman, Milton. (1962). *Capitalism and Freedom*. Chicago: University of Chicago Press.

Grzinic, Barbara. (2022). *9th Circuit Aligns with SmileDirectClub's Antitrust Claims*. Reuters. www.reuters.com/legal/litigation/9th-circuit-aligns-with-smi ledirectclubs-antitrust-claims-2022-03-18/.

Hicks, John. (1939). The Foundations of Welfare Economics. *Economic Journal* 49: 696–712.

Just, Richard E., Darrell L. Hueth, and Andrew Schmitz. (2004), *The Welfare Economics of Public Policy*. Northampton, UK: Edward Elgar.

Kaldor, Nicholas. (1939). Welfare Propositions in Economic and Interpersonal Comparisons of Utility. *Economic Journal* 49: 549–552.

Kleiner, Morris M. (2015). Reforming Occupational Licensing Policies. The Hamilton Project. www.brookings.edu/wp-content/uploads/2016/06/thp_klei nerdiscpaper_final.pdf.

National Conference of State Legislatures. (2017). The State of Occupational Licensing: Research, State Policies and Trends. www.ncsl.org/Portals/1/ HTML_LargeReports/occupationallicensing_final.htm.

National Conference of State Legislatures. (2020). Occupational Licensing Final Report: Assessing State Policies and Practices. www.ncsl.org/research/labor-and-employment/occupational-licensing-final-report-assessing-state-policies-and-practices637425196.aspx.

Norris, Conor, and Edward J. Timmons. (2020). Restoring Vision to Consumers and Competition to the Marketplace: Analyzing the Effects of Required Prescription Release. *Journal of Regulatory Economics* 57: 1–19.

Obama White House. (2015). Occupational Licensing: A Framework for Policymakers. https://obamawhitehouse.archives.gov/sites/default/files/docs/ licensing_report_final_nonembargo.pdf.

PART III Monopsony

In this section, we will discuss monopsony and its welfare effects on health care markets. A monopsonist is the single buyer of a good or service. For antitrust purposes, a dominant buyer that accounts for 70–75 percent of purchases will be characterized as a monopsonist. In Chapter 2, we learned that the monopsonist can decrease the price it pays by reducing the quantity it buys. The monopsonist's suppliers are harmed and social welfare is reduced. Additionally, by reducing the quantity that it buys, the monopsonist reduces the quantity that it produces for the output market, which leads to higher prices for consumers. Although the effects on the output market may be insignificant, the harmful effects of monopsony on the input market can be substantial.

A hospital may function as a monopsonist in the local nurse labor market if it is the only employer of nurses. But pure monopsonies – single buyers – are generally rare. The exercise of monopsony power, however, is quite common and occurs in markets with dominant buyers or oligopsonies. In Chapter 11, we introduce models of monopsony, dominant buyers, and oligopsony. In a market with a dominant buyer, a dominant firm buys a significant share of the goods or services. The dominant buyer will set a price by taking into account the supply functions of the other, smaller firms in the market. Although the dominant buyer exercises its monopsony power, the influence of the fringe firms mitigates that power.

When multiple similarly sized firms buy goods in a marketplace, they may act as Cournot or Bertrand oligopsonists. When they act as Cournot oligopsonists, the firms compete on quantity. The firms will pay a price that is lower than the competitive price but higher than the monopsony price. When firms act as Bertrand oligopsonists, the firms compete on price and the competitive solution is reached. In both the dominant buyer model and the oligopsony model, the firms act unilaterally. Therefore, no antitrust remedy exists to mitigate the harmful effects to society.

Health insurers control policies for thousands of policyholders, which gives them substantial monopsony power in negotiating reimbursement rates with health care providers. Organizations with little bargaining power, such as small physician groups, may see their reimbursement rates fall to very low levels. Some physicians have therefore sought legal permission to collectively bargain; that is, physicians would cooperate to negotiate better rates with large health insurers. Through collective bargaining physicians would create a market structure that resembles a bilateral monopoly, which occurs when a monopsonist buys a good or service from a monopolist. This market structure is an improvement from monopsony or monopoly alone, since each firm counters the market power of the other. In Chapter 12, we discuss collective bargaining and how it can benefit consumers when health insurers wield considerable market power. But such bargaining should be regulated by the government to ensure that physicians do not cooperate to fix prices for uninsured patients.

Finally, in Chapter 13, we discuss group purchasing organizations (GPOs). Hospitals often procure their supplies from GPOs, which are entities that consolidate the purchases of their members in order to leverage their monopsony power. GPOs therefore control a large book of business and can use this market power to negotiate better rates with suppliers. Antitrust policymakers are concerned about GPOs because of their monopsony power, their ability to exclude rivals, and their funding mechanism.

Monopsony, although less common than monopoly, is just as harmful. The Agencies can promote competition by mitigating the effects of monopsony in health care industries.

11 Monopsony, Dominant Buyers, and Oligopsony

11.1 INTRODUCTION

Monopsony is the inelegant term that refers to a market in which there is a single buyer (or employer) of a well-specified good or service.[1] For example, a rural hospital may be the only employer of nurses in the local nurse labor market. By definition, that rural hospital would be a monopsonist in the nurse labor market. Provided that the supply of hospital nurses is positively sloped, the hospital will have monopsony power, which is the ability to control the wages of nurses by adjusting their employment. Relative to the employment level under competitive conditions, the monopsonist increases its profit by curtailing employment that reduces the wages paid to the nurses. Although it is somewhat counterintuitive, this apparent cost saving does *not* result in lower hospital charges. As we will see, the exercise of monopsony power has deleterious economic effects on both the input market and the output market.

Monopsony and the exercise of monopsony power are not confined to nurse labor markets in rural areas. We observe monopsony in many health insurance markets. Dominant health insurers generally represent a large share of business for health care providers. This allows the insurer to depress reimbursement rates for health care providers by adjusting the quantity of the services that it buys. Those lower reimbursement rates may lead to a reduction in the availability and quality of care for patients. In later chapters, we explore (1) potential monopsonistic abuses by group-purchasing organizations, (2) monopsonistic exploitation in nurse labor markets, (3) collusive

---

[1] This chapter borrows heavily from Blair and Durrance (2008), Blair and Harrison (2010), and Blair and Romano (1997).

monopsony in the oocyte market, and (4) no-poaching agreements among employers.

In this chapter, we focus on the economics of monopsony. We begin with the basic monopsony model in Section 11.2 and explore its impact on the monopsonist's cost functions and social welfare. In Section 11.3, we discuss the dominant buyer model and its effects on social welfare. In Section 11.4, we discuss both Cournot and Bertrand oligopsony. We turn our attention to monopsonistic abuses in health insurance markets in Section 11.5. Section 11.6 discusses the antitrust policy that governs monopsony and offers suggestions for mitigating negative consequences of monopsonistic behavior. We close with concluding observations in Section 11.7.

11.2   BASIC MODEL

A brief review of economic theory reveals the effect of monopsony on the prices consumers pay, the quantity of workers employed, and the nature of the social welfare loss.[2] If the supply of an input is positively sloped, a monopsonist can depress the wage that it pays by restricting the quantity of inputs that it employs.[3] It is a common misconception that the exercise of monopsony power will make consumers better off. After all, if an input price falls, the employer's cost would fall – which would normally lead to an expansion of output with a corresponding reduction in the output price. This result would seem to make consumers better off. But the economic results are quite different when the input price falls due to monopsony. In fact, since employment falls, the monopsonist's output also falls, which will lead to adverse economic consequences in the output market.[4] In the short run at least, the reduced total output produced will cause the price to rise

---

[2] Bhaskar, Manning, and To (2002) explore the pervasive presence of monopsony in the economy.

[3] Jacobson and Dorman (1991) and Jacobson (2013) show that if supply is perfectly elastic, then a single buyer will have no monopsony power.

[4] Angerhofer and Blair (2020).

and consumer welfare to fall.[5] In general, the adverse economic effects of monopsony will be more pronounced in a local input market relative to those in a broader output market.

In order to make the exposition less abstract, consider the market for acute care hospital services. A hospital hires nurses to produce acute care services. If the output market is competitive, the hospital will consider the price of health care services to be exogenously determined by supply and demand. In our scenario, acute care services are produced with nurse labor (L) and capital inputs (K) according to the production function, $Q = Q(L, K)$. In the absence of monopsony power in any input market, the hospital's profit function (Π) can be written as $\Pi = P \cdot Q(L, K) - wL - rK$, where P is the market-determined price, w is the wage rate, and r is the price of capital.

In order to maximize profit, the hospital will hire nurses such that $P \cdot MP_L = w$, where MP_L is the marginal product of labor, which is the increase in acute care services resulting from a unit increase in the employment of nurses. Multiplying the marginal product of labor by the price translates the marginal product of labor into dollar units. This term, $P \cdot MP_L$, is the value of the marginal product of labor (VMP_L).

In Figure 11.1, the derived demand for labor in the local labor market is shown as VMP_L.[6] The supply of labor is shown as the positively sloped line, S_L. The competitive solution occurs where these two curves intersect, resulting in an employment of L_1 and wage of w_1. Employer surplus is captured by the triangular area abw_1, and employee surplus by the triangular area w_1bc. The sum

---

[5] The magnitude of the effect depends on the structure of the output market. The more concentrated the output market, the larger will be the effect of a quantity reduction induced by a monopsony.

[6] The employer's demand for labor is derived from the consumer's demand for the acute care hospital services produced by the employer. For a competitive firm, the value of the marginal product of labor is its derived demand for labor. The derived demand for labor in the local labor market is the horizontal sum of the derived demands of the individual employers in the labor market.

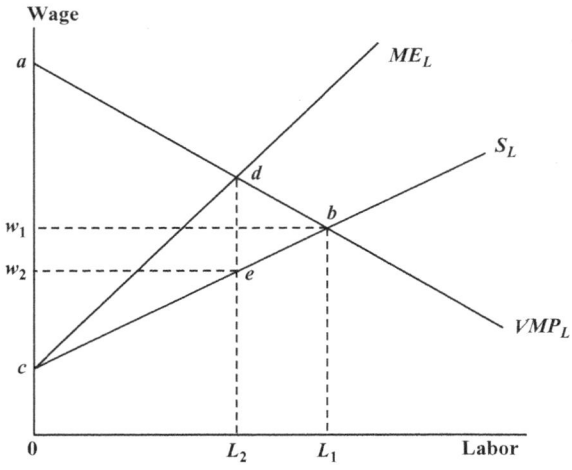

FIGURE 11.1 The basic monopsony model

of employer and employee surplus, area abc, is a measure of social welfare.

Suppose that the hospital is a monopsonist in the nurse labor market. The wage rate now depends upon the quantity of labor services employed. In other words, w is now a function of L. Since labor supply is positively sloped, the wage rises with employment, that is, $\frac{dw}{dL} > 0$.[7] Accordingly, the profit function changes to $\Pi = P \cdot Q(L, K) - w(L)L - rK$. To maximize profits, the hospital employs labor such that $\frac{\partial \Pi}{\partial L} = P \cdot \frac{\partial Q}{\partial L} - w - L\frac{dw}{dL} = 0$.[8] The first term, $P \cdot \frac{\partial Q}{\partial L}$, is the VMP_L while the sum of the next two terms, $w + L\frac{dw}{dL}$, is the marginal expenditure on labor, ME_L. Consequently, a profit-maximizing employer will employ labor such that the VMP_L is equal to the ME_L. As shown in Figure 11.1, profit maximization by the monopsonist leads to a reduction in the employment of

---

[7] The supply of labor is positively sloped since workers have different reservation wages. Some workers are willing to work for very low wages. Others need a higher wage to entice them to contribute their labor.

[8] Normally, we would simultaneously solve the first-order conditions for both labor and capital. Since we focus on labor, we hold capital constant.

labor from L_1 to L_2, with a corresponding reduction in the wage paid from w_1 to w_2.

Employer surplus increases from area abw_1 to area $adew_2$, but employee surplus falls from area w_1bc to area w_2ec. There is a transfer of surplus; employee surplus equal to $(w_1 - w_2)L_2$ is redistributed to the employer. Total surplus shrinks by the triangular area dbe due to allocative inefficiency – too few units of labor are being employed. For the units of labor between L_1 and L_2, the reservation wage (as measured by the height of the supply curve) is less than the value of the output that the employment would have generated to society (as measured by the height of the VMP_L curve). In a social sense, these units of labor should have been employed. But they were not employed because it was profit maximizing for the employer to limit employment to L_2:

The economic effects of monopsony are not confined to the nurse labor market. They also extend to the output market. Since labor is reduced, the hospital has reduced its productive capacity and must produce fewer acute care hospital services.[9] The reduction in services results in increased prices and thereby leads to a social welfare loss in the acute care hospital services market. The effect on price increases with higher levels of concentration in the acute care hospital services market. If the hospital also functions as a monopolist, the effect on price can be quite substantial. If the hospital is part of a competitive acute care services market, the effects will be negligible. It can be shown that the social welfare loss depicted in Figure 11.1 is equivalent to the corresponding social welfare loss in the output market.[10]

In the simple economic model displayed in Figure 11.1, we confined our attention to the effect of monopsony on employment, wages, and social welfare. This bare-bones model does not capture the

---

[9] Alternatively, the hospital could maintain the quantity but reduce the quality. This reduction could expose the hospital to malpractice suits should the reduced quality lead to unfortunate outcomes.

[10] For a mathematical derivation, see Blair and Romano (1997).

full array of economic consequences that may result from monopsony in the local labor market. Monopsony can lead to lower benefits, such as reduced family leave, sick leave, paid vacations, health and dental insurance, retirement plans, and employer contributions to employee educational programs. Additionally, enhanced monopsony power could result in the elimination of bonus plans or profit-sharing plans. Finally, there could be an adverse effect on working conditions that affect employee health and safety. Qualitatively, these deleterious effects are analogous to the economic results that we have captured in our simple model of monopsony.

Lerner Index of Monopsony

The essence of monopsony power is the ability of a large buyer to influence prices by restricting its purchases. The monopsonist recognizes that the supply function is positively sloped and that it can slide along that supply curve to a lower price by decreasing its purchases. In this way, the monopsony price deviates from the competitive price. A measure of monopsony power should reflect this deviation. One way to do this is to adapt the Lerner index of monopoly power to the case of monopsony.[11]

Accordingly, the Lerner index of monopsony is defined as the percentage deviation from the competitive result:

$$\lambda = \frac{VMP_L - w}{w}. \tag{11.1}$$

In other words, λ represents the gap between the value of the marginal product and the wage being paid divided by the wage. In order to maximize profit, the monopsonist will employ L where the value of the marginal product is equal to the marginal expenditure:

$$VMP_L = ME_L = w + L\frac{dw}{dL}.$$

---

[11] Lerner (1934). For an adaptation to monopsony, see Blair and Harrison (1992a).

After substitution into Equation (11.1), we have

$$\lambda = \frac{L(dw/dL)}{w}.$$

Since the elasticity of supply is $\varepsilon = (dL/dw)(w/L)$, we see that the Lerner index is the reciprocal of the elasticity of supply of L:

$$\lambda = \frac{1}{\varepsilon}.$$

Increases in the supply elasticity decrease monopsony power: $d\lambda/d\varepsilon < 0$. This makes economic sense because the greater the quantity response of the nurses to changes in their wage, the less influence on wage the monopsonist will have. We demonstrate the effect of supply elasticity on the magnitude of monopsony power with a few examples. If the supply elasticity is 0.5, then the monopsony power is 2.0. In that event, the wage paid may be $10 while the value of the marginal product is $30. If the supply elasticity is 5, then monopsony power is only 0.2. In this case, if the wage paid is $10, the value of the marginal product will be $12. When the supply elasticity approaches infinity, there is no monopsony power. Therefore, when supply is inelastic ($\varepsilon < 1$), there is a substantial deviation from the competitive result. But the more elastic the supply, the smaller the deviation. In the limit, when $\varepsilon = \infty$, the buyer is essentially in a competitive market and the deviation is zero.[12]

Impact of Monopsony on Cost Functions

In Figure 11.1, we see that the competitive employment and wage is L_1 and w_1, respectively. The exercise of monopsony power reduces the wage from w_1 to w_2. In ordinary circumstances, this appears to be a good outcome for everyone except the suppliers of L. After all, lower input prices ordinarily lead to lower costs, which in turn lead to lower

---

[12] Jacobson and Dorman (1991) make the point that if supply is flat (i.e., $\varepsilon = \infty$), there is no monopsony power because the wage cannot be depressed.

prices for consumers of the monopsonist's output. As a result, it appears that the monopsonist makes more profit and consumers are better off. So why is there an economic objection to monopsony?

The rosy scenario just described is wrong; it is based on a fundamental misunderstanding of the relationship between the exercise of monopsony and the resulting cost curves. In reality, monopsony leads to lower *average* cost at the profit-maximizing employment level, which provides the profit incentive for monopsonistic behavior, but monopsony causes *marginal* cost to shift upward, which leads to reduced output and a consequent decrease in consumer surplus.[13] We believe that it is important to understand these effects if antitrust policy is to be sound.

Impact on Marginal Cost

First, recall that the marginal product of L, MP_L, measures the increase in output resulting from a small increase in the employment of L. As a result, the increase in the quantity of L necessary to expand output by one unit is given by the inverse of MP_L, that is, $1/MP_L$. Absent monopsony power, the wage of L is w, which is the market-determined wage for one unit of labor. The expenditure on L necessary to increase output by one unit will be w/MP_L. This, of course, is marginal cost:

$$MC = \frac{w}{MP_L}.$$

But this marginal cost changes with the exercise of monopsony power. The monopsonist recognizes that the supply of L has a positive slope and, therefore, the increase in expenditures on L accompanying a one-unit increase in employment is the marginal expenditure:

$$ME_L = \frac{d(w \cdot L)}{dL} = w + L\frac{dw}{dL}.$$

---

[13] Analogous results can be found in Blair and Romano (1997).

The increase in cost necessary to expand output by one unit for a monopsonist is therefore

$$MC' = \frac{ME_L}{MP_L} = \frac{w + L(dw/dL)}{MP_L}.$$

Since $L(dw/dL)$ is positive, we can see that

$$\frac{w}{MP_L} < \frac{w + L(dw/dL)}{MP_L}.$$

In other words, $MC < MC'$, so monopsony causes marginal cost to shift upward!

Whether the firm has market power in the output market or not, an upward shift in the firm's marginal cost curve leads to a reduction in its optimal output. Accordingly, there is no improvement in consumer welfare. In fact, the opposite will be the case if the firm has any degree of market power, that is, if the firm faces a negatively sloped demand curve. In those instances, the firm's reduced output causes output price to rise and thereby leads to a loss in consumer surplus.[14]

Impact on Average Cost

In spite of the shift in marginal cost, the monopsonist enjoys higher profits as a result of curtailing its employment of L. This results from a shift downward and to the left of the minimum point on the average cost curve. For a firm that competes in all input markets, the average cost is

$$AC = \frac{wL + rK}{Q(L, K)},$$

where the quantities of L and K minimize the cost of producing the quantity of output. For the monopsonist, however, the average cost is

---

[14] Angerhofer and Blair (2020).

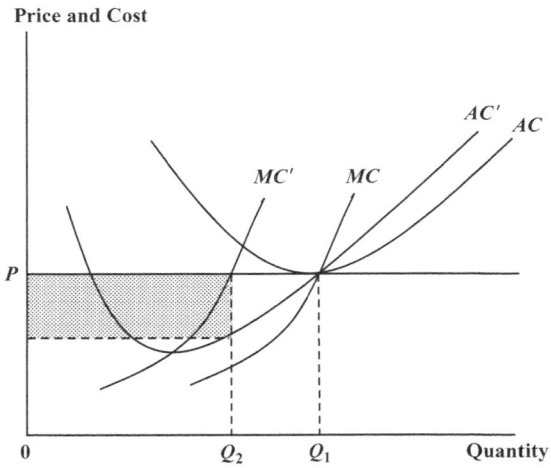

FIGURE 11.2 The impact of monopsony on marginal and average cost

$$AC' = \frac{w(L)L + rK}{Q(L,K)}.$$

Since the supply of L is positively sloped, $w(L)$ will exceed w_1 (the competitive wage) when L exceeds L_1. In contrast, $w(L)$ will be less than w_1 when L is less than L_1. As a result, $AC > AC'$ when output is below the competitive level and $AC < AC'$ when output is above the competitive level. The reduction in average cost resulting from reduced employment of L and the corresponding decrease in output provides the profit incentive for the monopsonist's restricted employment of L.

Figure 11.2 shows these results. To maximize profits, a firm in a competitive market produces Q_1 and sells it at the competitive price, P. Since $P = MC = AC$ at Q_1, the competitive firm earns no excess profit. If the firm enjoys monopsony power, however, the marginal cost shifts from MC to MC' and the optimal output declines to Q_2, which is sold at the market price of P. At the same time, average cost shifts from AC to AC'. Note that $AC = AC'$ at Q_1, $AC > AC'$ for $Q < Q_1$, and $AC < AC'$ for $Q > Q_1$. At the reduced output, $P = MC'$, but $P > AC'$.

So profits rise above the competitive level to $(P - AC')Q_2 > 0$, which is depicted as the shaded rectangle in Figure 11.2. Similar results hold for a monopsonist that enjoys some market power in its output market.

For antitrust policy purposes, it is important to understand that the reduced input prices flowing from an exercise of monopsony power are *not* socially beneficial. While they result in lower *average* cost and, therefore, higher profits for the monopsonist, they result in higher *marginal* cost. This, in turn, leads to no benefit for the consumer. On the other hand, if input prices are reduced due to greater efficiency, both marginal and average cost will fall, output will expand, and consumer welfare will increase.

11.3 DOMINANT BUYER MODEL

We have examined the basic monopsony model and its impact on the monopsonist's cost functions and social welfare. We now consider the dominant buyer model.

Basic Model

The dominant buyer is a close cousin of the pure monopsonist. In this model, a single large buyer shares an input market with a collection of small buyers, which are termed *fringe firms*. Due to its size, the dominant firm recognizes that its purchases will influence the market price. As a result, this firm will act as a price setter. Each fringe firm is small enough that it acts as a price taker because its purchases are too small to influence price in the market. In essence, the fringe of competitive buyers accepts the price that the dominant firm pays as the market-determined price. Behaving competitively, the fringe firms will buy the input up to the point where their collective demand equals the price set by the buyer. Now, the dominant buyer's problem lies in adjusting its purchases to maximize profit subject to the competitive behavior of the fringe buyers.

The dominant buyer model is depicted in Figure 11.3, where VMP_f represents the demand for nurse labor of the competitive fringe,

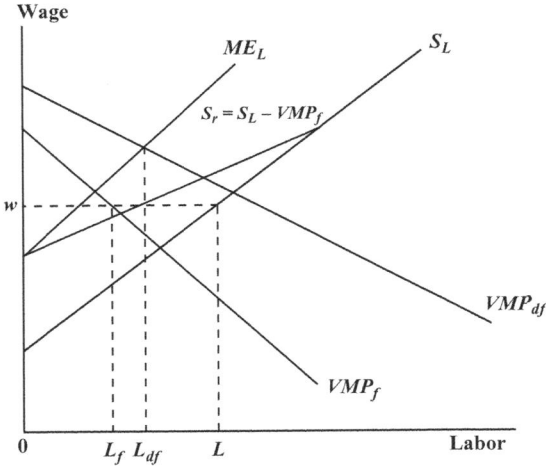

FIGURE 11.3 The dominant buyer model

VMP_{df} represents the demand for labor of the dominant firm, and S_L is the labor supply curve. The dominant firm recognizes that the fringe will purchase the quantity where VMP_f equals the wage that it sets. The dominant employer incorporates this behavior into its decision calculus by subtracting VMP_f from S_L to obtain the residual supply, which is denoted by S_r in Figure 11.3.[15] The curve marginal to S_r, which is labeled ME_L, represents the marginal expenditure for the dominant buyer. The balance of the analysis is familiar: The dominant employer purchases L_{df} where ME_L equals VMP_{df}, which determines the wage (w) from the residual supply. At w, the fringe will purchase L_f where w equals VMP_f. At w, the nurses will provide L, which is equal to the sum of L_f and L_{df}.

The profit-maximizing behavior of the dominant buyer leads to the same sort of allocative inefficiency that results from pure monopsony. Since ME_L exceeds w, the value created by employing one more unit of labor exceeds the social cost of doing so. As a consequence,

---

[15] We subtract the curves horizontally since we want to subtract quantity, not wage.

dominant buyer behavior leads to a deadweight social welfare loss analogous to that of pure monopsony.

Lerner Index

The buying power of a dominant firm is mitigated by the demand response of the competitive fringe. The Lerner index can be adapted to this case. The Lerner index of monopsony for a dominant buyer is

$$\lambda = \frac{s}{\varepsilon_L - (1 - s)\eta_f},$$

where s represents the dominant buyer's share of the market, ε_L is the elasticity of supply, and η_f is the elasticity of demand of the fringe buyers, which is negative.

In order to evaluate monopsony power, we consider how each variable influences λ.[16] First, we observe that $\partial\lambda/\partial s > 0$. This makes economic sense and is consistent with our intuition. The higher the dominant buyer's share of the market, the greater is its buying power, and the greater is its ability to curtail quantity and depress price.

Second, increases in ε_L will decrease λ since $\partial\lambda/\partial\varepsilon_L < 0$. The elasticity of supply measures the relative responsiveness of the quantity supplied to changes in price. As the quantity supplied becomes more responsive to changes in price (i.e., as ε_L increases), the market power of the dominant buyer falls. This occurs because the suppliers can redirect their efforts to other products where prices may be higher. In the limit, the elasticity of supply goes to infinity (i.e., the supply curve is flat and, therefore, perfectly elastic) and the value of λ goes to zero.[17]

Finally, we may examine the influence of the demand elasticity of the fringe buyers. As this elasticity increases, the buying power of the dominant firm falls since $\partial\lambda/\partial\eta_f > 0$. This follows because any

[16] Several numerical examples are provided in Blair and Harrison (1992b).
[17] This is the point that Jacobson and Dorman (1991) were making when they expressed some skepticism regarding the empirical importance of monopsony problems.

reduction in price implemented by the dominant buyer's curtailed purchases is offset to some extent by the enhanced purchases of the fringe. The more responsive the fringe firms are to price decreases, the more difficult it is for the dominant buyer to make such a decrease stick. In the limit, the elasticity of fringe demand goes to infinity and the dominant buyer's power goes to zero.

11.4 OLIGOPSONY

Oligopsony refers to a market structure in which there are a few relatively large buyers of a good or service. In such markets, the ability to depress the input price is more circumscribed than under monopsony. The exertion of oligopsony power relies on the mutual interdependence of firms' price and quantity decisions. Depending upon whether the firms compete on quantity or on price, the oligopsony equilibrium price will be between the monopsony and competitive prices.

If the buyers behave as Cournot rivals, they compete on the basis of the quantity that they employ. In this event, the equilibrium quantity is above the employment level of a monopsonist but below the competitive level. Accordingly, the resulting price will be above the monopsony price but below the competitive price. In the case of Bertrand competition, buyers compete on the basis of the price paid. In that case, the price will equal the competitive input price even when only two buyers are present.

In this section, we examine both Cournot duopsony and Bertrand duopsony. We also consider generalizations to more buyers and discuss the implications for the exercise of oligopsony power.

Cournot Oligopsony

If firms independently and simultaneously choose the quantity of labor (L) to employ, they will behave as Cournot oligopsonists. For ease of exposition, we assume that supply is linear, $w = a + bL$, and the two firms are identical. Since both firms are identical, the values of their marginal product curves are identical.

The profit function of Firm 1 (Π_1) is

$$\Pi_1 = PQ_1(L_1, K_1) - L_1(a + b(L_1 + L_2)) - rK_1,$$

where P is the market-determined output price, $Q_1(L_1, K_1)$ is the production function with labor (L) and capital inputs (K), $L_1(a + b(L_1 + L_2))$ is the total expenditure on labor, and rK_1 is the total expenditure on capital. Since Firm 1 and Firm 2 are identical, Firm 2 will have a similar profit function (Π_2):

$$\Pi_2 = PQ_2(L_2, K_2) - L_2(a + b(L_1 + L_2)) - rK_2.$$

Both firms recognize their ability to affect the wage rate by adjusting their employment levels. Accordingly, the firms choose the quantity of labor to employ while recognizing that the wage rate increases in their own employment and the employment of others. The profit-maximizing quantities of labor are found by solving the following first-order conditions simultaneously:

$$\frac{\partial \Pi_1}{\partial L_1} = P(\partial Q_1/\partial L_1) - (a + 2bL_1 + bL_2) = 0,$$

$$\frac{\partial \Pi_2}{\partial L_2} = P(\partial Q_2/\partial L_2) - (a + bL_1 + 2bL_2) = 0.$$

Since both firms have the same value of the marginal product and face the same supply curve, the equilibrium employment levels will be the same: $L_1 = L_2$. Then, in equilibrium, the Cournot duopsonists employ labor such that

$$L_1 = \frac{P(\partial Q_1/\partial L_1) - a}{3b},$$

$$L_2 = \frac{P(\partial Q_2/\partial L_2) - a}{3b},$$

$$w = \frac{a}{3} + \frac{2}{3}P(\partial Q_1/\partial L_1),$$

$$L = \frac{2(P(\partial Q_1/\partial L_1) - a)}{3b}.$$

These results generalize to the case of n employers. The equilibrium in a Cournot oligopsony is then characterized by the following three equations:

$$L_i = \frac{P(\partial Q_i/\partial L_i) - a}{b(n+1)},$$

$$w = \frac{a}{n+1} + \frac{n}{n+1}(P(\partial Q_i/\partial L_i)),$$

$$L = nL_i = \frac{n(P(\partial Q_i/\partial L_i) - a)}{b(n+1)}.$$

In the first equation, we note that the quantity of labor employed by each firm is decreasing in the number of firms. In the second, we can see that the extent of oligopsony power is decreasing as the number of firms increases by looking at the wage rate. As $n \to \infty$, $w \to P(\partial Q_i/\partial L_i)$, which is the competitive outcome. Therefore, the more concentrated a market is, the more monopsony power the firms in that market may have. This power can lead to the depression of the wage and a reduction in the employment level.

Bertrand Oligopsony

Oligopsony can also be analyzed as a Bertrand oligopsony in which firms compete for labor by offering a wage, w. When the decision variable is the wage, the competition between even two firms will drive the wage up to the competitive level. To show this result, we begin by analyzing a Bertrand duopsony with homogeneous labor services. If Employer 1 offers a lower wage than Employer 2, it will be unable to hire any labor and vice versa.[18] If both employers offer the same wage, they will each employ half of the labor supplied at that wage. This wage will be the competitive wage. Since the employers buy labor at the competitive wage, there is no allocative inefficiency and no competitive concerns.

---

[18] This assumes there are no capacity constraints on the part of the employers.

11.5   MONOPSONY IN HEALTH INSURANCE MARKETS

Health care costs can be prohibitive for consumers, especially when a three-day hospital stay can cost thousands of dollars.[19] Therefore, many consumers elect to purchase health insurance either through their employer or in the individual market to mitigate the risk of an unexpected large medical bill. In so doing, the consumer transfers the cost of his or her risk of injury to the insurance company. When an insured patient requires medical attention for an illness or injury, his or her insurance firm will pay a portion of the medical bill to the provider on behalf of the patient. In many local markets for health care provider services, the major health insurance firms wield considerable monopsony power. They can leverage their large number of policyholders to depress the prices that they pay to health care providers.

The more concentrated the insurance market, the more leverage health insurers have over health care providers, which results in lower reimbursement rates. When concentration is high, a single health insurer may represent a large number of policyholders in a single area. If hospitals, physicians, and other health care providers do not accept the health insurer's payment offers, they would be foreclosed from providing care to that insurer's large number of policyholders.[20] The insurer, therefore, has significant leverage to depress the price of health care when it manages the policies of a large portion of health care consumers in a local market.

There is reason to believe that health insurance markets are dominated by large health insurers that wield considerable monopsony power. A recent study by the American Medical Association

---

[19] In 2020, the list price of the operating room in a Florida hospital was $2,500 for the first minute plus $250 per minute thereafter. So the use of the operating room for an hour would be $2,500 + $250(59) = $17,250. One of the authors discovered this pricing scheme through firsthand experience.

[20] United Healthcare allegedly excluded anesthesiologists in Texas and Colorado from its network by pressuring hospitals and surgeons to refer their patients to other anesthesiologists (Abelson 2021).

quantified market concentration of health insurers using the Herfindahl-Hirschman Index (HHI).[21] The average HHI was 3,473, and about 74 percent of metropolitan statistical area markets had an HHI above 2,500.[22] The DOJ and the FTC consider an HHI above 2,500 as a dangerous level of concentration since firms may hold considerable market power.[23] These large health insurers represent a large number of policyholders, which increases their bargaining power with health care providers.

Two key reasons help explain concentration in the market for health insurance. First, opportunities for economies of scale may incentivize health insurers to grow bigger. The larger the pool of policyholders, the more predictable is the cost of health care, which reduces firm risk. Some experts claim that a pool of at least 50,000 individuals is necessary to keep a health insurer financially sound.[24] Some local markets may be unable to sustain more than one or two health insurers, leading to higher concentration. Second, insurers may be consolidating to increase their market power, which would increase their bargaining power over health care providers. With fewer insurers, health care providers have fewer options if they are dissatisfied with the reimbursement rates offered.

In our theoretical models, firms with monopsony power are able to manipulate quantity in order to depress wages and thereby increase prices. In the same way, we would expect health insurers to reduce the quantity of claims that they pay in order to depress payments and increase profits. But the ability of insurers to manipulate quantity is not as clear-cut. The quantity of health care services demanded is controlled by the policyholders, not the insurers. It would be inconceivable for a policyholder to receive no insurance coverage on a broken arm simply because an insurer was trying to reduce quantity to depress claim payments. But insurers play a numbers game. By

---

[21] We discuss the HHI in more detail in Chapter 18.

[22] American Medical Association (2020).

[23] Department of Justice and Federal Trade Commission (2010).

[24] Austin and Hungerford (2010).

manipulating their policies, they are able to reduce the health care services demanded by their pool of policyholders.

An insurer's main avenue for manipulation is its insurance policy. In this policy, the insurer determines what health care services it will cover. The insurer can decide which hospitals and physician groups will be in-network for its policyholders as well as the services that are covered. For example, the insurance company usually covers a yearly physical for each of its policyholders. If an insurer wanted to reduce routine appointments, it could require patients to pay an extra copayment for attending another routine appointment in that year. Additionally, it could change the yearly threshold and cover the price of physicals only once every 15 months. Manipulating the insurance policy may incentivize patients to get less care.

Expensive health care visits, prescriptions, or medical devices, such as continuous positive airway pressure (CPAP) machines that treat sleep apnea, generally require insurer permission before reimbursement. By being more restrictive in what prescription drugs or medical devices it covers or by charging higher copayments for more expensive options, the insurer may also reduce the quantity of health care services it provides. Using these tactics, health insurers can reduce their policyholders' demand for services, which will allow them to depress the price that they pay for those services.

In summary, the oligopsony model predicts that as a health insurance market becomes more concentrated, the quantity and quality of health care services will be reduced, which will lower the fees health care providers receive for the services they provide. Due to the higher insurance premiums and lower costs to health care providers, insurers make a profit that enriches themselves. In Chapter 12, we discuss countervailing power, which can be used to check the monopsony power of health insurers.

11.6 ANTITRUST TREATMENT OF MONOPSONY

As we have seen, the structural conditions of monopsony, dominant buyer, and oligopsony involve social welfare losses due to allocative inefficiency. In each case, too few resources are employed. But market structure alone is not an antitrust violation. Unilateral employment decisions may not be efficient, but they are seldom unlawful. Only when competitively unreasonable conduct is used to attain or maintain a noncompetitive market structure can the Agencies and victims of the conduct cry foul.

A useful example can be found in *Weyerhaeuser* v. *Ross-Simmons Hardwood Lumber Company.*[25] A small lumber mill had accused Weyerhaeuser of engaging in predatory bidding in an effort to monopsonize the market for hardwood sawlogs. Predatory bidding occurs when a firm offers a price above the value of the marginal product of the input in question in order to deny access to rivals. Weaker rivals would not be able to stay in business if their input costs were more than the revenue they received from selling their output. Presumably, after these rivals were forced to exit the market, Weyerhaeuser could act as the sole buyer and recoup its losses. If it had been proven that Weyerhaeuser had engaged in predatory bidding, then its conduct would have violated Section 2 of the Sherman Act.[26] The Court, however, concluded that the conduct was not predatory bidding, and the Court also set important precedent stating that monopsony and monopoly were economically similar and should share similar judicial treatment.

The economic objection to monopsony is analogous to the economic objection to monopoly: Too few resources are employed, resulting in a social welfare loss. The structural condition of monopoly is not unlawful and neither is the exercise of monopoly power; when the monopoly itself is lawful. Consistency requires analogous treatment for monopsony. The *Grinnell* test for unlawful monopoly can be adapted to the case of monopsony:

> The offense of [monopsony] under §2 of the Sherman Act has two elements: (1) the possession of [monopsony] power in the relevant

---

[25] *Weyerhaeuser* v. *Ross-Simmons Hardwood Lumber Company*, 127 US 1068 (2007).

[26] For an extensive analysis of the economic issues in this case, see Blair and Lopatka (2008).

market and (2) the willful acquisition or maintenance of that power [through predatory or exclusionary practices] that are competitively unreasonable.[27]

A plaintiff would therefore have to define a relevant market and prove that the defendant had monopsony power in that market to satisfy the first prong of the *Grinnell* test. In addition, the plaintiff would have to prove that the defendant attained or maintained its monopsony through exclusionary or predatory means. This can be quite difficult.

Similarly, in the absence of proof that a dominant buyer has engaged in some form of predatory or otherwise exclusionary conduct, there is no antitrust violation. If oligopsonists act independently in setting their prices and quantity, they will also be spared any antitrust troubles.[28]

But there are other ways to curb monopsony power. Monopsony power can be offset by countervailing power, which we discuss in Chapter 12. Additionally, government agencies can reject mergers that would substantially increase concentration. We discuss horizontal mergers in Chapter 18.

11.7 CONCLUDING REMARKS

The economic objection to monopsony is analogous to the economic objection to monopoly: Too few resources are employed, resulting in a social welfare loss. Although single-firm monopsonists are rare, dominant buyers and Cournot oligopsonists are ubiquitous and can exercise their monopsony power to reduce the quantity of inputs supplied and thereby depress prices. In so doing, the firms harm both input suppliers and consumers. Although the exercise of monopsony power in itself is not illegal, the antitrust Agencies should make an effort to mitigate its prevalence.

---

[27] *Weyerhaeuser* v. *Ross-Simmons Hardwood Lumber Company*, 127 US 1068 (2007).

[28] Overt collusion among firms that form a buyer cartel is a violation of Section 1 of the Sherman Act. We discuss buyer cartels in detail in Part IV.

REFERENCES

Abelson, Reed. (2021). Doctors Accuse United Healthcare of Stifling Competition. *New York Times.* www.nytimes.com/2021/04/01/health/unitedhealthcare-lawsuit.html.

American Medical Association. (2020). *Competition in Health Insurance: A Comprehensive Study of US Markets.* www.ama-assn.org/system/files/2020-10/competition-health-insurance-us-markets.pdf.

Angerhofer, Tirza J., and Roger D. Blair. (2020). *Collusion in the Labor Market: Intended and Unintended Consequences.* CPI Antitrust Chronicle: May II. www.competitionpolicyinternational.com/collusion-in-the-labor-market-intended-and-unintended-consequences/.

Austin, D. Andrew, and Thomas L. Hungerford. (2010). *The Market Structure of the Health Insurance Industry.* Congressional Research Service. https://fas.org/sgp/crs/misc/R40834.pdf.

Bhaskar, V., Alan Manning, and Ted To. (2002). Oligopsony and Monopsonistic Competition in Labor Markets. *Journal of Economic Perspectives* 16: 155–174.

Blair, Roger D., and Christine Piette Durrance. (2008). The Economics of Monopsony. In W. Dale Collins, ed., *Issues in Competition Law and Policy.* Chicago: American Bar Association, 393–408.

Blair, Roger D., and Jeffrey L. Harrison. (1992a). Cooperative Buying, Monopsony Power, and Antitrust Policy. *Northwestern University Law Review* 86: 331–367.

Blair, Roger D., and Jeffrey L. Harrison. (1992b). The Measurement of Monopsony Power. *Antitrust Bulletin* 37: 133–150.

Blair, Roger D., and Jeffrey L. Harrison. (2010). *Monopsony in Law and Economics.* New York: Cambridge University Press.

Blair, Roger D., and John E. Lopatka. (2008). Predatory Buying and the Antitrust Laws. *Utah Law Review* 2: 415–469.

Blair, Roger D., and Richard E. Romano. (1997). Collusive Monopsony in Theory and Practice: The NCAA. *Antitrust Bulletin* 42: 681–719.

Department of Justice and Federal Trade Commission. (2010). Horizontal Merger Guidelines. www.ftc.gov/system/files/documents/public_statements/804291/100819hmg.pdf.

Jacobson, Jonathan. (2013). *Monopsony 2013: Still Not Truly Symmetric.* The Antitrust Source. www.wsgr.com/a/web/191/jacobson-0413.pdf.

Jacobson, Jonathan, and Gary Dorman. (1991). Joint Purchasing, Monopsony, and Antitrust. *Antitrust Bulletin* 36: 1–79.

Lerner, Abba. (1934). The Concept of Monopoly and the Measurement of Monopoly Power. *Review of Economic Studies* 1: 157–175.

12 Countervailing Power

Physician Collective Bargaining

12.1 INTRODUCTION

In some situations, it may be advantageous for a government to allow buyers or sellers to cooperate on prices and output to keep a lawful monopolist or a lawful monopsonist, respectively, in check. Although it may seem anticompetitive at first, allowing this behavior is a way to level the playing field and can lead to a socially optimal solution.[1] This cooperation increases the bargaining power of the buyers or sellers such that the monopolist or monopsonist cannot abuse its market power.

The parties will first agree on the quantity of the good or service to be transacted. They will find it in their mutual self-interest to select the quantity that maximizes the surplus, which is the competitive quantity. Moreover, the agreed-upon price serves only as a mechanism for dividing the surplus and is irrelevant as a rationing device, as it does not influence the quantity transacted. This market structure, with actors on both sides acting as a single monopolist and single monopsonist, is known as *bilateral monopoly*.

In many local markets for physician services, reimbursement rates (i.e., payment for services) are dictated by large health insurers acting on behalf of their policyholders, as shown in Chapter 11. These health insurers may wield monopsony power in dealing with physicians, who are independent professionals or members of small practice groups with little bargaining power of their own. In an effort to blunt the buying power enjoyed by the health insurer, physicians have tried to join forces for the sole purpose of negotiating

---

[1] The solution is socially optimal given the presence of a lawful monopolist or lawful monopsonist. The true optimum requires competition on both sides of the market.

reimbursement rates. This, however, would appear to be a price-fixing agreement, which violates the antitrust laws. Although there is an antitrust exemption for organized labor, this exception is not available to most physicians since they are self-employed professionals who cannot unionize.[2] As a result, they have turned to the legislature for relief. In this chapter, we examine the case for collective bargaining by physicians. We also examine the requirement for state legislation that displaces the antitrust laws in favor of regulation.

In Section 12.2, we explore the bilateral monopoly solution and show how surplus is maximized with this market structure. We apply these results in Section 12.3 to physician collective bargaining. In Section 12.4, we consider some of the competitive concerns raised by the Federal Trade Commission about physician collective bargaining. We close with some concluding remarks in Section 12.5.

12.2 BILATERAL MONOPOLY

A bilateral monopoly exists when a single supplier of a well-defined product has only one customer. In this setting, the single customer is a monopsonist while the single seller is a monopolist. Together, they form a bilateral monopoly. The monopolist's effort to maximize profit by restricting output and thereby raising the price it receives conflicts with the monopsonist's effort to maximize profit by restricting purchases and thereby lowering the price it pays. As a consequence, it is difficult to identify the equilibrium price and quantity.

Bowley (1928) recognized that there is a profit motive for cooperation to emerge between the upstream monopolist and the downstream monopsonist. This profit incentive arises because joint profits are not maximized at either the monopoly solution or the monopsony solution. The two trading partners can do better, but only

---

[2] Workers who are defined as employees are permitted to unionize. Independent contractors are not employees and, therefore, may not unionize. See *Federal Trade Commission* v. *Indiana Federation of Dentists*, 476 US 447 (1986). Physicians who are employed by hospitals would qualify for unionization pursuant to the National Labor Relations Act, but physicians who are self-employed would not.

if they cooperate with one another. Such cooperation may take the extreme form of vertical integration, which is the joint ownership of the upstream and downstream entities.[3] Alternatively, this cooperation may emerge from the bargaining process. For the latter, it is important to realize that the negotiation involves the optimal quantity in the first stage. That is, agreement on the quantity is essential if joint profits are to be maximized. After maximizing the joint profits, the parties can then negotiate the shares of profit.

A Simple Model of Bilateral Monopoly

Suppose that the final good (Q) is produced according to a production function

$$Q = Q(x, y), \tag{12.1}$$

where x is the intermediate good traded under bilateral monopoly conditions and y represents the other inputs supplied competitively at a constant price of p_y. The total cost of producing the intermediate good x is given by $C(x)$.

If the intermediate good monopolist and its sole customer were vertically integrated, the profit function of the integrated firm would be

$$\Pi = P(Q)Q(x, y) - C(x) - p_y \cdot y, \tag{12.2}$$

where $P(Q)$ is the final good demand function. The firm will maximize its profits by selecting quantities of x and y such that the first partial derivatives of the profit function are equal to zero.[4] It should be noted that this is the only quantity at which the joint profits are maximized.

Now suppose that the single buyer and single seller had not vertically integrated. These firms will conduct arm's-length

---

[3] We discuss vertical integration in Chapters 19 and 20.

[4] Integrated profits are maximized where the marginal revenue products of the inputs are equal to their respective marginal costs. Thus, $\frac{\partial \Pi}{\partial x} = \left(P + Q\frac{dP}{dQ}\right)\frac{\partial Q}{\partial x} - \frac{dC}{dx} = 0$ and $\frac{\partial \Pi}{\partial y} = \left(P + Q\frac{dP}{dQ}\right)\frac{\partial Q}{\partial y} - p_y = 0$.

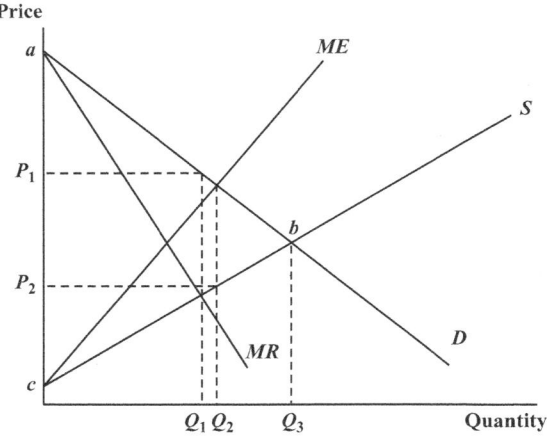

FIGURE 12.1 The bilateral monopoly solution

negotiations on the price and quantity of x. Bowley (1928) argued that under these market conditions, the negotiations will inexorably lead to the very same employment decisions as those that a vertically integrated firm would reach. The same joint profit-maximizing quantities of inputs x and y will be employed. This, of course, will lead to the same quantity of the final good being produced. Thus, a determinate quantity of the intermediate good will be transacted. Moreover, the price and quantity of the final good will also be determinate. Only the price of x remains indeterminate, but this is not allocatively significant because this price does not influence the quantity of x purchased. The price of x is just a means of dividing the jointly maximized profit.

Figure 12.1 illustrates the indeterminacy of the bilateral monopoly equilibrium. The demand and corresponding marginal revenue are shown as D and MR, respectively. The supply (or marginal cost) is displayed as S, and marginal expenditure is displayed as ME. In order to maximize its profit, the monopolist would like to produce Q_1, where marginal revenue and marginal cost are equal, and sell it for a price of P_1. The monopsonist, however, would like to maximize its profit by buying Q_2, where its demand equals the marginal expenditure, and paying a price of P_2. But neither outcome is feasible.

The monopolist wants to curtail production to raise price, whereas the monopsonist wants to curtail purchases in order to depress price. But the monopolist cannot sell the good at a price different from what the monopsonist pays for the good. If the two firms merged, the solution would involve a quantity of Q_3, which is larger than both Q_1 and Q_2. Selling or buying this quantity would maximize the total surplus, which would be equal to the triangular area abc. Therefore, it is in the firms' best interests to agree to this quantity. Since the firms are not vertically integrated, however, there must be a price. Since the price will be determined by bargaining, it will be indeterminate. But price indeterminacy, however, is of no allocative significance since the quantity has already been determined. Consequently, the price serves only as a means of sharing the profit. The higher the price, the greater will be the monopolist's share; the lower the price, the greater will be the monopsonist's share.

There are, however, limits on the indeterminacy of the input price. We can bound the price range by considering the demand (D) and the supply (S) shown in Figure 12.2.[5]

At quantity Q_3, P_{max} is the maximum price the monopolist can command. At this price, all of the consumer surplus has been extracted by the monopolist since area abP_{max} is equal to area bcd. Analogously, at Q_3, P_{min} is the minimum price because that price allows the monopsonist to extract the entire producer surplus since area $P_{min}eg$ is equal to area def. These maximum and minimum prices determine the bargaining range. The price is in that range, but there is nothing that particularly recommends that price as a solution.

Although the actual price is indeterminate, there are some likely price effects. If buyers join forces in the presence of a monopoly,

---

[5] The all-or-none demand schedule represents price–quantity combinations that leave no consumer surplus. Analogously, the all-or-none supply schedule depicts price–quantity pairs that yield no producer surplus.

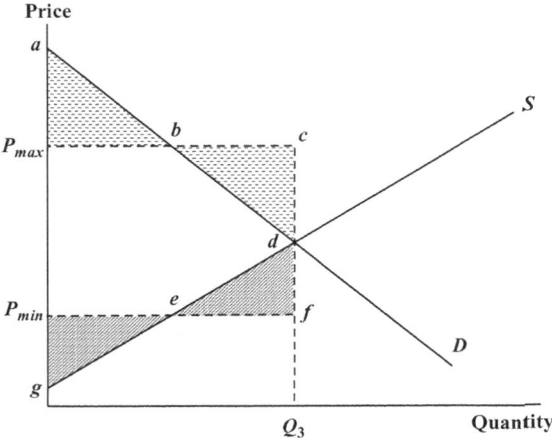

FIGURE 12.2 The bargaining range from P_{min} to P_{max}

one would expect the price to fall below P_{max} since the purpose of joining forces is to get a better deal. Analogously, if competing sellers merge in response to monopsony, the price is apt to rise above P_{min} – again, because the firms merged in pursuit of a better deal. These price movements, however, have no competitive significance since quantity does not respond to such price changes. The price movement does have distributive consequences, but these have no impact on social welfare.[6]

Caveats

To the extent that the formation of countervailing power improves social welfare, the effort to create countervailing power should go unimpeded. If, however, the monopoly is illegal, it should be challenged and then countervailing power becomes unnecessary. Similarly, competitive sellers may band together in the face of an unlawful monopsony. This collaboration might well be challenged

---

[6] There are, of course, many complicated market structures that have some elements of bilateral monopoly, but with results that may deviate from those of pure bilateral monopoly. See, for example, Crémer and Riordan (1987), Horn and Wolinsky (1988), and Chen (2003).

under Section 1 of the Sherman Act, but it would be procompetitive. The appropriate antitrust policy, however, would be to disband the unlawful monopsony so that countervailing power is unnecessary. Thus, it is vital to ascertain the presence of lawful monopoly or monopsony on one side of the market before embracing cooperation on the other side.

Additionally, there is a risk associated with the formation of countervailing power in response to a lawful monopoly. Firms that buy the same inputs very often sell their output in competition with each other. Thus, the cooperation among these firms as buyers may spill over into cooperation as sellers of their output, which is illegal. Consequently, the net social welfare of permitting their collusion as buyers could be negative.

It is important to note that the possibility that these buyers may become price-fixing sellers can quickly offset the gains made possible by allowing the monopolist and the collusive monopsonist group to determine the joint profit-maximizing level of output. Once the firms begin to act as a collusive monopoly, they will raise prices, restrict output, and consequently demand less of the input. The increase in consumer welfare, which was the justification for permitting the buyers to cooperate in the first place, could be quickly eliminated.

More subtle is the selling price stability that may result if the parties do not agree on a selling price but price individually with knowledge of the input price their competitors pay.[7] It is always possible that input cost uniformity will lead to uniformity in the pricing of outputs. And, in industries in which production techniques and input mixes are standardized, one would not expect a great variance in price. This would be true even in highly competitive markets. On the other hand, if the market is oligopolistic and these buyers cooperate, the knowledge that they all have paid the same amount for a major input can reduce competitive pressure.

---

[7] We discuss various forms of tacit collusion in Chapter 9.

12.3   PHYSICIAN COOPERATIVE BARGAINING

In some cases, countervailing power can reduce anticompetitive effects and maximize social welfare. In this section, we discuss how the notion of countervailing power can be used by physicians to offset the monopsony power of health insurance companies.

Unions

One of the clearest examples of countervailing power is a union. According to the National Labor Relations Act (NLRA) of 1935, private-sector employees may collectively bargain in the form of unions. Suppose a hospital is the only employer of nurses in a local area. It stands to reason that this hospital would exercise its monopsony power by reducing the number of nurses employed to depress their wages. Each individual nurse has little bargaining power since he or she would not have other employment opportunities. The nurse could threaten to quit working, but this is an empty threat. The hospital could merely hire another worker to replace the nurse.

But if all the nurses joined together and formed a union, their collective bargaining power would be much greater. The union could make credible threats. The union could organize strikes, where nurses refuse to work unless they get better employment conditions and benefits. The union also has the resources to sue the hospital if it treats its workers unfairly. With the balance in bargaining power, it is much more difficult for the local hospital to take advantage of its nurses.

Perceived Problem

Although many physicians are, in fact, employees, most are independent professionals who practice alone or in small groups. Independent contractors, managers, and supervisors are exceptions to the NLRA, and thus many physicians cannot legally collectively bargain. In most communities of any size, there are many physicians; therefore, the structure of the supply side appears to be competitive. The demand side of the market also appears to be competitive since there are many patients. This, however, is not the case since a substantial number of patients are covered by health insurance. The health insurers buy physician services on behalf of their policyholders. In other words, patient demand for health services is consolidated by the insurance companies. As a result, health insurers may often wield substantial monopsony power in local markets.[8]

The monopsonistic exploitation of physicians leads to reduced quantities of services as well as reduced reimbursement rates relative to the competitive outcome. From a policy perspective, two concerns emerge. First, the availability of health care services appears to be curtailed, which will have an adverse effect on public health. Specifically, physicians may devote less time to patients. Second, there is a concern that the depressed reimbursement rates will impair the quality of physician services. Quality may fall because physicians cannot afford to devote the resources necessary for the best quality of care. Moreover, the reduced reimbursement rates may put economic pressure on physicians to see even more patients, which necessarily means spending less time with each one.

The Medical Society of the State of New York highlighted insurer market dominance as a problem for the quantity and quality of care for patients.[9] This dominance has led to "ever-increasing health insurer pre-authorization and payment hassles, excessive regulation and enormous medical liability insurance costs, exacerbated by inadequate payments from health insurers and Medicaid, and huge patient cost-sharing responsibilities."[10] Due to these restrictions, many physicians find themselves with no options but to join hospital groups, where they have less freedom.[11] Additionally, these restrictions make New York a less attractive location for new doctors, which has contributed to shortages in primary care for patients.

---

[8] See Chapter 11 for more information on monopsony power wielded by insurance companies.

[9] For more examples of insurer market dominance, see Chapter 11.

[10] Medical Society of the State of New York (2019).

[11] Medical Society of the State of New York (2019).

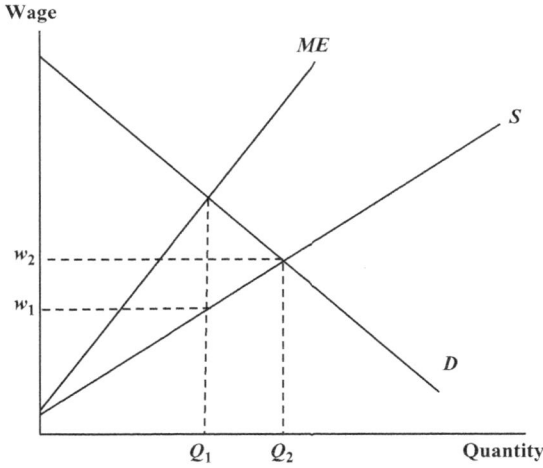

FIGURE 12.3 From monopsony to bilateral monopoly

These issues led the New York Senate to propose physician collective bargaining as a solution.[12] In most instances, two wrongs do not make a right, but collective negotiations may eliminate these ill effects.

Countervailing Power as a Solution

Cooperative bargaining by the physicians practicing in the monopsonized market may provide countervailing power. In essence, by providing a united front, the physicians alter the market structure from monopsony to bilateral monopoly. In that event, the parties have an incentive to maximize total surplus by supplying the competitive quantity of physician services and bargaining over its division. This economic solution will improve allocative efficiency, expand physician services, and reduce prices.

Figure 12.3 illustrates these results. If the physicians in the local market band together for the sole purpose of negotiating with health insurers over reimbursement rates, the market structure becomes one of bilateral monopoly. The parties should agree on the quantity that

[12] Astor (2011).

maximizes the sum of producer surplus and consumer surplus, or Q_2. Having already agreed on the quantity, the reimbursement rate will not affect the quantity. Instead, the negotiated reimbursement rate serves to share the surplus between the physicians and the insurers. One might expect the reimbursement rate to rise, say to w_2.[13] After all, the physicians sought collaboration because they were disgruntled over the reimbursement rates that the health insurers had been dictating to them. The higher rates, however, will not reduce the quantity of health care services supplied because the physicians and health insurers have already agreed upon quantity.

Opponents to this solution, which notably include the Federal Trade Commission (FTC), view physician collective bargaining as a price-fixing agreement that will raise prices for patients. Under certain assumptions, this view is correct. If insurance companies had no monopsony power, allowing physicians to cooperate would create a monopoly in a competitive market. Yet, with the assumption that insurance companies have monopsony power, it becomes clear that countervailing power will improve social welfare. In fact, prices may drop for patients. By introducing countervailing power, quantity increases would decrease prices for patients if the demand for services is negatively sloped.

Opponents are right to be wary of allowing physicians to form collective bargaining groups in any market without clear evidence of monopsony power among health insurers. In the absence of monopsony power, collective action by the physicians would result in cartel conduct: increased fees and reduced output. If collective action is warranted, however, the physicians may be immunized from antitrust prosecution by the state action doctrine. If handled improperly, this immunization could lead to anticompetitive outcomes, which we explore in Section 12.4. By using the state action doctrine properly, however, states can regulate physician groups and mitigate harm.

---

[13] There is nothing that particularly recommends w_2 as the agreed-upon reimbursement rate, but it is in the bargaining range.

The State Action Doctrine

Ordinarily, Section 1 of the Sherman Act prohibits cooperation among competing physicians in negotiating reimbursement rates with health insurers. If the state legislature is persuaded that physicians should be exempt from the Sherman Act's prohibitions, it may pass legislation that provides such an exemption under the so-called state action doctrine, which was discussed in Chapter 10. In order for the legislation to confer antitrust immunity, however, two conditions must be met. First, the state must clearly articulate its intention to displace market forces with regulation. Second, the state must actively supervise the conduct in question.[14]

Alaska, New Jersey, and Texas, which have authorized collective negotiations by health care providers with health insurers, have clearly articulated their concerns and their intention to displace competition.[15] In addition to these bills, legislatures in New York, Connecticut, Washington, and at least nine other states have developed similar collective bargaining proposals.[16] In a very real sense, the active state supervision requirement has also been met, albeit in a somewhat novel way – by altering the market structure.

Clear Articulation

The Alaska, New Jersey, and Texas legislatures appreciated the virtues of competitive market forces in the provision of health care

---

[14] *California Retail Liquor Dealers Association* v. *Midcal Aluminum, Inc.*, 445 US 97 (1980).

[15] New Jersey's bill expired in 2008, but physician collective bargaining proposals have been introduced.

[16] New York Assembly Bill A00336, An Act to Amend the Public Health Law, in Relation to Requirements for Collective Negotiations by Health Care Providers with Certain Health Benefit Plans (2016); Connecticut H.B. No. 6343, An Act Concerning Health Cooperative Health Care Arrangements (2011); and Washington H.B. 2360, An Act Relating to the Regulation of Negotiations between Health Providers and Health Carriers (2001). Additionally, in 2001, similar acts were introduced in California, Florida, Illinois, Louisiana, Missouri, Montana, Pennsylvania, Rhode Island, and Tennessee (Hellinger and Young 2001).

services. They recognized that competition among health care providers usually leads to high-quality health care services at reasonable fees. The New Jersey legislature, for example, explicitly found that

> Active, robust and fully competitive markets for health care and dental services provide the best opportunity for the residents of this State to receive high-quality health care and dental services at an appropriate cost.... [I]t is the intention of the Legislature to authorize independent physicians and dentists to jointly negotiate with carriers and to qualify such joint negotiations and related joint activities for the State-action exemption to the federal antitrust laws thoroughly articulated State policy and active supervision provided under this act.[17]

Although the Alaska and Texas statutes are not as clearly articulated, both reveal an understanding that collective negotiations represent a departure from competition.[18] Moreover, the departure was deemed necessary to preserve health care quality and patient access to health care services.

All three states recognized that health benefit plans may enjoy substantial market power in their negotiations with independent physicians. The Alaska, New Jersey, and Texas legislatures were persuaded that in some local markets, the managed care plans exerted so much downward pressure on reimbursement rates that they

---

[17] See legislative finding of New Jersey Assembly Bill 2169 (2001).

[18] "There are, however, instances in which a health plan dominates the market to the degree that fair negotiations between physicians and the health benefit plan are not possible in the absence of joint action on behalf of the physicians. In those circumstances, the health plan can virtually dictate the terms of the contract that it offers to physicians." Legislative finding (b) of Alaska Senate Bill 37, Physician Negotiations with Health Insure (2001). "Although the legislature finds that joint negotiations over fee-related terms may in some circumstances yield anticompetitive effects, it also recognizes that there are instances in which health plans dominate the market to such a degree that fair negotiations between physicians and the plan are unobtainable absent any join action on behalf of physicians." Texas Senate Bill 1468, Art. 29.01 (1999).

jeopardized the availability and quality of health care services. The New Jersey statute, for example, found that

> Inadequate reimbursement and other unfair payment terms offered by carriers adversely affect the quality of patient care and access to care by reducing the resources that physicians and dentists can devote to patient care and decreasing the time that physicians and dentists are able to spend with their patients.[19]

These ill effects are attributed to a perceived imbalance in bargaining power between independent physicians or small practice groups and large managed care plans. Using nearly identical language, each state observed that a large health benefit plan "can virtually dictate the terms of the contracts that it offers to physicians."[20] Physicians complained that non-fee terms as well as fee-related terms were abusive and curtailed the medical services that could be offered to their patients.

Persuaded by the physicians' complaints, Alaska, New Jersey, and Texas have all enacted legislation that allows physicians to bargain collectively with managed care plans over both fee and non-fee terms. But the physicians have not been given carte blanche in this regard. All three states have tried to restrict collective bargaining to those situations in which market conditions warrant collective bargaining. Although these efforts have not always been satisfactory from an economic perspective, the intent was clearly to provide an antitrust exemption in limited circumstances when necessary to achieve the state's legislative goals. In New Jersey, for example, two or more

---

[19] Legislative finding (h) of New Jersey Assembly Bill 2169 (2001). The Alaska and Texas statutes refer to procompetitive effects of collective bargaining. See Alaska Senate Bill No. 37, Sec. 23.50.010 (2001); see also Texas Senate Bill No. 1468, Art. 29.01 (1999).

[20] Alaska Senate Bill No. 37, Sec. 23.50.010 (b) (2001). Texas Senate Bill No. 1468, Art. 29.01 (1999), uses identical language. In New Jersey, the legislature found that "[c]arriers are often able to virtually dictate the terms of the contracts that they offer physicians and dentists and commonly offer these contracts on a take-it-or-leave-it basis." New Jersey Assembly Bill 2169, C.52:17B-196.e (2001).

physicians are authorized to negotiate jointly with an insurance carrier provided that "the carrier has substantial market power in its service area and that any of the terms or conditions of the contract with the carrier pose an actual or potential threat to the quality and availability of patient care among covered persons."[21] The clear purpose of these legislative efforts is to balance the bargaining power of physicians and managed care plans. Accordingly, collective bargaining is authorized only in geographic areas where an insurance carrier has some (unspecified) degree of market power in purchasing health care services. In all three states, the attorney general is responsible for identifying those geographic areas in which carriers have such market power.[22]

The central legislative purpose of these statutes is to protect patient access to high-quality health care services. The legislatures hope to accomplish this by authorizing collective negotiations rather than by directly regulating market transactions. As a safeguard, the statutes limit what may result. For example, the New Jersey and Texas statutes forbid negotiations that limit health care being provided to patients.[23] Moreover, the authorized negotiations may not result in a reduction in health care quality. These limitations are clearly sensible given the underlying purpose of the legislation.

Active State Supervision

It is not enough for a state to clearly articulate its understanding that it is displacing competitive market forces with some alternative. For antitrust immunity, a state must also actively supervise the resulting economic conduct. In this way, the state, through its regulatory body, acts as a surrogate for the market. It is imperative that the regulatory

---

[21] New Jersey Assembly Bill 2169, C.52:17B-199, 4 (a) (2001). There are similar limitations in the Alaska and Texas statutes. See Alaska Senate Bill No. 37, Sec. 23.50.010 (b) (2001); see also Texas Senate Bill No. 1468, Art. 29.01 (1999).

[22] New Jersey Assembly Bill 2169, C.52:17B-207:12A(1) (2001); Texas Senate Bill No. 1468, Art. 29.10 (1999).

[23] New Jersey Assembly Bill 2169, C.52:17B-207:12A(1) (2001); Texas Senate Bill No. 1468, Art. 29.10 (1999).

body act in the public interest rather than the private interest of those who are to be regulated. In *North Carolina Dental*,[24] for example, the Supreme Court found that the North Carolina Board of Dentistry, which regulated the profession, was dominated by dentists who had an economic conflict of interest. The Court found that since the State of North Carolina failed to actively supervise the board's conduct, its members did not enjoy antitrust immunity.

In Alaska, New Jersey, and Texas, physician collective bargaining does not need active state supervision in the usual sense. In general, supervision usually manifests itself as a regulatory agency that protects the public interest, such as a public service commission that regulates natural monopolies (e.g., electric power or local telephone providers). Physician collective bargaining is different since it is not inherently anticompetitive in the context of a bilateral monopoly market structure. State supervision, therefore, involves identifying markets where collective negotiation can be beneficial rather than directly regulating groups. The latter is unnecessary since bargaining will lead to the optimal economic solution without state intervention. What is needed is periodic review of the market structure. As long as the buying side remains monopsonistic, collective action by suppliers remains warranted.

The attorney general of each state acts as a gatekeeper by allowing collective bargaining only in markets dominated by monopsonistic health insurers. His or her specific role regarding physician collective bargaining, however, can vary from state to state. For example, the Texas bill requires the attorney general to determine that health insurers are using monopsony power to impose unfair contracts before granting approval to a group to begin negotiations.[25] Then collective bargaining is allowed over fees for services, reimbursement factors, discounted fees for services, and payment to

---

[24] See *North Carolina State Board of Dental Examiners* v. *Federal Trade Commission*, 574 US 494 (2015), which is discussed in detail in Chapter 10.
[25] Texas Senate Bill No. 1468, Art. 29.09 (b) (1999).

physicians from health benefit plans.[26] The attorney general limits countervailing power to market structures where it increases social welfare, while preventing it in cases where it could lead to social welfare losses, price increases in insurance premiums, and availability decline. If the attorney general gets it right, there is no need to micromanage the bargaining process. If he or she errs, no amount of micromanaging will correct the mistake. It is critical, therefore, that the attorneys general have full information and follow a sound analytical process in deciding whether to authorize collective negotiations.

Available Information

When a group of physicians wants to negotiate collectively with a managed care plan, they must select a cooperative bargaining representative. This representative is required to file a petition with the attorney general seeking approval. The petition must identify the physicians who will be in the group, along with their business addresses. It must also reveal (1) the percentage of all physicians in the insurance carrier's service area who are in the group, (2) the identity of the carrier, (3) the subject matter of the proposed negotiations, (4) the expected benefits of the cooperative negotiations, and (5) the anticipated effects on the quality and availability of health care services. In addition, the attorney general may request further information or data. To aid the attorney general in analyzing the market structure on the buying side, New Jersey allows that official to collect market share data for each carrier in the state.

The attorney general must act on the proposed group's petition within 30 days. New Jersey's statute instructs the attorney general to approve the petition if he or she finds that the proposed benefits outweigh the costs of any reduction in competition that cooperative negotiations may involve. As seen in Section 12.2, if the market

---

[26] Texas Senate Bill No. 1468, Art. 29.05, 29.06 (1999). Texas lists 16 other *non-fee* issues that physicians may collectively bargain over without such limitations. Texas Senate Bill No. 1468, Art. 29.04 (1999).

structure warrants cooperative negotiations, there will be only benefits and no costs.

12.4 COMPETITIVE CONCERNS

The FTC has filed many complaints against physician groups that "fix
prices" by cooperatively negotiating with insurance companies.[27] In
the matter of *Southwest Health Alliances, Inc., dba BSA Provider
Network*, a Texas physician hospital organization, the FTC alleged
that the group was acting together to fix fees for health care services.[28]
The FTC alleged that this behavior would (1) "unreasonably [restrain]
price among physicians"; (2) "[increase] price for physician services";
(3) "[deprive] payers, including insurers and employers, and individual
consumers, of the benefits of competition among physicians"; and (4)
"[deprive] consumers of the benefits of competition among payers."[29]
The FTC, however, opposes the claim that insurers have monopsony
power. In that event, their advice would be well-founded since
cooperative bargaining would lead to higher fees. If the insurance
companies are exerting monopsony power, however, the FTC's concerns are no longer so troubling. Fees for services should increase,
which will expand output. This will lower prices in the output market
(at least for insurance premiums), and consumers will be better off.
Consequently, it is crucial to determine whether health insurers hold
monopsony power.[30] The attorney general, however, should be aware
of certain caveats.

First, the attorney general must ensure that physicians' new-
found countervailing power does not become monopoly power.
Consider the extreme case where every physician in a state is part of
the same collective bargaining group. Then the market structure

---

[27] Federal Trade Commission (2019).

[28] In this case, the group negotiated unilaterally with insurance companies to increase
compensation for the physicians in its group.

[29] *In re Southwest Health Alliances, Inc., dba BSA Provider Network*, Docket No. C-
4327 (2011).

[30] See Chapter 11 for more information on this topic.

would be one of monopoly on one side and oligopsony on the other side. In other words, the bargaining power is still unequal. Since insurance companies are prohibited from colluding, the physicians can exert their monopoly power to lower quantity and increase fees for physician services, which would lead to higher prices for consumers. A careful analysis of the market structure and the expected market power of the physician group is important to prevent undue monopoly power.

The attorney general should review the genesis of any physician collective bargaining group. In this way, the attorney general can review the market structure and ensure that there will not be an imbalance. Another solution is to place restrictions on the number of physicians who can belong to a certain group, as was done in the Alaska bill. Setting restrictions on the physician specialty may also serve to increase the checks on physician collective bargaining units. But the lack of flexibility in the number of members could be troubling depending on changes in the health insurer market.

Now suppose that the market power of insurance companies declines over time due to entry. Consequently, the exertion of monopsony power may no longer be applicable to physicians. If physician groups continue to exert their countervailing power, they may very well be acting anticompetitively and harming consumers. Thus, the attorney general must periodically appraise the insurance market to ensure that there have been no major changes to the market structure.

The FTC, in its letter to the Alaska legislature warning against collective bargaining legislation, was unconvinced that the attorney general would have enough information or time to determine what constituted "substantial market power." The FTC also criticized the Texas bill on similar grounds. They did not believe the Texas attorney general had set adequate standards to determine substantial market power. To some extent, determining market structure may be challenging. However, the attorneys general can use the same tools that the FTC employs to determine the likelihood of anticompetitive issues. These tools, such as the Herfindahl-Hirschman Index, associate market concentration with the likelihood of anticompetitive behavior.[31] If these concerns become valid, legislation can be revised accordingly. Currently, both Texas and Alaska have not considered this a problem in the more than 20 years since they introduced physician collective bargaining.

Attorneys general should also be aware that allowing joint negotiation with insurance companies can create an opportunity to illegally fix the prices of other goods. Although not part of the collective bargaining agreement, physicians may fix fees of services for uninsured patients or fix input prices since bargaining in one market facilitates unlawful collusion in another. Uninsured patients are unorganized and have no monopsony power. Consequently, they are particularly vulnerable to a price-fixing conspiracy that would reduce quantity and increase prices. Physicians could also illegally fix the prices of inputs, harming suppliers. The harm to uninsured patients and input suppliers could soon be larger than the harm to physicians due to insurance monopsony power, which would cause countervailing power to be counterproductive.

One way to mitigate this concern is to use a hub-and-spoke system with a single representative. Rather than bringing all physicians in a collective bargaining group together to argue over base fees, each physician would contract individually with a representative. The representative would compile the information gained from each physician and would negotiate with payers on their behalf. Although this does not necessarily preclude price fixing, this system would minimize fee discussions between physicians and therefore mitigate anticompetitive pricing.

12.5   CONCLUDING REMARKS

In this chapter, we applied the economics of bilateral monopoly to pleas from physicians for permission to bargain collectively with health insurers over reimbursement rates. When the health insurer

---

[31] We review these tools in Chapter 18.

has monopsony power, allowing collective bargaining alters the market structure to that of bilateral monopoly. The results will be greater access to health care services and improved patient welfare. If, as the FTC has warned, the health insurer does not have monopsony power, physician collective bargaining will result in higher costs, reduced access, and a reduction in patient welfare. Thus, it is apparent that a careful analysis of market structure is crucial for sound public policy.

Empirical research must still be done to evaluate the long-term effects of physician collective bargaining on the quality, quantity, and price of care. State legislative proposals in New York, Washington, and Connecticut that would allow physician collective bargaining, however, indicate that the practice may become more prevalent in the future.

REFERENCES

Astor, Will. (2011). Senate OKs Letting Doctors Bargain Collectively. *Rochester Business Journal*. https://rbj.net/2011/07/01/senate-oks-letting-doctors-bargain-collectively/.

Bowley, A. L. (1928). Bilateral Monopoly. *Economic Journal* 38: 651–658.

Chen, Zhiqi. (2003). Dominant Retailers and the Countervailing-Power Hypothesis. *RAND Journal of Economics* 34: 612–625.

Crémer, Jacques, and Michael H. Riordan. (1987). On Governing Multilateral Transactions with Bilateral Contracts. *RAND Journal of Economics* 18: 436–451.

Federal Trade Commission. (2019). Overview of FTC Actions in Health Care Services and Products. www.ftc.gov/system/files/attachments/competition-policy-guidance/overview_health_care_june_2019.pdf.

Hellinger, Fred J., and Gary J. Young. (2001). An Analysis of Physician Antitrust Exemption Legislation: Adjusting the Balance of Power. *Journal of the American Medical Association* 286: 83–88.

Horn, Henrick, and Asher Wolinsky. (1988). Bilateral Monopolies and Incentives for Merger. *RAND Journal of Economics* 19: 408–419.

Medical Society of the State of New York. (2019). 2019 Legislative Procedure. www.mssnyenews.org/wp-content/uploads/2018/10/LegProgramC91a-2.pdf.

13 Group Purchasing Organizations, Monopsony, and Antitrust Policy

13.1 INTRODUCTION

Hospitals use group purchasing organizations (GPOs) to purchase medical supplies, devices, and other inputs rather than purchasing directly from a manufacturer.[1,2] GPOs consolidate the purchasing power of their members and negotiate contracts with input suppliers on their behalf. In the pursuit of lower input prices and reduced transaction costs, most hospitals have joined GPOs.[3]

The consolidation of purchasing power by GPOs has raised several public policy concerns. In 2004, the Department of Justice (DOJ) and the Federal Trade Commission (FTC) identified three major public policy concerns related to GPOs.[4] First, to be successful in reducing input prices, a GPO must represent a sufficient volume of purchases and therefore will have some measure of buying power. Since the exercise of monopsony power reduces social welfare, this may be a real competitive concern. Recall that monopsony power, as discussed in Chapter 11, is the power to depress price below the competitive level by restricting purchases. Second, GPOs employ a variety of contractual provisions that may limit the sources of supply to their members, which raises antitrust concerns about the exclusion of equally efficient competitors. The third concern involves the

---

[1] This chapter draws heavily on Blair and Durrance (2014).

[2] A hospital can freely choose to use a GPO or to contract directly with the manufacturer. Hospitals reportedly purchase approximately 25 percent of their health care supplies without using the services of a GPO (Healthcare Supply Chain Association 2016).

[3] GPOs are not confined to the health care sector. State and local government agencies, fast-food franchisees, and retail grocers have found GPOs beneficial (Department of Justice and Federal Trade Commission 2004).

[4] Department of Justice and Federal Trade Commission (2004, 34–46).

GPO's funding mechanism. In its role as an intermediary between manufacturers and hospitals, the GPO creates value by reducing transaction costs and (possibly) input prices. The GPO can extract some (or even all) of this value through membership fees from the hospitals or by charging the suppliers for contracting services. Concerns have surfaced that the GPO may not actually decrease hospital costs due to these funding mechanisms. Moreover, there is some risk that the GPO's pursuit of its own self-interest may lead to incentive compatibility problems, where GPOs may not secure the best price for their hospitals when it is profitable to do so.

This chapter provides an economic analysis of the competitive consequences of GPOs. It also addresses the economic effects of the funding mechanism. In Section 13.2, we provide an overview of what we know about GPOs. We examine the competitive impact of GPOs in Section 13.3. As we will see, the standard monopsony model is not particularly useful, and, therefore, we propose the all-or-nothing monopsony model. The economic results depend upon the market structure on the supply side. In Section 13.4, we address how the GPO's contracting practices appear to result in the exclusion of some suppliers, and in Section 13.5, we examine the GPO funding mechanism and its impact on hospital costs. Section 13.6 contains an analysis of the enforcement policy of the antitrust agencies and suggests some improvements. We present our concluding remarks in Section 13.7.

13.2 WHAT DO WE KNOW ABOUT GPOS?

GPOs are pervasive in health care. There are more than 600 GPOs in the United States that account for some 90 percent of all hospital purchases.[5] In 2014, 98 percent of hospitals used a GPO for some purchases.[6] Although the vast majority of these GPOs are relatively small, the four largest GPOs – Vizient, Premier, HealthTrust,

---

[5] Health Industry Group Purchasing Association (HIGPA; 2011a, 2011b) and Burns (2002). There were some GPO mergers in the 1990s (Government Accountability Office 2002).
[6] Bruhn, Fracica, and Makary (2018).

and Intalere – accounted for more than \$189 billion in annual spending volume.[7]

GPOs can be procompetitive by providing lower input prices for hospitals through buyer aggregation and reduced transaction costs.[8] Specifically, GPOs can provide cost savings for providers and health care consumers, operate in competitive markets, and utilize a vendor funding model that is more efficient than other funding options.[9] GPOs are estimated to generate cost savings of between 10 and 18 percent of hospital supply expenses and save the US health care industry approximately \$36 billion per year.[10] The majority of US hospitals that participate in GPOs report satisfaction and cost savings.[11] GPOs, however, have raised some antitrust concerns due to their anticompetitive potential, including their funding mechanism and its implications for hospital costs.[12] Specifically, GPO contracts may not always secure the best price for their members.[13] GPOs should be aware of the antitrust risks associated with any type of collaboration among their members.[14]

13.3   GPOS AND THE EXERCISE OF MONOPSONY POWER

Although it is undeniable that a GPO consolidates the demands of its members,[15] the economic consequences of that consolidation depend on the market structure before and after the GPO's formation.

---

[7] Gooch (2017).   [8] Lindsay (2009).   [9] O'Brien, Leibowitz, and Anello (2017).

[10] Goldenberg and King (2009); Schneller (2009).

[11] Burns and Lee (2008); Burns and Yovovich (2014).

[12] Elhauge (2002, 2003) and Hovenkamp (2002, 2004) have each analyzed the competitive effects of GPO contracting practices and the likelihood of exclusion. Elhauge criticized GPOs for adopting exclusionary agreements that essentially foreclose some rival manufacturers, observing that foreclosure can result from sole-source contracting, minimum purchase requirements, volume-based discounting, and loyalty rebates. In contrast, Hovenkamp is largely supportive of GPOs and their ability to reduce prices and increase output, noting that sole-source contracting and other contracting practices are only anticompetitive under narrow conditions.

[13] Government Accountability Office (2002, 2003, 2010); Litan and Singer (2010).

[14] Lindsay (2009).

[15] There are some hospitals that have joined more than one GPO. In those cases, the consolidation by any one GPO is necessarily incomplete.

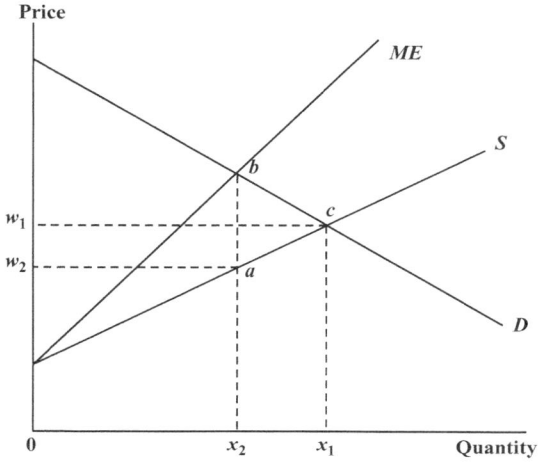

FIGURE 13.1 The monopsony model

We consider two alternative scenarios to illustrate the range of outcomes. First, we analyze a competitive market in which the formation
of a GPO does not alter the market structure or, in other words, where
the market remains competitive. Second, we explore the case of a
GPO that converts a competitive market into one with monopsony
power. Here, we reject the standard monopsony model in favor of its
all-or-nothing alternative.[16]

GPOs with No Monopsony Power

We begin with a competitively structured market, one in which there
is neither monopoly power nor monopsony power. This market is
depicted in Figure 13.1, where D is demand, S is supply, and the
competitive price and output are w_1 and x_1, respectively. If a GPO is
formed but it has no buying power, the economic results will be either
competitively neutral or procompetitive. Unless the formation of the
GPO is simply a failed attempt to achieve monopsony, the only

---

[16] The all-or-nothing model was applied to the health insurance market by Herndon
(2002).

sensible explanation for the existence of a GPO is the realization of some efficiency. Transaction costs, for example, may be reduced by the GPO. These cost savings will lead to an increase in total purchases, which improves both consumer welfare and producer welfare.[17] This case poses no antitrust concerns and would be ignored by the antitrust Agencies.

GPO Monopsony with Competitive Supply

Suppose that the GPO consolidates the demands of its members and thereby acquires monopsony power while the supply remains competitive. In the usual exercise of monopsony power, the monopsonist maximizes its profit by restricting purchases to the point where the marginal expenditure (ME) equals the marginal revenue product, which is the derived demand for x labeled D. In Figure 13.1, this exercise of power would require a reduction in quantity from x_1 to x_2. The price paid will fall below the competitive level (w_1) to w_2. The resulting loss in social welfare is captured by the triangular area abc. In this case, the average cost for the members falls, which leads to increased profits. With reduced purchases, output of the members falls as well. If they have any appreciable market share, this will result in higher output prices. These are clearly legitimate competitive concerns that should attract the attention of the antitrust Agencies.

In practice, especially in the hospital sector, the traditional monopsony model is of limited usefulness in analyzing GPO behavior. Ordinarily, the GPO cannot exercise its monopsony power in the usual way because its members do not want fewer purchases. Instead, they want to buy the same amounts at lower prices. A GPO can hardly expect its hospital members to reduce their use of everyday items such as latex gloves, bandages, syringes, and plastic cups. Nor can the GPO expect a hospital to forgo the purchase of much-needed medical devices such as pacemakers so other members can enjoy

---

[17] This case, which is analyzed by Blair and Harrison (1991) in some detail, poses no competitive concerns and should be applauded.

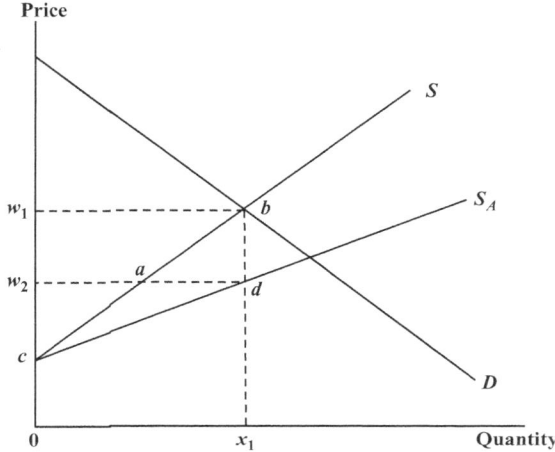

FIGURE 13.2 The all-or-nothing model

lower prices. The hospital's service quality would be compromised if it curtailed the use of the inputs necessary to produce acute care hospital services. This could lead to unfortunate patient outcomes and consequently invite medical malpractice claims. Far from encouraging its members to curtail purchases, a GPO will want to enhance its importance as a customer. GPO members, therefore, may be encouraged to keep their purchases up. Thus, the GPO must find another way to exploit its monopsony power. One avenue is to offer all-or-nothing contracts to input suppliers.

Instead of reducing its total purchases below x_1 and sliding along the supply curve to a lower price, the GPO could offer to buy x_1 at a price below w_1 or buy nothing at all. This all-or-nothing offer converts producer surplus into buyer surplus by pushing the supplier off the usual supply curve and onto the all-or-nothing supply curve, which is represented by S_A in Figure 13.2. Points on S_A are price and quantity combinations that yield no producer surplus. In the profit-maximizing all-or-nothing offer, the offer would be to purchase the competitive quantity x_1 at a price of w_2 or not buy anything at all. At this point, all of the producer surplus will have been extracted by the

GPO. If the seller refuses, it sells nothing and the GPO turns to another seller for its purchases of x_1. This strategy, therefore, can only work if there is another seller to whom the GPO may turn. In other words, the threat to go elsewhere must be credible.

With the all-or-nothing strategy, the quantity is equal to the competitive output. As a result, this outcome does not involve any allocative inefficiency, which is the usual economic objection to departures from competition. The outcome does, however, involve a significant distributional impact. Before the formation of the GPO, there was producer surplus of w_1bc, but after the emergence of the GPO, all of the producer surplus was converted to buyer surplus. It is not completely clear that this redistribution of surplus is an antitrust problem. Policy arguments can be made on both sides. One can certainly argue that the purpose of antitrust policy should be to promote social welfare. In that case, the distributional consequences are irrelevant. But one could also argue that the antitrust laws should preserve competition. In that event, monopsony is objectionable even when it results in no allocative inefficiency.

A Caveat

The use of all-or-nothing offers does not cause allocative inefficiency in the short-run static model that we analyzed, but it may have serious, adverse effects in the long run. Consider a firm's investment decision. When a firm must incur research and development (R&D) costs prior to realizing any operating profit, the decision to go forward depends on the expected net present value (NPV) of the project. The NPV can be written as

$$NPV = -\sum_{t=1}^{\tau} \frac{(R\&D)_t}{(1+i)^t} + \sum_{t=\tau+1}^{T} \frac{\Pi_t}{(1+i)^t},$$

where the research and development expenditures in year t are denoted as $(R\&D)_t$, Π_t are the expected operating profits in year t, i is the discount rate, τ is the time period after which the R&D costs have all been incurred, and T is the final year of the project.

Obviously, the *NPV* must be positive or the project will not be undertaken.

Once the R&D costs have been incurred, they are considered sunk costs. If a GPO extracts all of the producer surplus, the operating profits, Π_t, will be zero and the firm's investment would become a total loss. The possibility of this happening will reduce the expected *NPV* and will lead to reduced investments in some forms of R&D. Consequently, social welfare may be reduced in the future even though there is no allocative inefficiency in the present.

13.4 FORECLOSURE OF SUPPLIERS

GPOs negotiate contracts with input suppliers on behalf of their members. Some of these contracts contain provisions that raise the specter of anticompetitive foreclosure.[18] Perhaps the most obvious candidate for criticism is the sole-source contract. In such contracts, one manufacturer has the exclusive right to sell its product pursuant to the GPO contract.[19,20] Some GPO contracts offer minimum volume purchase requirements to a specific supplier. A close cousin is the requirements contract, which obligates members to buy at least a specified percentage of their requirements from that supplier. Bundled discounts provide another example of a contractual provision

---

[18] Some of these provisions amount to exclusive dealing, which may be anticompetitive (Frech 2008). In the present case, however, the GPO is offering to deal exclusively in exchange for lower prices. This would seem to be procompetitive.

[19] Legal challenges to sole-source contracts have not fared well. In *Allied Orthopedic* v. *Tyco Health Care*, 592 F.3d 991 (9th Cir. 2010), for example, a group of hospitals challenged Tyco's sole-source status with several GPOs that excluded generic substitutes. The trial court found that Tyco received sole-source status because it offered a superior product at reduced prices.

[20] In *Retractable Technologies, Inc.* v. *Becton Dickinson and Company*, No. 01-cv-036 (E.D. Tex. 2013), the plaintiff alleged that it was foreclosed from the market due to unlawful monopolization. Retractable Technologies created a retractable syringe aimed at reducing needle sticks but allegedly experienced difficulty marketing its new product as a result of GPO agreements that favored other manufacturers. After suing the two largest syringe manufacturers and the two largest GPOs for monopolization of the syringe market, Retractable Technologies settled its suit.

that tends to exclude rivals.[21] When discounts are bundled, purchase volumes on product X influence the discount on product X and on products Y and Z as well. Tiered or loyalty discounts provide increased discounts as the hospital buys increased percentages of its requirements for a specific product. There have been a number of antitrust cases involving these discounts. We discuss two examples.

First, C.R. Bard, Inc., sold its branded catheters to hospitals pursuant to a GPO contract negotiated with Novation. The contract in question contained provisions for making Bard the sole source of these catheters. The contract also provided tiered (or loyalty) discounts and bundled discounts that deterred substitution. St. Francis Medical Center sued Bard, alleging that it had abused its dominance in the catheter market. The trial court granted summary judgment in favor of Bard because the hospitals were not bound to purchase under the contract. Since they could purchase off-contract, they must have purchased from Bard because Bard offered the best terms. Thus, there could be no injury to the hospitals.[22]

Second, *Kinetic Concepts, Inc.* v. *Hillenbrand Industries, Inc.*, was also a bundling case that required a GPO to buy a certain percentage of supplies. In this case, Kinetic and Hillenbrand each manufactured and sold standard as well as specialty hospital beds. Kinetic argued that Hillenbrand offered additional discounts on standard hospital beds if a customer was willing to purchase at least 90 percent of its specialty beds from Hillenbrand. Kinetic was allegedly unable to match the discounted price and sued for illegal tying. Ultimately, Kinetic prevailed with a $521 million verdict.[23]

---

[21] Bundled discounting was found to be a monopolizing business practice in *LePage's Inc.* v. *3M*, 324 F.3d 141 (3rd Cir. 2003). The competitive consequences of bundled discounts were refined in *Cascade Health Solutions* v. *PeaceHealth*, 515 F.3d 973 (9th Cir. 2008). For more on this topic, see the discussion on bundled discounts in Chapter 5.

[22] For additional details, see *Southeast Missouri Hospital* v. *C.R. Bard, Inc.*, 616 F.3d 888 (8th Cir. 2010), and *Southeast Missouri Hospital* v. *C.R. Bard, Inc.*, 642 F.3d 608 (8th Cir. 2011).

[23] *Kinetic Concepts, Inc.* v. *Hillenbrand Industries, Inc.*, 95-cv-0755 (W.D. Tex. 2000).

The competitive impact of GPO contractual provisions has been the subject of some debate.[24] Critics argue that these contracts have the potential for anticompetitive foreclosure. In each instance, there is a tendency for one supplier to thrive while its rivals are excluded entirely or marginalized, as evidenced by the following examples.

In *In re Benco Dental Supply Company et al*,[25] the FTC filed a complaint against the three largest dental supply companies – Benco, Henry Schein, and Patterson – alleging the three had conspired to refuse to offer discounts to buying groups comprised of small dental practitioners. GPOs in this setting would consolidate buying power for small dental practitioners and negotiate lower prices for these dental providers. There was no evidence to prove Schein's involvement, but Benco and Patterson were found to have violated Section 5 of the FTC Act, which prohibits unfair and deceptive business practices. In this case, large dental suppliers excluded joint purchasing groups of small members.

In 2007, the DOJ challenged a GPO that allegedly required its member hospitals to contract with approved nursing staff agencies who agreed to lower wages set by the GPO. The case settled in the same year, with an agreement that the GPO and hospital would not agree on contract terms with nursing staff agencies.[26]

Finally, *Marion HealthCare, LLC* v. *Becton Dickinson and Company* involved allegations of a conspiracy between a manufacturer and GPO. Marion is a group of health care providers who purchase medical products from many manufacturers, including Becton, through GPOs that negotiate the contracts. Marion alleged that Becton, in collusion with the GPO, conspired to set prices for its

---

[24] In response to some of these concerns, the Health Industry Group Purchasing Association, a trade association representing 16 GPOs, has created a code of conduct regulating GPO behavior (HIGPA 2002). See also Elhauge (2002, 2003) and Hovenkamp (2002, 2004).

[25] *In re Benco Dental Supply Company et al.*, Docket No. 9379 (FTC 2018).

[26] *United States and State of Arizona* v. *Arizona Hospital and Healthcare Association*, No. CV07–1030-PHX (D. Ariz. 2007).

medical products at anticompetitive levels. Becton was alleged to have incentivized the GPO by paying high administrative fees in exchange for exclusionary contracting with Marion, including long-term exclusive contracts and disloyalty or low-volume penalties.[27]

The competitive concerns, however, are largely an optical illusion when the suspect provisions are viewed in the correct light. The issue is not whether a supplier is at a postcontractual disadvantage in competing for sales to the GPO member. Instead, the issue is whether rival suppliers can compete for the GPO contract. The locus of competition shifts from the members to the GPO.

Consider the sole-source contract provision. A GPO negotiates contract terms with several input suppliers on behalf of its members. Once the deals are made, the GPO then offers its members a list of the products that they can purchase pursuant to the contract. For some inputs, a specific manufacturer is the sole source of that input. For a hospital to buy from another source, it must buy off-contract, which the GPO may discourage.[28] Rival suppliers that are not included in the GPO's list may object that they have been foreclosed from access to the GPO's members. This allegation may, of course, be true *ex post*, but it does not mean that those suppliers could not have competed for the contract. The locus of competition is simply different. The GPO selects the supplier that offers the best deal, so rival suppliers can compete to be the sole source. If all suppliers are equally efficient producers, then the "winner" will be the firm willing to accept the lowest return on this book of business. There is no public policy reason to object to this outcome. The identity of the winner among equally efficient rivals has no policy relevance. If the suppliers are not equally efficient, it is the most efficient supplier who can offer the

---

[27] *Marion HealthCare, LLC* v. *Becton Dickinson and Company*, No. 18-3735 (7th Cir. 2020).

[28] A GPO can negotiate lower prices when it can promise increased volumes. In an effort to assure suppliers of the promised increase, some GPOs may insist that their members not join other GPOs. Other GPOs may include provisions that deter switching.

lowest price to the GPO. In this case, the "right" firm is the sole source because it expends fewer resources in providing GPOs with that input. Sole-source contracts, therefore, are the product of competition among rival input suppliers at the contracting level. Consequently, they are procompetitive rather than anticompetitive.

There are two further points to consider. First, a sole-source contract will make sense only if the winning firm can supply all of the GPO's needs at a lower price than the GPO could obtain by relying on multiple supply sources. Second, our argument assumes that there is only one GPO, when in fact there are some 600 GPOs. Consequently, a rival that is foreclosed from the market must be excluded everywhere. Moreover, it is possible for suppliers to make sales to hospitals that are willing to buy off-contract.

The other contractual provisions are more obviously procompetitive. All of those provisions involve suppliers offering lower input prices for increased volume that GPOs promise. At least in principle, all input suppliers can compete on this basis. When a GPO wants to contract only with suppliers that can fill all orders by its members,[29] small suppliers may not be able to compete for the contract. But there are at least two reasons why this is not the death knell for those small suppliers. First, there are hundreds of GPOs, and many of them are small. Second, most GPOs do not require their members to buy 100 percent of their requirements on the GPO contract. Small manufacturers can approach hospitals directly to compete for some of their business.

Volume-based discounts are usually procompetitive because (1) they permit a manufacturer to exploit economies of scale and thereby reduce its average cost, and (2) in a world of uncertainty, the discount structure can provide some predictability. To the extent that some firms may be excluded by the volume discounts, there is probably

---

[29] This restriction must be driven by cost considerations. The GPO will contract with one large supplier rather than several small suppliers only when it is more profitable to do so. The combination of input price and transaction costs must be lower with a single supplier.

excess capacity. Some firms may fall by the wayside as a result, but it is socially desirable to eliminate excess capacity. Presumably, the least efficient firms will be the ones that fail.

In short, any *ex post* foreclosure is the product of the *ex ante* competitive process. The result is lower prices and more efficient production. Thus, the fear of anticompetitive foreclosure seems to be misplaced.

13.5   GPO FUNDING MECHANISMS

In the preceding section, we ignored the fact that the GPO and its members are separate business entities each with its own profit function. Some GPOs, however, are owned by their member hospitals and providers.[30] GPOs do not purchase medical products directly, but rather negotiate contracts for purchase on behalf of their member hospitals. GPO members then choose which products to buy and in what volumes at the GPO-negotiated contract terms. To the extent that the GPO is successful in exploiting the combined purchasing power of its members, it converts some producer surplus into buyer surplus. In doing so, the GPO incurs costs that must be covered through its funding mechanism. In this section, we examine two funding mechanisms: (1) membership fees paid by the hospitals and (2) administrative fees paid by the suppliers.

Membership Fees

The GPO can be compensated through membership fees that the hospitals pay for the privilege of buying inputs pursuant to the GPO-negotiated contract.[31] Consider the all-or-nothing contract described in Figure 13.2. By exercising monopsony power in this fashion, the GPO increases buyer surplus by the rectangular area $w_1 b d w_2$. For the hospitals to maintain their interest in being a GPO member, they

---

[30] O'Brien, Leibowitz, and Anello (2017).

[31] This funding mechanism is far less prevalent than the second one that we will consider. As will become apparent, the main difference between the two is distributional rather than allocative.

must share that surplus. Precisely how that surplus is shared is indeterminate since it depends on the GPO market structure. At one extreme, suppose that GPOs compete among themselves for members by offering larger shares of the surplus. Assuming that the GPOs are equally efficient, the net surplus available for sharing will be area w_1bdw_2 minus the costs of operating the GPO. In the long run, competition will lead to the hospitals getting all of this net surplus, with the GPO earning only a competitive return on its investment. In this case, the membership fees will equal the average cost of the GPO operation.

At the other extreme, suppose there is a single GPO, that is, a monopoly middleman of sorts. In that event, there will be no competition for members and the GPO will be able to retain the entire net surplus. Between the two extremes, there may be varying amounts of competition for members. In this case, there will be some division of the surplus between the GPO and its hospital members.

Administrative Fees

The second, and far more prevalent, funding mechanism involves administrative fees that the manufacturers pay the GPO. In this case, the GPO negotiates contracts with the manufacturers on behalf of its members. The hospitals then buy whatever they require from the manufacturers based on the GPO-negotiated contract. The administrative fee is paid by the manufacturer to the GPO for its contracting services.[32] The negotiated contract stipulates the administrative fee, which is a percentage of the sales revenue. In 2010, average administrative fees were reported to be approximately 1.22 to 2.25 percent of purchase costs.[33]

---

[32] As long as certain provisions have been met, these fees will not be deemed kickbacks, which would violate the federal anti-kickback statute. Medicare and Medicaid Patient Protection Act of 1987 (42 USC 1320a-7b).

[33] Government Accountability Office (GAO; 2010).

The economic results of this funding mechanism are not as dissimilar from membership fees paid by the hospitals as they appear. Consider the all-or-nothing case examined in Figure 13.2. The input supplier enjoys the producer surplus of w_1bc when it sells x_1 at a price of w_1. If the firm has no access to the GPO's members, the GPO can charge an access fee of w_1bc. The members pay w_1 and buy x_1. The difference between this outcome and the one in which hospitals pay membership fees is cosmetic. The GPO gets all of the surplus in either case. For the hospitals, total expenditures are equal to w_1x_1 when the suppliers pay administrative fees. When they pay membership fees, their total expenditures will be w_2x_1 to the supplier and w_1bdw_2 to the GPO, for a total of w_1x_1. Thus, in principle, there is no difference between the two funding mechanisms.

GPOs can provide valuable service, but payments by suppliers may appear to be kickbacks. As a result, policymakers have responded with legislation. For example, the Social Security Act of 1935 makes it illegal to receive compensation for the referral of products or services that are reimbursed under federal health care programs. In 1987, Congress enacted the Medicare and Medicaid Patient Protection Act,[34] which provided an exemption for GPOs allowing them to collect administrative fees from medical product manufacturers while negotiating contracts for hospitals. In 1991, the Department of Health and Human Services adopted "safe harbor" provisions with respect to the anti-kickback policies that require additional transparency in the payment of fees from the manufacturer to the GPO.[35] First, the GPO and hospital must have a written agreement that explicitly states the rate at which the manufacturer will compensate the GPO based on the volume of products sold. The threshold should not exceed 3 percent, but it has been reported to be higher in special cases.[36] Second, the GPO is required to annually disclose to the hospital the dollar amount received from each manufacturer as a result of hospital

---

[34] Medicare and Medicaid Patient Protection Act of 1987 (42 USC 1320a-7b).
[35] 56 Fed. Reg. 35952.   [36] GAO (2003).

purchases from the GPO contract. In 2002 and 2003, Congress initiated Senate hearings to investigate concerns regarding GPOs and possible conflicts of interest. In response to this line of inquiry, in 2003 GPOs adopted a code of conduct that applies at the industry level.[37] The code of conduct has resulted in limits to the establishment of sole-source contracts. The Department of Health and Human Services (HHS) as well as the DOJ and FTC have oversight over the anti-kickback rule, but there is no routine monitoring of GPO agreements.[38]

13.6   ANTITRUST ENFORCEMENT POLICY

In 1996, the DOJ and FTC jointly issued their *Statements of Antitrust Enforcement Policy in Health Care*. GPOs appear to be covered by Statement 7, "Enforcement Policy on Joint Purchasing Arrangements among Health Care Providers." GPOs and joint purchasing agreements among health care providers are not precisely the same thing.[39] By definition, the latter involves a horizontal agreement among competitors. In contrast, a GPO simply bargains on behalf of its members. Nonetheless, the structural approach of Statement 7 seems to be relevant for GPOs. Statement 7 outlines market share thresholds related to two competitive concerns: (1) the exercise of monopsony power by the GPO in the input markets and (2) the possibility of tacit or overt collusion among GPO members in their output markets.[40] These concerns would appear to be more serious for joint purchasing agreements that involve organization and operation by the hospitals themselves than for a GPO representing the consolidated demands of its member hospitals. Joint purchasing agreements necessarily involve more direct interaction among competing hospitals and, therefore, create more opportunities for competitive mischief than would a GPO.

[37] HIGPA (2020); O'Brien, Leibowitz, and Anello (2017).   [38] GAO (2010).
[39] Carstensen (2010).
[40] American Bar Association Section of Antitrust Law (2017).

Monopsony Power

There is a presumption that a GPO that accounts for less than 35 percent of the total sales of a product in the relevant market is unlikely to have monopsony power, but that shares above 35 percent could be problematic. Consequently, the DOJ and FTC are not apt to challenge GPOs with market shares below 35 percent. The structural approach of Statement 7 can be evaluated by considering the relationship between monopsony power and market share.

Monopsony power is the power to depress price below the competitive level by restricting purchases.[41] One measure of monopsony power is the Lerner index, which measures deviation from the competitive outcome. The dominant buyer variant of the Lerner index (λ) is

$$\lambda = \frac{S}{\varepsilon + \eta_f(1 - S)},$$

where S is the share of total purchases accounted for by the dominant buyer, ε is the elasticity of supply, and η_f is the elasticity of the competitive fringe demand.[42] While it is true that $\partial\lambda/\partial S$ is positive, which implies that higher shares increase monopsony power, the index shows that relying on market share alone is misguided.[43] For any given value of S, $\partial\lambda/\partial\varepsilon$ is negative, so the more elastic the supply, the lower is the Lerner index. Thus, supply conditions cannot be ignored in assessing the competitive significance of a GPO. Similarly, $\partial\lambda/\partial\eta_f$ is also negative; therefore, the more elastic the competitive fringe demand, the lower is the dominant buyer's ability to

----

[41] This conception of monopsony power may be inappropriate as applied to GPOs. Far from encouraging its members to curtail purchases, a GPO may encourage them to maintain their purchases, as that will enhance the GPO's importance to the suppliers.

[42] Blair and Harrison (1991).

[43] In assessing the monopsony power a particular GPO possesses, it is also important to define the market properly. Shares do not mean much if the product market or the geographic market is not defined correctly, as indicated in Landes and Posner (1981) and Blair and Harrison (1991).

depress price. Thus, the purchasing reactions of the other buyers also must be considered in inferring the competitive effects of GPOs. To see this, consider the following numerical example. In one case, suppose $S = 0.25$, $\varepsilon = 0.50$, and $\eta_f = 1.0$. In this case, the GPO would enjoy the safe harbor afforded by Statement 7's 35 percent threshold. The value of λ is 0.20, which means that there is a 20 percent deviation from the competitive price. Now suppose that $S = 0.50$, $\varepsilon = 2.0$, and $\eta_f = 1.0$. In this case, the GPO falls outside the safe harbor and would be suspect. But the value of λ is 0.20 again even though the market share is twice as much as in the first case.

Potential Collusion

The second threshold for monopsony power involves the similarity of hospital costs that may emerge from the similarity of input prices. A GPO is unlikely to be challenged if the expenditures on inputs purchased pursuant to the GPO contract amount to no more than 20 percent of the total revenues from the hospital's sales of hospital services. The competitive concern is that if the member hospitals are all paying the same input prices, costs will become standardized across all hospitals. With similar cost structures, collusion on price in the output market becomes easier. While it is certainly true that reaching an agreement on output prices is easier when costs are identical, this concern is peculiar. After all, if all firms employ the same production functions and they pay the same input prices, then their cost functions will be identical. The logic of this threshold would seem to imply that cost dissimilarity is procompetitive. It is not clear that this follows, however, since the hospitals with higher costs will be at a competitive disadvantage.

Countervailing Power

Implicit in Statement 7 is the assumption that input markets are competitive on the supply side, but this need not be the case. There may be some medical devices for which there are no reasonably close substitutes, and, therefore, some monopoly power exists. This market

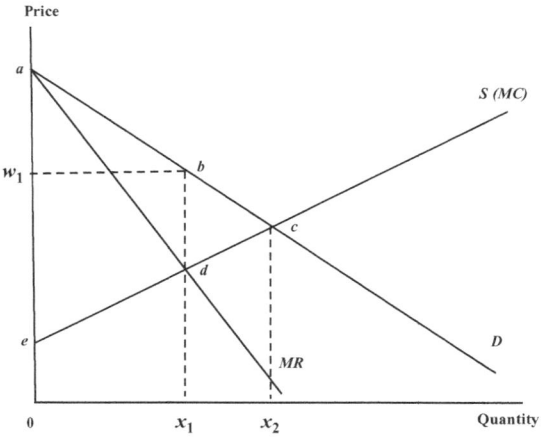

FIGURE 13.3 The bilateral monopoly model

structure is not contemplated in Statement 7 but deserves analysis. To avoid unnecessary complications, we assume that the manufacturer has a lawful monopoly due perhaps to a valid patent.[44] If the hospitals are not part of a buying group, then the manufacturer can exercise its monopoly power in the usual way, which is illustrated in Figure 13.3. The monopoly price and quantity are w_1 and x_1, respectively. The formation of a GPO that includes all hospitals would far exceed the 35 percent threshold. Such a GPO, however, creates a bilateral monopoly market structure. Under conditions of bilateral monopoly, the GPO and the manufacturer should reach an agreement on the quantity that maximizes the total surplus, which is, of course, the competitive output equal to x_2 in Figure 13.3.[45] The expanded purchase of the input leads to an increase in output with a corresponding decrease in the output price, which obviously improves consumer welfare. The price, which no longer acts as a rationing device, is indeterminate.[46]

---

[44] If the monopoly were not lawful, the appropriate antitrust policy prescription would be to prohibit the unlawful monopoly behavior.

[45] See Chapter 12 for a discussion of countervailing power.

[46] The price can neither exceed the height of the all-or-nothing demand at x_2 (because that price extracts all of the consumer surplus) nor fall below the height of the all-or-

The monopoly solution generates consumer surplus of abw_1 and producer surplus of w_1bde. The bilateral monopoly increases the total surplus by bcd to a total of ace. Precisely how the surplus will be split is indeterminate, but that is of no competitive significance. The price will act as a means of sharing the maximized surplus and will be determined through bilateral bargaining. Since the input quantity is not determined by the price, the output will not be influenced by the price. Consequently, the output price will be unaffected by the input price.

In the static model presented in Figure 13.3, it is clear that the formation of a GPO will improve social welfare. Consequently, it poses no competitive concerns and should be applauded rather than condemned by the antitrust Agencies. But the world is not static, and the monopolist may soon face competition in the medical device market. In that event, the GPO could reduce social welfare if it exercises its monopsony power in the usual way.[47] Accordingly, some forecast of future competition is necessary to advance a sound antitrust policy proposal.[48]

13.7 CONCLUDING REMARKS

As we have seen, GPOs raise some competitive issues that may arouse antitrust scrutiny. In some cases, GPOs are procompetitive; in others, they may be anticompetitive. Care must be exercised to determine the actual competitive consequences of GPOs according to the particular circumstances. The structural approach embraced by the antitrust agencies is prone to error for at least two reasons. First, the emphasis on market share can lead to incorrect inferences

nothing supply at x_2 (because that price extracts all of the producer surplus). The precise value of the price is subject to bargaining and, therefore, cannot be determined on an a priori basis (Blair, Kaserman, and Romano 1989).

[47] It is unlikely that a GPO could exercise monopsony power in the usual way because it would have to impose purchase quotas on its members.

[48] There may be a trade-off between the immediate gains in social welfare and possible welfare losses in the future. Evaluating the trade-off necessarily requires present value calculations that are fraught with uncertainty.

regarding market power because supply and demand elasticities are ignored. Second, the structural approach focuses only on the GPO while presuming that supply is competitive. This focus ignores the possibility of countervailing power, which could be procompetitive.

GPO contracts often include terms that appear at first blush to be exclusionary or anticompetitive. Upon closer examination, however, these terms may be the quid pro quo for lower prices. Condemning such terms can lead to perverse results, such as higher prices. Again, care must be exercised to avoid errors. Finally, the GPO funding mechanism may suggest conflicts, but these too may well be more apparent than real. The actual impact depends on market structure and, therefore, cannot be determined through a priori reasoning.

Per se rules and structural safe harbors are appealing because enforcement resources are reduced. But errors, potentially serious errors, can creep in and thereby lead to perverse decisions and outcomes. Policymakers must proceed cautiously to minimize or prevent errors.

REFERENCES

American Bar Association Section of Antitrust Law. (2017). *Antitrust Law Developments*. 8th ed. Chicago: American Bar Association.

Blair, Roger D., and Christine Piette Durrance. (2014). Group Purchasing Organizations, Monopsony, and Antitrust Policy. *Managerial & Decision Economics* 35: 433–443.

Blair, Roger D., and Jeffrey L. Harrison. (1991). Cooperative Buying, Monopsony Power and Antitrust Policy. *Northwestern University Law Review* 86: 331–367.

Blair, Roger D., David L. Kaserman, and Richard E. Romano. (1989). A Pedagogical Treatment of Bilateral Monopoly. *Southern Economic Journal* 55: 831–841.

Bruhn, William E., Elizabeth A. Fracica, and Martin A. Makary. (2018). Group Purchasing Organizations, Health Care Costs, and Drug Shortages. *Journal of the American Medical Association* 320: 1859–1860.

Burns, Lawton R. (2002). *The Health Care Value Chain: Producers, Purchasers, and Providers*. 1st ed. San Francisco: Jossey-Bass.

Burns, Lawton R., and J. Andrew Lee. (2008). Hospital Purchasing Alliances: Utilization, Services, and Performance. *Health Care Management Review* 33: 203–215.

Burns, Lawton R., and Rada Yovovich. (2014). Hospital Supply Chain Executives' Perspectives on Group Purchasing: Results from a 2014 National Survey. www.supplychainassociation.org/wp-content/uploads/2018/05/AHA_AHRMM_Wharton_2014_Surve.pdf.

Carstensen, Peter. (2010). Buyer Cartels versus Buying Groups: Legal Distinctions, Competitive Realities, and Antitrust Policy. *William & Mary Business Law Review* 1: 1–46.

Department of Justice and Federal Trade Commission. (2004). *Improving Health Care: A Dose of Competition.* Washington, DC: Federal Trade Commission.

Elhauge, Einer. (2002). The Exclusion of Competition for Hospital Sales through Group Purchasing Organizations. Report to US Senate. https://scholar.harvard.edu/files/einer_elhauge/files/gpo_report_june_02.pdf.

Elhauge, Einer. (2003). Antitrust Analysis of GPO Exclusionary Agreements. Comments Regarding Hearings on Health Care and Competition Law and Policy – Statement for DOJ-FTC Hearing on GPOs. www.ftc.gov/os/comments/healthcarecomments2/elhauge.pdf.

Frech, Ted. (2008). *Some Thoughts on Bundled Rebates Exclusionary Policies.* GCP: The Online Magazine for Global Competition Policy 1–10.

Goldenberg, David E., and Roland King. (2009). A 2008 Update of Cost Savings and a Marketplace Analysis of the Health Care Group Purchasing Industry. www.supplychainassociation.org/wp-content/uploads/2018/05/goldenberg_king.pdf.

Gooch, Kelly. (2017). 4 of the Largest GPOs: 2017. *Becker Hospital Review.* www.beckershospitalreview.com/finance/4-of-the-largest-gpos-2017.html.

Government Accountability Office. (2002). Group Purchasing Organizations: Pilot Study Suggests Large Buying Groups Do Not Always Offer Hospitals Lower Prices. www.gao.gov/products/GAO-02-690T.

Government Accountability Office. (2003). Group Purchasing Organizations: Use of Contracting Processes and Strategies to Award Contracts for Medical-Surgical Products. www.gao.gov/products/GAO-03-998T.

Government Accountability Office. (2010). Group Purchasing Organizations: Services Provided to Customers and Initiatives Regarding Their Business Practices. www.gao.gov/products/GAO-10-738.

Herndon, Jessica B. (2002). Health Insurer Monopsony Power: All-or-None Model. *Journal of Health Economics* 21: 197–206.

Health Industry Group Purchasing Association. (2002). Health Industry Group Purchasing Association Code of Conduct Principles. www.higpa.org/pressroom/2002/7-29HIGPACode.pdf.

Health Industry Group Purchasing Association. (2011a). A Primer on Group Purchasing Organizations. www.supplychainassociation.org/resource/resmgr/research/gpo_primer.pdf.

Health Industry Group Purchasing Association. (2011b). Group Purchasing: An Examination of the Growing Group Purchasing Business Model across Multiple Industries. www.higpa.org/?page=GPO101.

Hovenkamp, Herbert. (2002). *Competitive Effects of Group Purchasing Organizations' (GPO) Purchasing and Product Selection Practices in the Health Care Industry.* Prepared for the Health Industry Group Purchasing Association. www.novationco.com/pressroom/industry_info/HovenkampGPOStudy.pdf.

Hovenkamp, Herbert. (2004). *Group Purchasing Organization (GPO) Purchasing Agreements and Antitrust Law.* Prepared for the Health Industry Group Purchasing Association. http://higpa.site-ym.com/resource/resmgr/press_releases_2004/2004hovenkampgposandantitrus.pdf.

Healthcare Supply Chain Association. (2016). A Primer on Group Purchasing Organizations: Questions and Answers. www.supplychainassociation.org/resource/resmgr/research/gpo_primer.pdf.

Landes, William M., and Richard A. Posner. (1981). Market Power in Antitrust Cases. *Harvard Law Review* 94: 937–996.

Lindsay, Michael. (2009). Antitrust and Group Purchasing. *Antitrust* 23: 66–73.

Litan, Robert E., and Hal J. Singer. (2010). Do Group Purchasing Organizations Achieve the Best Prices for Member Hospitals? An Empirical Analysis of Aftermarket Transactions. www.medicaldevices.org/node/795.

O'Brien, Daniel, Jon Leibowitz, and Russell Anello. (2017). *How Group Purchasing Organizations Reduce Healthcare Procurement Costs in a Highly Competitive Market.* Antitrust Source. www.davispolk.com/files/antitrust_source_how_group_purchasing_organizations_reduce_leibowitz_anello.pdf.

Schneller, Eugene S. (2009). *The Value of Group Purchasing in the Health Care Supply Chain.* Novationco. www.novationco.com/pressroom/industry_info/GroupPurchasing.pdf.

PART IV   Buyer Cartels

The exercise of monopsony power is not confined to single buyers. Many buyers cooperating with one another can collude to yield similar deleterious results. By depressing the quantity of goods or services that it buys, a buyer cartel can impose price reductions that increase its profits at the expense of suppliers and society. Such coordinated conduct, however, violates antitrust laws. Victims who have suffered from buyer collusion are therefore entitled to sue and recover damages for their loss.

The nurse labor market has been marked by a persistent shortage. Many positions go unstaffed, and many nurses are overworked. Generally, a shortage could be resolved by increasing wages to induce an increase in the number of nurses willing to work. The absence of this remedy suggests that hospitals may be exercising their monopsony power to keep employment low in order to reduce the wages they must pay. Indeed, a number of nurses have sued their hospital employers for just that reason. We discuss monopsony in the nurse labor market and relevant litigation in Chapter 14.

In Chapter 15, we discuss another example of a buyer cartel. Fertility clinics and donor centers pay donor women for their oocytes, which can be used for in vitro fertilization. But these clinics colluded by agreeing to fix compensation below the competitive level, which harmed donors. The reduced compensation also likely reduced the number of donor eggs available for those who needed them.

We discuss no-poaching agreements in Chapter 16. Employers may collude by agreeing not to hire one another's employees. This type of collusion is essentially an agreement between employers to not compete, which makes it difficult for employees who are dissatisfied with their job or compensation to move to another employer. We discuss the case of a no-poaching agreement between the medical schools of Duke University and the University of North Carolina at Chapel Hill.

Like pure monopsonies, buyer cartels cause similar harm to society. But buyer cartels are formed through the collusive activity of multiple firms. When this collusion is overt, victims can sue for damages. Additionally, the threat of antitrust enforcement and prosecution can serve as a deterrent to collusion before it occurs.

14 Collusion in the Nurse Labor Market

14.1 INTRODUCTION

Acute care hospitals require nurses. In addition to providing patient care, nurses monitor the progress of patients, report to physicians, and keep patients informed about their case. Unfortunately, a chronic shortage of nurses in the United States, which has been exacerbated by the COVID-19 public health crisis, translates into suboptimal care for patients. In 2020, there were approximately 3.1 million nurses in the United States.[1] The nursing shortage was estimated to be 154,018 nurses in 2020 and has been projected to grow to a shortage of 500,000 nurses by 2030.[2]

An important economic question is why the nursing shortage has persisted over time. Usually, a shortage is remedied with increased prices (or wages), which would induce an increase in the quantity of labor supplied that resolves the shortage. Since the shortage has persisted for decades, hospital administrators appear to be unwilling to raise salaries for nurses. Vacancies are both ubiquitous and persistent. Unfortunately, this means that patients may not receive the quality of care that a fully staffed hospital could provide.

The exercise of monopsony power may be one explanation for the persistent shortage. Employers of nurses often have substantial monopsony power, which allows them to increase their profits by reducing the number of nurses they hire. This quantity reduction leads to reduced wages that must be paid.[3] Having and exercising monopsony power, however, is not per se illegal. In this chapter, we focus on a possible alternative explanation for the nursing shortage:

---

[1] Bureau of Labor Statistics (2019).   [2] Zhang et al. (2017)
[3] Chapter 11 discusses the economics of monopsony.

collusive monopsony in the nurse labor market, which occurs when firms conspire with one another to depress wages. Recent antitrust litigation in several states has indicated that there may be pervasive collusion and information sharing among hospitals aimed at depressing the salaries of nurses. Collusive behavior among employers of nurses is per se illegal and a violation of Section 1 of the Sherman Act.

In Section 14.2, we document the nurse shortage in the United States. In Section 14.3, we present a relatively simple model of collusion, which we apply to employers of nurses. As we will show, collusion leads to a shortage of nurses relative to the ideal staffing level. In Section 14.4, we turn our attention to several recent antitrust class actions that alleged collusion among hospitals. In Section 14.5, we review the damage claims of the nurses. We then examine the antitrust treatment of buyer cartels in Section 14.6. Concluding comments are in Section 14.7.

14.2   THE SHORTAGE OF NURSES

Registered nurses can be employed in a number of settings, including hospitals, physician offices, home health care, assisted living facilities, and outpatient clinics, as well as in education and industry, where they can provide valuable expertise to pharmaceutical firms and medical device manufacturers. Registered nurse (RN) is one of the fastest-growing professions in the United States, with a projected growth rate of 7 percent between 2019 and 2029 according to the US Bureau of Labor Statistics.[4] This growth is fueled by increased demand for medical care as well as reduced supply due to increases in the retirement of current nurses.

In this section, we examine four factors that help explain why the demand for nursing services has grown over the past few decades: an aging population, a reorganization of health care, health care reform, and the turnover rate of nurses.

---

[4] Bureau of Labor Statistics (2019).

An Aging Population

The American population is aging quickly as the number of baby boomers (Americans born between 1946 and 1964) over age 65 grows. Over the past decade, the United States has seen a 34 percent increase in its 65-and-older population,[5] creating strain on the health care system since the elderly require more services.[6] Additionally, people are living longer as a result of advances in medical treatment and healthier lifestyles. At the same time, chronic diseases that require regular care, such as diabetes and heart disease, are increasing. Diseases that would have killed people decades ago are now being managed by the health care system, which increases the demand for health care services.[7]

Reorganization of Health Care

The demand for nursing services is increasing due to reorganization of health care. Due to a physician shortage, which is in part due to the increase in demand for health services, nurses are expected to take on various roles that were traditionally left to doctors. For example, some state scope of practice regulations permit nurse practitioners to practice independently and/or prescribe medication. Also, many nonserious medical services are being offered on an outpatient or ambulatory basis. This minimizes the amount of downtime that patients spend in facilities, allowing hospitals to offer more medical services to patients. The patients that are in the facilities, however, require more intensive care, which increases the workload of the nurses. Additionally, patient intensity has increased because of invasive procedures, more powerful medications, and increases in the number of patients with acute illness. Hence, more nurses are needed per bed in order to maintain the appropriate quality of care.

---

[5] US Census Bureau (2020).

[6] The United States will see 55 percent growth from 2015 to 2030 in its number of senior citizens (Buerhaus et al. 2017).

[7] Buerhaus et al. (2017).

The Affordable Care Act

The Patient Protection and Affordable Care Act (ACA) legislation, passed in 2010, led to 20 million more people enrolling in health insurance plans. With newly insured individuals in private health plans and Medicaid, there is additional strain on an already strained health care system.

Turnover Rate of Nurses

The nursing shortage has also been affected by reduced supply of nurses. One issue is the need to replace nurses who have left the profession. Some 60,000–70,000 nurses retire each year.[8] Exacerbating the issue is the high turnover rate for nurses, often due to poor working conditions. Even before the COVID-19 public health crisis, nurses would often work long hours in understaffed hospitals in jobs that could be both physically and mentally taxing. The public health crisis only caused conditions to decline further as coronavirus patients overwhelmed hospitals, increasing workloads, mental loads, and health risks for nurses.[9] The national turnover rate increased from 17.8 percent in 2019 to 25.9 percent in 2021.[10]

Additionally, nursing schools face capacity constraints that limit the flow of new nurses into the workforce. In 2019, approximately 80,400 qualified applicants were turned away from nursing schools due to space constraints.[11] Satisfying the higher demand for nurses requires consistently training a large enough cohort of nurses each year to replace departures and accommodate the increased need.

Consequences of the Nursing Shortage

Understaffing has two major negative consequences for health policy outcomes. First, understaffing leads to overworked nurses, which reduces job satisfaction. Indeed, understaffing is one of the major causes of nurse burnout and increased nurse turnover. Thus,

---

[8] Buerhaus et al. (2017).   [9] Jacobs (2021).   [10] Nursing Solutions Inc. (2022).
[11] American Association of Colleges of Nursing (2020).

understaffing creates a negative feedback loop that leads to more nurses leaving the nurse labor market. Second, understaffing leads to a lower quality of care for patients. Overworked nurses are not as efficient and may make mistakes. Additionally, they may be spread too thin across their job responsibilities and may not be able to give the best care to all the patients assigned to them. In one Massachusetts hospital, union nurses threatened to strike over staffing shortages, a problem that has been exacerbated by the COVID-19 public health crisis.[12]

Yet, understaffing of nurses continues to be a problem in the United States. One other potential cause of the nurse shortage, which has been espoused by academics, is monopsonistic exploitation. In this scenario, hospitals exert monopsony power and hire fewer nurses than the competitive amount in order to suppress nurse wages. In the short run at least, nurses can be subjected to monopsony exploitation by employers.[13] In the next section, we discuss the economics of buyer cartels and apply it to the nurse labor market.[14]

14.3   A SIMPLE ANALYSIS OF AN EMPLOYER CARTEL

In this section, we examine the economic consequences of collusion in the nurse labor market.[15] We begin with the competitive benchmark and then introduce collusion. We show how collusion decreases both the quantity of nurses employed and their wages. Additionally, the monopsony power wielded by the cartel reduces social welfare.

---

[12] Kullgren (2021).   [13] Hirsch and Schumacher (2005).

[14] See Chapter 11 on the economics of monopsony. Although we focus on the impact of collusion by employers of nurses in this chapter, a cartel is not necessary for hospitals to exert monopsony power. Since hospitals often wield substantial monopsony power in local markets, they may reduce their employment of nurses even without colluding with other hospitals.

[15] Hirsch and Schumacher (2005) provide empirical evidence of monopsony in the nurse labor market. They find that although monopsonistic effects can be seen in the short run, they are most likely not sustained in the long run. The latter conclusion is belied by the chronic shortage.

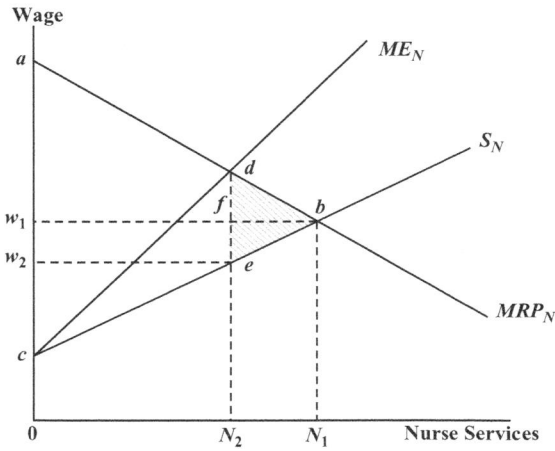

FIGURE 14.1 Monopsonistic exploitation of nurses

Competitive Benchmark

Under competitive conditions in the market for RNs, supply and demand determine the number of nurses employed and the wage paid. Figure 14.1 depicts the competitive solution where the derived demand for nurses (MRP_N) and supply (S_N) are equal. At that point, the competitive wage is w_1 and the number of nurses employed is N_1. In this competitive equilibrium, every nurse who is willing to work at the competitive wage will be employed. Similarly, at the competitive solution, every hospital willing to pay the competitive wage is able to employ nurses. The competitive employment level is the optimal level of staffing. The marginal value of the nursing services is equal to their marginal cost, which is the wage paid, and social welfare is maximized.

Collusive Monopsony

Now suppose that the hospitals agree among themselves to act together as though they were a single employer, that is, a monopsonist. By acting collusively, the hospitals can depress the wage, but they must curtail employment to do so. In order to maximize their collective profits, the hospitals restrict employment to the point where the marginal value of employing an additional nurse is just equal to the marginal expenditure of that additional nurse.

The marginal value is given by the height of the demand curve in Figure 14.1. The total wage bill for nurses is the product of the wage paid (w) and the number of nurses employed (N). Since the supply of nurses is positively sloped, the hospitals must raise the wage to induce the hire of an additional nurse. Absent wage discrimination, however, the hospital must pay that increased wage to all nurses; therefore, the marginal impact on the wage bill is equal to the wage paid to the added nurse *plus* the change in the wage paid to all the nurses previously employed.[16] This sum is called the *marginal expenditure*, which is shown as ME_N in Figure 14.1. Consequently, the colluding hospitals will employ N_2 nurses and pay the wage on the supply curve at N_2, which is w_2. Thus, collusive monopsony leads to lower wages for the nurses and reduced employment. If N_1 is the optimal staffing level, notice that the reduced staffing at N_2 is suboptimal. This necessarily means that the quality of patient care may be compromised for the sake of enhanced profit. In an economic sense, the gap between N_1 and N_2 measures the shortage. As one can see, the nurse shortage is a predictable consequence of collusion. The hospitals enjoy increased profits at the expense of the nurses.

Welfare Implications of Collusive Monopsony

Figure 14.1 illustrates the effect of collusive monopsony on economic welfare. For the hospitals, employer surplus is the difference between their willingness to pay as reflected in the demand and the wage that the market requires. At the competitive solution, the employer surplus is given by area abw_1. For the nurses, employee surplus is the difference between the minimum wage at which the nurses will work

---

[16] The total wage bill is $E = w(N) \cdot N$, so the marginal expenditure will be $\frac{dE}{dN} = w + N\frac{dw}{dN}$.

as reflected in the supply curve and the wage that the market dictates. At the competitive solution, the employee surplus is given by area w_1bc in Figure 14.1.

Competition in this market leads to the maximum sum of employer and employee surplus, which is area abc in Figure 14.1. No other wage and employment level will generate a larger total surplus. The sum of employer surplus and employee surplus is a measure of social welfare. The economic foundation for an antitrust policy that promotes and protects competition is the maximization of social welfare that results from competition.

Collusive monopsony has an adverse effect on the welfare of the nurses and on social welfare. Profit maximization by the colluding hospitals results in a reduction in employee surplus of w_1bew_2. Part of this reduction, area w_1few_2, is converted into employer surplus (or profit) and part of it, area fbe, is simply lost. The net effect on social welfare is a loss equal to the triangular area dbe. As Figure 14.1 illustrates, the social cost of hiring the nurses between N_2 and N_1, as measured by the height of the supply curve, is below the value that these nurses provide, as measured by the height of the demand curve. From a social perspective, too few nurses are being employed. The collusive monopsony solution is allocatively inefficient due to under-employment. This allocative inefficiency is what causes the reduction in social welfare.

Impact on Hospital Costs

Since there is widespread concern over burgeoning health care costs, one might suppose that the reduced wages will reduce the hospitals' costs and thereby benefit patients. This, however, is not the case. It is consistent with our intuition that the reduced wages will reduce the average cost of producing acute care hospital services. This average cost reduction improves hospital profits and thereby provides an incentive for collusion. But the effect of monopsony is to raise marginal cost. Since marginal cost is what drives price and output decisions, the increase in marginal cost leads to a reduction in the hospitals' output and higher hospital charges.[17] In other words, since there are fewer nurses employed, fewer nursing services can be offered. A reduction in the quantity of services in the output market equates to an increase in price for patients. Thus, collusive monopsony has no redeeming virtues.

Empirical Evidence

For decades, the nurse labor market has been held up as a prime example of monopsony power and could therefore be a ripe environment for collusive monopsony. Indeed, a number of empirical studies that estimate labor supply elasticity conclude that nurses face substantial monopsony power from hospitals. For example, Sullivan (1989) estimated supply elasticities of 0.79 in the short run and 0.26 in the long run.[18] Staiger, Spetz, and Phibbs (2010) estimated a supply elasticity of 0.1 for nurses; Hirsch and Schumacher (2005) similarly found evidence of monopsony in the nurse labor market, identified by comparing nurse wages to hospital concentration.[19] Later studies by DePasquale (2018) and Prager and Schmitt (2021) showed that mergers that increase concentration in nurse labor markets tended to decrease wages after consummation. The empirical literature largely corroborates the existence of monopsony power in the nurse labor market, with effects on wages at least in the short run. The presence of monopsony power indicates that collusive monopsony may be profitable. We argue that collusive monopsonistic behavior among hospitals, at least in part, can explain some of the shortage in the nurse labor market.

14.4 RECENT ANTITRUST LITIGATION

There have been several class action antitrust suits filed by nurses alleging collusion in local nurse labor markets, including suits filed in

---

[17] For further analytical details, see Blair and Durrance (2014) and Chapter 11.

[18] For a discussion of the Lerner index of monopsony, see Chapter 11.

[19] Although the authors found evidence of monopsony power in the short run, they did not necessarily find monopsony power in the long run.

Albany (New York),[20] Chicago,[21] Detroit,[22] Memphis,[23] and San Antonio.[24] In these cases, nurses alleged that the defendants wielded collusive monopsony power in the local markets for hospital nurses and conspired to use that power to further depress the wages of nurses in violation of Section 1 of the Sherman Act.[25] Second, the nurses alleged that the defendants had entered into a conspiracy to regularly exchange "detailed and non-public information about compensation being paid or to be paid to their RN employees," which facilitated suppression of RN compensation.[26] The plaintiff nurses alleged that the area hospitals eliminated, or at least impaired, competition for nurses, avoided competition in the nurse labor market, and thereby depressed RN wages below the non-collusive level.

In *Cason-Merenda*, there were allegations of frequent telephone exchanges of competitively sensitive information by hospital human resources (HR) professionals regarding RN compensation as well as third-party surveys about compensation that were circulated among the hospitals. The plaintiffs collected various emails, transcripts, and other documents that clearly showed how HR professionals interchanged wage information directly. Even though evidence of an overt conspiracy to depress prices was lacking, the courts ruled that the wage information sharing was conclusive enough to allow the plaintiffs to pursue their case on those grounds.

---

[20] *Fleischman* v. *Albany Medical Center*, No. 06-cv-0765 (N.D. N.Y. 2010).

[21] *Reed* v. *Advocate Health Care*, No. 06C3337 (N.D. Ill. 2009).

[22] *Cason-Merenda et al.* v. *Detroit Medical Center et al.*, No. 2:06-cv-15601 (E.D. Mich. 2006).

[23] *Clarke* v. *Baptist Memorial Healthcare Corporation*, 264 F.R.D. 375, 377 (W.D. Tenn. 2009).

[24] *Maderazo* v. *VHA San Antonio Partners, L.P.*, No. 5:06-cv-00535 (W.D. Tex. 2006).

[25] Antitrust allegations of wage fixing are not limited to the market for nurses. For example, there have been similar allegations in the labor market for physical therapists and physical therapist assistants (Department of Justice 2021).

[26] *Fleischman* v. *Albany Medical Center*, No. 06-cv-0765 (N.D. N.Y. 2010). In addition to wages, some of the plaintiffs alleged that the information-sharing agreements included signing bonuses, merit raises, certification bonuses, work schedules, and the like.

Since the information sharing was allegedly designed to decrease nurse compensation, it can be considered a violation of Section 1 of the Sherman Act. There was no doubt that this information could tip the scales and give the hospitals more leverage over nurse wages.

Of the five cases, only two, in Albany and Detroit, settled for substantial sums.[27] Albany's plaintiffs received a total of $14 million from the five hospital defendants, whereas the RNs in Detroit received $90 million from the defendants. The remaining three class action lawsuits were not certified, and the cases settled for small sums.

Class Certification

When a large group of antitrust victims has suffered antitrust damages that are individually small, a class action, which combines all plaintiffs, may be the only feasible way for them to proceed. The court, however, must first certify the class. Class certification allows the class action lawsuit to proceed. Before certifying the proposed class, the court must be convinced that the small number of class representatives will adequately reflect the interests of everyone in the class. The injury experienced by the class representatives must be the same as the injury suffered by the class members. If there is any conflict of interest, the class will not be certified.

It is also essential that common proof will be sufficient to prove both liability and the fact of injury. This means that proof for one is proof for all. Otherwise, the court might have to conduct a large number of mini-trials within the overall litigation. When it comes to individual damage awards, the court will be less concerned about common proof. In a class action, the damage award goes to the class. This sum must be distributed to the class members on some sort of

---

[27] As shown in the Appendix of Chapter 8, most cases settle before they reach the trial stage. Settlements ensure that the plaintiffs recover some damages while reducing the costs of the defendants. At the same time, settlements reduce the need for lengthy trials and improve the efficacy of the court system.

formulaic basis, which may prove to be problematic. In most instances, however, the court does not care much about this at the class certification stage. The class actions for Chicago, Memphis, and San Antonio were not certified by the courts on the basis of common proof,[28] conflicts of interest,[29] and feasibility of the claim.[30]

14.5   ANTITRUST DAMAGES

In most circumstances, an antitrust violation has many victims. But only some of them are entitled to recover treble damages. Although Section 4 of the Clayton Act appears to confer a private right of action upon literally anyone who is an antitrust victim,[31] the Supreme Court has placed limits on those who have standing to pursue damages. First, a would-be plaintiff must have suffered *antitrust injury*.[32] This means that the injury must flow from the anticompetitive consequences of the antitrust violation. In the case of collusion in the nurse labor market, the anticompetitive consequences are the depression of wages and/or salaries below the competitive level and the reduction in the number of nurses employed. Since these consequences flow from the unlawful agreement, the nurses would appear to have suffered antitrust injury.

Second, a plaintiff must have been injured *directly* by the unlawful conduct. This requirement is meant to avoid duplicative damages or the need for complex apportioning. In the case of collusion in the nurse labor market, the nurses are the direct victims of the collusion.

[28] In the Chicago case, the judge determined that the damages model was not accurate enough since it relied on averages, which would have overcompensated some nurses and undercompensated others.

[29] The class representatives in the Memphis case were not considered appropriate for the class since one had ties to a nurse union and another was filing for bankruptcy. Their conflicts of interest would not have accurately portrayed the wider class.

[30] In San Antonio, the class was denied since the court determined that there was not enough evidence to conclude that the conspiracy would have resulted in wage depression.

[31] Section 4 of the Clayton Act, 15 USC §15, provides that "any person who shall be injured in his business or property by reason of anything forbidden in the antitrust laws may sue therefor ... and shall recover threefold the damages by him sustained."

[32] *Brunswick Company* v. *Pueblo Bowl-O-Mat*, 429 US 477 (1977).

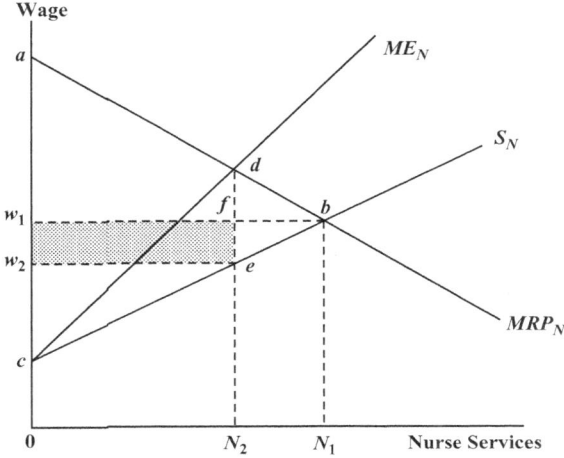

FIGURE 14.2 Antitrust damages

Third, the damage estimate may not be speculative. To avoid charges of speculation, the damages claimed must be based on a just and reasonable inference rather than mere guesswork. In Section 14.4, some of the classes discussed were not certified due to the lack of a reliable method for calculating damages.

The Measure of Damages

Assuming that the collusion among the hospitals is impermissible, the nurses will have standing to sue for damages. The measure of damages is the underpayment suffered by the victims of the conspiracy, in this case, the nurses. Consequently, the appropriate measure of damages (Δ) is the difference between the wage but for the collusion (w_{bf}) and the actual wage (w_a) times the number of nurses actually employed (N_a):

$$\Delta = (w_{bf} - w_a)N_a.$$

In Figure 14.2, we can see that the damage will be equal to the difference between w_1, which is the but-for wage, and w_2, which is the actual (collusive) wage, times N_2, which is the actual number of nurses employed.

There are nurses who would have been employed but for the collusion – in fact, there are $N_1 - N_2$ of them. They have suffered antitrust injury because the competitive wage (w_1) exceeds their reservation wages. They are essentially priced out of the market by the collusion among the hospitals. These nurses, however, cannot be part of the class because it would be difficult to prove that they would have worked at the competitive wage, since there is an incentive to misrepresent their willingness to participate. In addition, the damage to these nurses would be the difference between the competitive wage and the reservation wage, which is the height of the supply curve. This gap narrows as one slides along the supply curve to point b in Figure 14.2. Proving (or disproving) each nurse's reservation wage along that segment of the supply curve is ordinarily not feasible.

Proving the amount of damages for those nurses who are actually employed can be an econometric challenge because an estimate of antitrust damages requires a reliable estimate of the but-for wage. In order to determine the but-for wage, we must reliably estimate the supply of and demand for nurses. These are typically difficult, but not impossible, to estimate. In the absence of a reliable estimate, however, we are left with speculation and guesswork. These do not provide the necessary foundation for an admissible estimate of damages.

Standard of Precision

As a general proposition, the courts are demanding when it comes to proving the fact of injury but far less so when it comes to estimating the amount of the damages suffered. The logic is fairly straightforward. If a nurse claims to have been injured, he or she will have to prove it. For a defendant to be liable, the preponderance of the evidence must support the plaintiff's allegation. Once the jury has found a defendant liable, however, the standard of precision in measuring the damages is relaxed. In order to estimate damages due to a buyer cartel, the plaintiff must estimate the difference between the wage that would have been received if there had been no conspiracy and the actual wage that was received. While a plaintiff can be expected to present accurate evidence of the cartel wage, the but-for wage is not observable because the but-for wage did not actually occur and therefore must be estimated. There is an unavoidable element of uncertainty surrounding such estimates due to data limitations. Consequently, the estimated underpayment may be imprecise.

In general terms, the US Supreme Court explained that whenever damages are estimated, there is some unavoidable element of uncertainty involved. In the antitrust arena at least, we have learned to live with uncertainty. Once an antitrust plaintiff has proved the fact of injury with reasonable certainty, the burden of proof in estimating the amount of damages is somewhat relaxed. In *Story Parchment*, the Supreme Court explained the different standards of proof for the fact of damages and the amount of the damages: "The rule which precludes the recovery of uncertain damages applies to such as are not the certain result of the wrong, not to those damages which are definitely attributable to the wrong and only uncertain in respect of their amount."[33] Once a plaintiff proves the fact of the damages, "it will be enough if the evidence show[s] the extent of the damages as a matter of just and reasonable inference."

Although the jury can rely on reasonable inferences, there is a difference between drawing reasonable inferences and speculation or guesswork. Charges of speculation can be avoided by the proper use of modern econometrics that yield reasonable inferences. Using these methods, the impact of the cartel can be isolated by controlling for other factors that may influence wages. The plaintiff should be able to provide a just and reasonable estimate of the damages that he or she suffered. Such estimates should not be deemed speculative.

---

[33] *Story Parchment Company* v. *Paterson Parchment Paper Company*, 282 US 555 (1931).

Estimating Antitrust Damages

Imprecision may remain with relevant data and rigorous econometric examination. Nonetheless, the estimated price differential is still the most reliable damage estimate that the plaintiff can produce.

One way to estimate the damages suffered by the nurses who were actually employed is to estimate a reduced-form wage equation:

$$w = w(MRP_N, S_N, C),$$

where w is the nurse's wage, MRP_N is a vector of demand variables, S_N is a vector of supply variables, and C is a dummy variable that takes a value of one for cartel period observations and zero otherwise.[34] Using panel data before, during, and after the cartel, the coefficient on C is a measure of $(w_{bf} - w_a)$. This estimated underpayment can be applied to the number of nurses actually employed (N_a) to estimate the total underpayment.

Proving Damages on a Class-Wide Basis

In our stylized model, each nurse is paid precisely the same amount. When the hospitals compete in the nurse labor market, each nurse is paid w_1. When the hospitals collude, each nurse is paid w_2. In this simple model, a nurse's damage claim is relatively straightforward: The underpayment is the difference between the competitive wage (w_1) and the collusive wage (w_2). In most cases, however, antitrust damage estimation is far more complicated. For one thing, the successful plaintiff is only entitled to recover the underpayment that is attributable to the antitrust violation.[35] The damage methodology

---

[34] If the expert had data from only cartel members, then C would present the time period of the cartel observations relative to a time period before and/or after the conspiracy. If, however, the expert had data from cartel and non-cartel members, C could represent the time period during the conspiracy for the cartel participants.

[35] In *Bigelow* v. *RKO Radio Pictures*, 327 US 251, 264 (1946), the Supreme Court found that antitrust damages must be found "by comparison of profits, prices and values as affected by the [antitrust violation], with what they would have been in its absence under freely competitive conditions."

must control for all other factors that could contribute to a reduction in employment and the wage paid.

In most cases, the damage claim will span several years. Although there is a four-year statute of limitations on damage claims, by the time of trial the damage period may be six or seven years. During that time, much can happen that can influence nurse wages, including normal inflation, hospital mergers or acquisitions, changes in technology or protocols, or shifts in demand.

The discussion above implicitly assumes that the nursing services are homogenous. In an actual hospital, compensation across nurses may vary due to factors including experience, tenure, specialization, educational achievement, or shift differentials.

There is another complication: Wages are not just the take-home pay. The actual compensation of a nurse includes benefits such as health and life insurance, retirement contributions, paid vacation and sick leave, and bonuses. These benefits vary across hospitals and over time. It is, however, necessary to account for non-wage benefits in the damage analysis.

The bottom line is that damage estimation for a single nurse is complicated. Estimation for a class of nurses is necessarily more complicated, but it is not impossible. Fortunately, most cases where class certification has been approved settle before a rigorous measure of damages is needed.

14.6 ANTITRUST POLICY

Since the Supreme Court's 1948 decision in *Mandeville Island Farms v. American Crystal Sugar Company*, collusion among buyers has been condemned as a violation of Section 1 of the Sherman Act. Although the case involved collusion among sugar beet refiners who conspired to reduce the price that they paid to sugar beet farmers, the logic would seem to apply to employers of labor generally and nurses in particular. In 2016, the DOJ and the FTC made it clear that they would protect employees from colluding employers.

Antitrust Agency Guidance

In October 2016, the antitrust Agencies issued their *Antitrust Guidance for Human Resources Professionals* in an effort to forestall inadvertent collusion in labor markets.[36] The Agencies began by pointing out that Section 1 of the Sherman Act applies to all firms that compete in the labor market. A horizontal agreement among ostensible competitors that "limits or fixes the terms of employment for potential hires" is suspect under Section 1. If firms agree on wages or salaries, benefits, terms of employment, or job opportunities, it is apt to be a per se violation of Section 1.

The Agencies cautioned that "[i]t is unlawful for competitors to expressly or implicitly agree not to compete with one another even if they are motivated by a desire to reduce costs." This caution, of course, makes sense because the cost savings will improve the profits of the colluding employers, but they will not be passed on to consumers in the form of lower prices.[37] Additionally, the Agencies observed that naked wage-fixing agreements and no-poaching agreements are unlawful per se under the antitrust laws.[38] Consequently, such agreements are vulnerable to criminal prosecution and private damage claims.

Although it may not seem anticompetitive to answer and distribute results of a survey with sensitive wage data or to discuss hiring prospects with a colleague who works at a different hospital, these actions serve to illegally enhance the monopsony power of the competing hospitals. By issuing the *Guidance*, the antitrust Agencies ensure that HR professionals have no excuse for engaging in anticompetitive behavior.

Criminal Sanctions

The antitrust Agencies also made it crystal clear that collusion in the labor market that continued after the *Guidance* was published or

---

[36] Department of Justice and Federal Trade Commission (2016).   [37] See Chapter 11.
[38] See Chapter 16 for a discussion of no-poaching agreements.

began after that date would be met with criminal prosecution. For human resource professionals as well as their superiors, this decision meant the DOJ could impose personal fines and prison sentences. As for the fines, the maximum per offense is \$1 million. The maximum prison sentence is 10 years.[39]

14.7   CONCLUDING REMARKS

There seems to be little doubt that there is a persistent shortage of nurses. Economists would expect that competition in the nurse labor market would bid up the wages until supply and demand are equal, which would eliminate that shortage. This, however, has not happened. The question is why not? One answer may be collusion – either overt or tacit – among hospitals. Such collusion has predictable consequences: reduced employment, which is consistent with the observed shortages, depressed wages, and a loss in social welfare.

The Department of Justice and the Federal Trade Commission have expressed concern about collusion in labor markets. They promised vigorous enforcement of the Sherman Act and have admonished human resource professionals to avoid unlawful agreements with other employers regarding wages and/or other terms of employment.

REFERENCES

American Association of Colleges of Nursing. (2020). Nursing Shortage. www .aacnnursing.org/News-Information/Fact-Sheets/Nursing-Shortage.

Blair, Roger D., and Christine Piette Durrance. (2014). The Economics of Monopsony. In W. Dale Collins, ed., *Issues in Competition Law and Policy*. Chicago: ABA, 393–408.

Buerhaus, Peter, Lucy Skinner, David Auerbach, and Douglas Staiger. (2017). Four Challenges Facing the Nursing Workforce in the United States. *Journal of Nursing Regulation* 8: 40–46.

Bureau of Labor Statistics. (2019). Occupational Outlook Handbook, Registered Nurses. www.bls.gov/ooh/healthcare/registered-nurses.htm.

---

[39] No one has gotten the maximum yet. So far, the longest sentence was five years.

Department of Justice. (2021). Former Health Care Staffing Company Executives Charged in Superseding Indictment with Wage Fixing and Obstruction. Press Release, Eastern District of Texas US Attorney's Office. www.justice.gov/usao-edtx/pr/former-health-care-staffing-company-executives-charged-superseding-indictment-wage.

Department of Justice and Federal Trade Commission. (2016). Antitrust Guidance for Human Resource Professionals. www.justice.gov/atr/file/903511/download.

Depasquale, Christina. (2018). Monopsonistic Exploitation: Theory and Evidence. Working Paper.

Hirsch, Barry, and Edward Schumacher. (2005). Classic or New monopsony? Searching for Evidence in Nursing Labor Markets. *Journal of Health Economics* 24: 969–989.

Jacobs, Andrew. (2021). "Nursing Is in Crisis": Staff Shortages Put Patients at Risk. *New York Times*. www.nytimes.com/2021/08/21/health/covid-nursing-short age-delta.html.

Kullgren, Ian. (2021). *Nurses Plan to Strike Over Staffing at Massachusetts Hospital*. Bloomberg Law. https://news.bloomberglaw.com/daily-labor-report/nurses-plan-to-strike-over-staffing-at-massachusetts-hospital.

Nursing Solutions, Inc. (2022). 2022 NSI National Health Care Retention & RN Staffing Report. www.nsinursingsolutions.com/Documents/Library/NSI_National_Health_Care_Retention_Report.pdf.

Prager, Elena, and Matt Schmitt. (2021). Employer Consolidation and Wages: Evidence from Hospitals. *American Economic Review* 111: 397–427.

Staiger, Doug, Joanne Spetz, and Ciaran Phibbs. (2010). Is There Monopsony in the Labor Market? Evidence from a Natural Experiment. *Journal of Labor Economics* 28: 211–236.

Sullivan, Daniel. (1989). Monopsony Power in the Market for Nurses. *Journal of Law and Economics* 32: 135–178.

US Census Bureau. (2020). 65 and Older Population Grows Rapidly as Baby Boomers Age. www.census.gov/newsroom/press-releases/2020/65-older-popula tion-grows.html.

Zhang, Xiaoming, Daniel Tai, Hugh Pforsich, and Vernon W. Lin. (2017). United States Registered Nurse Workforce Report Card and Shortage Forecast: A Revisit. *American Journal of Medical Quality* 33: 229–236.

15 Collusion in the Oocyte Market

15.1 INTRODUCTION

Collusion among buyers is every bit as objectionable on social welfare grounds as collusion among sellers.[1] The Supreme Court recognized this economic fact in its *Mandeville Island Farms* decision.[2] The dispute in that case arose from an agreement among sugar beet refiners to depress the price paid to sugar beet farmers. The Court found this conduct to be in violation of Section 1 of the Sherman Act.[3] The farmers, therefore, could pursue damages under Section 4 of the Clayton Act.[4] Specifically, the Court held,

> It is clear that the agreement is the sort of combination condemned by the [Sherman] Act, even though the price fixing was by purchasers and the persons ... injured under the treble damage claim are sellers not customers or consumers, ... it does not follow that it is outside the scope of the Sherman Act.[5]

In this chapter, we focus on the antitrust claims in *Kamakahi* v. *American Society of Reproductive Medicine*,[6] which arose from collusion among buyers of human eggs (oocytes). Two closely related trade associations organized and orchestrated a price-fixing conspiracy aimed at depressing the fees paid to egg donors. The antitrust victims were women who were underpaid for the eggs that they

---

[1] This chapter relies heavily on Blair and Durrance (2021).
[2] *Mandeville Island Farms* v. *American Crystal Sugar Company*, 334 US 219 (1948).
[3] 15 USC §1.   [4] 15 USC §15.
[5] *Mandeville Island Farms* v. *American Crystal Sugar Company*, at 334.
[6] *Kamakahi* v. *American Society for Reproductive Medicine*, No. 3:11-cv-1781:16 (N.D. Cal. 2011).

donated[7] to fertility clinics or donor agencies. The collusion among fertility clinics would seem to warrant harsh treatment under Section 1 of the Sherman Act.[8] While this case raises important issues in medicine, public health, eugenics, and ethics, we focus our analysis on the merits of the antitrust claim and the effect on the competitive process.

In Section 15.2, we describe the conspiracy that was organized under the two trade associations. In Section 15.3, we describe the antitrust standards for impermissible agreements among buyers. We outline the economic effects of price ceilings in Section 15.4. In Section 15.5, we explore the possibility of a defense under the rule of reason. Section 15.6 outlines antitrust injury and damages in a collusive monopsony case, while Section 15.7 discusses the disposition of the *Kamakahi* case. We close with some concluding remarks in Section 15.8.

15.2   COLLUSION IN THE OOCYTE MARKET

In the United States, there are approximately 450 fertility clinics[9] dispersed across the country. A common method of assisted reproductive therapy (ART) is in vitro fertilization (IVF), which often requires the use of donor eggs. According to the Centers for Disease Control and Prevention (CDC), donor eggs were used in 24,300 ART cycles.[10] Egg donors must complete a screening process and medical history in advance of egg donation, which can include an intake process focused on eligibility requirements such as age, body mass index, health status, smoking status, education requirements, sexually transmitted disease history, alcohol/substance use history, and genetic factors. Donors may also be required to complete a psychological screening. This entire process can take six weeks. In fact, only about 10 percent of the individuals who begin the initial screening

---

[7] In the context of this market, *donated* and *donors* are euphemisms for *sold* and *sellers*.
[8] 15 USC §1.   [9] CDC (2020).   [10] CDC (2018).

process eventually donate their eggs.[11] The egg donation process itself (which can take two weeks) involves the donor receiving hormone injections to stimulate egg production, other medical visits and tests, and an egg retrieval procedure. There are medical risks associated with participating, such as abdominal pain, nausea, vomiting, diarrhea, bloating, or, in rare cases, death.[12] Individuals donate either through a fertility clinic or a donation agency and are compensated with a fee that is meant to account for their donation, time, and risk. Most egg donations are "fresh egg donations," meaning that the donor and the recipient are matched before the eggs are retrieved and the nonfrozen eggs are utilized in the recipient's IVF process.[13]

Compensation for donors is guided by two associations, the American Society for Reproductive Medicine (ASRM) and the Society for Assisted Reproductive Technology (SART). Guidelines for compensation through these organizations were informally understood as early as 1994 and formally stated in guidelines produced by the Ethics Committee in 2000 and reaffirmed in 2007. The rhetoric around egg donation focuses on altruism as a motivation and emphasizes that egg donor compensation should be "reasonable" and "not so substantial … that [it] will lead donors to discount risk."[14] The guidelines specify that compensation should not be a function of donor characteristics or number of eggs retrieved, and they outline maximum payments of $5,000, with payments above $5,000 requiring justification and payments above $10,000 prohibited.[15] Variation in the amount of compensation may be a function of local cost of living.[16] Approximately 400 fertility practices are members of SART, representing 90 percent of all practices.[17]

---

[11] Hsieh (2017).   [12] Hsieh (2017).   [13] Hsieh (2017).   [14] Krawiec (2009).

[15] In *Arizona* v. *Maricopa County Medical Society*, 457 US 332 (1982), the Supreme Court found that fixing compensation of medical services of differing quality was illegal.

[16] Hsieh (2017).   [17] www.sart.org/.

In *Kamakahi* v. *American Society for Reproductive Medicine*,[18] a class of women[19] who donated eggs beginning in 2007, filed suit against the two reproductive medicine associations, ASRM and SART, alleging horizontal collusion on the compensation for egg donations, a violation of Section 1 of the Sherman Act. The price-fixing scheme was accomplished through the use of the ethical guidelines and membership by fertility clinics and donor agencies to the association. As the price-fixing scheme could prove problematic without enforcement mechanisms, all fertility clinics who were members of SART were obliged to follow the ethical guidelines. In furtherance of the conspiracy, SART required member clinics to sign an agreement to follow the guidelines and published a list of those conforming clinics. SART stated that failure to comply would result in removal from the published list of clinics on the website. Self-reported clinic data suggested that the average amount of compensation for egg donation hovered close to the $5,000 maximum, between $4,217 and $5,200.[20]

15.3 ANTITRUST STANDARDS

For the last 130 years, collusive agreements that restrain trade have been unlawful. Section 1 of the Sherman Act provides that

> [E]very contract, combination in the form of trust or otherwise, or conspiracy, in restraint of trade or commerce among the several States, or with foreign nations, is declared to be illegal.[21]

This broad language has been interpreted by the judiciary to isolate competitively unreasonable agreements. At the end of its first half century of experience, the Court condemned all agreements that interfere with the competitive price mechanism. In its *Socony-*

---

[18] *Kamakahi* v. *American Society for Reproductive Medicine*, No. 3:11-cv-1781:16 (N.D. Cal. 2016).
[19] Class members include those who donated to a SART member clinic or donation agency.
[20] Krawiec (2009).   [21] 15 USC §1.

Vaccum Oil Company[22] opinion, the Supreme Court warned that any interference with the free market determination of prices was unlawful:

> Under the Sherman Act a combination formed for the purpose and with the effect of raising, *depressing*, fixing, pegging, or stabilizing the price of a commodity in interstate or foreign commerce is illegal per se.[23]

It is not clear that Justice William O. Douglas was issuing a warning against collusive monopsony when he included depressing prices, but it can certainly be read that way. In 1948, the Supreme Court's ruling in *Mandeville Island Farms*[24] made it clear that collusion among buyers is vulnerable to antitrust challenges under Section 1 of the Sherman Act.[25] Moreover, such conduct was also vulnerable to private damage actions under Section 4 of the Clayton Act.[26]

This holding makes it clear that (1) collusion among buyers is unlawful and (2) underpaid sellers have a right to sue for antitrust damages. Because only unreasonable restraints of trade violate Section 1 of the Sherman Act, defendants may argue that their agreement to refrain from competing is socially beneficial and thus not unreasonable. Put differently, defendants may argue that competition has some undesirable consequences, and, therefore, society should applaud rather than condemn agreements not to compete. The Supreme Court has made it clear that such a defense is a nonstarter.

---

[22] *United States* v. *Socony-Vacuum Oil Company*, 310 US 150 (1940).

[23] *United States* v. *Socony-Vacuum Oil Company*, 310 US 150 (1940), at 223–224, emphasis added.

[24] *Mandeville Island Farms* v. *American Crystal Sugar Company*, 334 US 219 (1948).

[25] 15 USC §1.

[26] 15 USC §15 provides that "any person who shall be injured in his business or property by reason of anything forbidden in the antitrust laws may sue therefor in any district court of the United States in the district in which the defendant resides or is found or has an agent, without respect to the amount in controversy, and shall recover threefold the damages by him sustained, and the cost of suit, including a reasonable attorney's fee."

Goldfarb[27] involved a minimum fee schedule for routine legal services such as title searches for prospective homeowners. The prescribed minimum fee was 1 percent of the price of the home. In its opinion, the Supreme Court correctly observed that imposing minimum fees for legal services was no different from imposing minimum fees for any other type of service. Adherence to the fee schedule was maintained with threats of disciplinary proceedings that could have resulted in suspensions or disbarments.

One might object that competition in the market for legal services must be tempered in the client's interest. Aggressive fee cutting might lead to low-quality, high-volume legal practice that produces shoddy legal services that could jeopardize the interests of those paying the low fees. In other words, high fees are necessary to ensure high-quality services. But there are less restrictive ways of deterring sloppy legal services, such as disciplining those lawyers who fail to meet minimum standards.

In *Professional Engineers*,[28] the antitrust issue involved a ban on competitive bidding by architects and engineers. The National Society of Professional Engineers tried to justify the ban as a way to promote the health and safety of the general public. According to the Society, competitive bidding would lead to low fees and an incentive for its members to do low-quality work, including, for example, over-engineered designs with high construction costs or poor designs that might lead to bridge failures.

As in *Goldfarb*, the Court rejected the notion that competition was bad. After all, the central premise of the Sherman Act is that competition is good because it results in the maximization of social welfare. Specifically, the Court observed that when a business practice is analyzed under the rule of reason, the goal is to determine the effect of the practice on competition. The inquiry is not to determine whether a policy favoring competition is in the public interest.

---

[27] *Goldfarb* v. *Virginia State Bar*, 421 US 773 (1975).
[28] *National Society of Professional Engineers* v. *United States*, 435 US 679 (1978).

That decision has been made by Congress. The Society's absolute ban on competitive bidding obviously limited competition. The Society argued that its ban on competitive bidding was socially beneficial because it reduced competitive pressures on engineers that may have resulted in expensive and possibly dangerous designs.

The Sherman Act precludes inquiry into the question of whether competition is good or bad for society. The presumption is that competition is good because it leads to lower prices, better quality, superior service, and innovation. In *Professional Engineers*, the Court concluded that "the Rule of Reason does not support a defense based on the assumption that competition itself is unreasonable."[29]

15.4   ECONOMIC EFFECTS OF PRICE CEILINGS

Collusion among buyers on the maximum price that will be paid has predictable, adverse consequences for social welfare and the distribution of wealth. In this section, we examine these economic effects.

In Figure 15.1, the demand for egg donations by fertility clinics is represented by D, while the supply of donors is denoted S. In the absence of collusion among the clinics, the number of donors would be N_1 and the fee paid to the donors would be F_1. The clinics would experience buyer surplus equal to the triangular area abF_1. The egg donors would enjoy donor surplus equal to the triangular area F_1bc. Social welfare is equal to the sum of buyer surplus and donor surplus, which is area abc.

When the buyers agree among themselves to limit the donation fee to a specified maximum, say F_2, the quantity supplied shrinks from N_1 to N_2. At the price ceiling, the quantity supplied will be equal to N_2, which is obviously smaller than N_1. The social welfare loss due to the collusive price agreement is equal to the triangular area ebf. Donor surplus falls from area F_1bc to area F_2fc. Part of this reduction,

---

[29] *National Society of Professional Engineers* v. *United States*, 435 US 679 (1978), at 696.

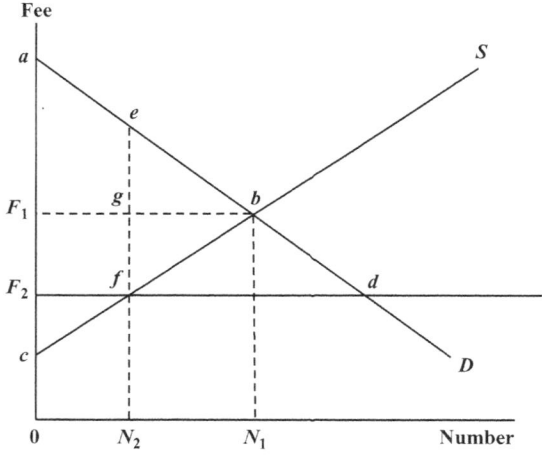

FIGURE 15.1 Economic impact of a price ceiling

area F_1gfF_2, is converted into profit for the clinics, and the rest is lost. Buyer surplus rises from area abF_1 to area $aefF_2$. The clinics are more profitable and, consequently, are better off. But the donors are clearly worse off. On balance, the gain to the clinics is smaller than the loss to the donors. In the absence of some procompetitive benefits flowing from the collusion, the clinics should be condemned for violating Section 1 of the Sherman Act and the undercompensated donors should have standing to pursue antitrust damages.

15.5 RULE OF REASON ANALYSIS

In most instances, price fixing, whether by sellers or buyers, is a per se violation of Section 1 of the Sherman Act. In rare cases, an unusual price-fixing agreement may be analyzed under the rule of reason.[30] A brief overview of that rule will demonstrate why the price ceiling adopted by ASRM and SART cannot survive a rule of reason analysis.

There are three phases in a rule of reason analysis of a challenged business practice. First, the plaintiff must make a prima facie

---

[30] The most thorough treatment of the rule of reason is provided by Areeda and Hovenkamp (2021, ¶1500–1512).

case that the challenged conduct is anticompetitive. In *Kamakahi*, the plaintiffs alleged that the two reproductive service organizations imposed ethical obligations on their members to limit compensation for egg "donations" to $5,000.[31] Thus, the actual and potential "donors" were deprived of the benefits of competition for their eggs. This would seem to be a prima facie case that Section 1 of the Sherman Act had been violated.

In the second phase, the ball is in the defendant's court. The defendant may respond to the plaintiff's allegation(s) in one of two ways. First, the plaintiff may dispute the allegations as being factually inaccurate. That is, the defendant may dispute the very existence of the challenged conduct. Alternatively, the defendant may offer a procompetitive justification for the challenged conduct. Given the prima facie case presented by the plaintiff, the defendant will have to prove that the alleged procompetitive benefits outweigh the negative effects of the conduct. In *Kamakahi*, the defendants could not rebut the plaintiff's challenge on factual grounds. The price limits were promulgated as ethical rules, and members of ASRM and SART were required to sign letters agreeing to abide by the ethical rules. Consequently, denying the existence of the collusive agreement would scarcely be credible. If the defendants had offered a cognizable procompetitive justification, the court would have had to weigh the conflicting effects in the third stage. The defendants could not do this, so they presented other justifications.

At this time, the defendants pointed to one or more ethical rationales for limiting payments. Donation of eggs was likened to donation of sperm as well as live donation of organs such as kidneys. It is worth noting that although the National Organ Transplant Act prohibits the sale of human organs, it does not apply to sperm or eggs

---

[31] In special cases, the ethical rules permitted compensation up to $10,000. Sums above $10,000 were deemed to be inappropriate. *Kamakahi* v. *American Society for Reproductive Medicine*, No. 3:11-cv-1781:16 (N.D. Cal. 2011), Order Regarding Motions to Exclude Expert Opinions and Motion for Class Certification, at 6.

because there is a legal market for both.[32] Sperm donation is marketed to potential donors as profit motivated,[33] and advertisements for sperm donation focus on the market potential of donating, indicating sperm is commodified. It is also important to note that sperm donation involves no risk. In contrast, egg donation is promoted as altruistic. That is, women can "give the gift of life" while men can sell it. The fertility clinic associations reportedly arrived at their maximum payments for egg donation by using the hourly rate for sperm donors and applying that to the estimated time involved in the egg donation procedure.[34] In other words, the compensation for egg donation was equated to the required compensation for sperm donation adjusting for the amount of time involved, without regard to risk.[35] In this way, eggs are incompletely commodified.[36]

Participation in activities such as research often involves incentives in the form of compensation. One issue is whether egg donation is considered a gift or a donation as opposed to the sale of a good or service. If the commodification status of human eggs is less than clear, the IRS tax rules should clarify the status. In fact, *Perez* v. *Commissioner*[37] resolved this outstanding question by stipulating that payment for donated eggs is taxable income, not payment for pain and suffering. This decision provides more evidence that the price fixing in this market is consistent with price fixing in other more traditional markets.

There is a literature focused on the ethics of participation in medical research and, in particular, how much compensation

---

[32] National Organ Transplant Act (1984, amended 1988 anf 1990), Pub. L. 98-507.

[33] Krawiec (2015).

[34] Sperm donors earned an average of $60–$75/hour in 2000. Egg donors spent approximately 56 hours per donor cycle, equating to approximately $3,300–$4,200 per donation cycle (Krawiec 2014).

[35] Krawiec (2015).   [36] Krawiec (2015).

[37] *Nichelle G. Perez* v. *Commissioner of Internal Revenue*, 144 T.C. 51 (2015). The court found, "We don't doubt that some portion of the compensation paid to all these people reflects the risk that they will feel pain and suffering, but it's a risk of pain and suffering that they agree to before they begin their work. And that makes it taxable compensation and not excludable damages."

individuals are due for their participation. Institutional review boards review research protocols including participants' informed consent, as well as the risks of participation. Compensation for participation is evaluated independently. Although compensation for research participation does not equate to *coercion* (i.e., a threat), ethicists express concern about whether compensation can exert *undue influence*.[38] Undue influence is said to potentially affect participant rational decision making or cause failure in appropriately valuing the risk of participating. In other words, an offer of payment might cause undue influence if it leads a participant to "unreasonably discount or fail to appreciate the risks."[39] It is important to note that individuals have different risk preferences; not all individuals value risk in the same way. Ethicists raise concerns that payment for participation may lead lower-income individuals to participate at higher rates, which could lead to the unfair distribution of risks or burden of research or donation.

Economists generally assume that individuals act rationally, using information about risks and benefits provided to them, before participating in market transactions. In this setting, *economic coercion* appears unlikely. If a thief points a gun at you and demands "your money or your life," the choice is unwelcome. Fearing for your life, you turn over your wallet. You are worse off than you were before the offer was made, but this coercion does not describe the situation potential egg donors face. If a woman is offered a choice between the status quo and donating her eggs for a fee, this offer does not make her worse off. If she donates her eggs, then it must be the case that the price for her discomfort, inconveniences, and perceived medical risks must be less than or equal to the fee that she has been offered. Otherwise, she can simply refuse the offer. If a woman rejected an offer of $5,000 or $10,000 but accepted an offer of $15,000, we cannot infer that this was the result of undue influence or economic coercion.

[38] Williams and Walter (2015).   [39] Gelinas et al. (2018).

In fact, the higher payment may have been necessary to compensate the woman for correctly perceived risks.

Limits on Paying for Quality

Fertility clinics and donor agencies screen women first to see who qualifies to donate. After screening, clinics collect and report detailed personal characteristics about the donor to prospective recipients of donor eggs. Recipients may prefer some personal characteristics to others, suggesting that donated eggs are heterogeneous. Through the ASRM and SART ethical guidelines, which restricted compensation to donors, fertility clinics were precluded not only from paying the market price for donated eggs but also from paying more for more "desirable" eggs. If, for example, a potential donor is exceptionally attractive, exceptionally intelligent, or gifted athletically, her eggs may be more desirable and, therefore, in greater demand. In fact, there is evidence that recipients of donated eggs value specific donor characteristics, such as higher SAT scores.[40] The ethical guidelines, however, preclude paying a premium for the eggs of preferred donors as well as tailoring compensation to specific donor characteristics. Thus, the maximum price restraint does not permit prices to respond to differences in demand due to perceived quality differences. It is also possible that restraints on payments could impact who donates. For example, higher-quality donors (or donors with more preferred characteristics) may not participate at the restrained payments.

The Supreme Court has frowned on restraints that limit market forces in this way. In *Arizona v. Maricopa County Medical Society*,[41] the Supreme Court encountered a novel effort to preserve fee-for-

---

[40] Levine (2012). This study includes advertisements in college newspapers for potential egg donors and identified advertisements containing suggested prices for egg donors well in excess of the ethical guideline maximums. Note that advertisements only indicate suggested payments, not the actual payments made to actual donors. Also, price-fixing conspiracies can be undermined in the presence of cheating. While these advertisements are suggestive of cheating on the agreement, the antitrust conclusions, however, remain unchanged.

[41] 4570 S. 352 (1982).

service medicine in the face of increasing competition from health maintenance organizations.[42] This effort required the participating doctors to accept maximum agreed-upon fees as full payment for certain medical services. In evaluating the economic consequences of maximum fees, the Court expressed concern that uniform adherence to the maximum fees allowed no distinction based on quality: "the price restraint ... tends to provide the same economic rewards to all practitioners regardless of their skill, their experience, their training, or their willingness to employ innovative and difficult procedures in individual cases.[43] From an economic perspective, it seems that price competition is valuable because it both appropriately compensates a potential donor and induces a greater number and quality of donors to enter the market. Paying for quality donors certainly opens separate social policy questions about eugenics and trait selection that we do not consider in this chapter.

15.6 ANTITRUST INJURY AND DAMAGES

Under Section 4 of the Clayton Act,[44] the victims of an antitrust violation have a private right of action which provides that

> Any person who shall be injured in his business or property by
> reason of anything forbidden in the antitrust laws may sue
> therefor ... and shall recover threefold the damages by
> him sustained.

This broad language has been clarified by the Supreme Court in two significant ways. First, "any person" has been severely restricted by the Supreme Court's rulings in *Hanover Shoe*[45] and *Illinois Brick*.[46] In order to have standing to pursue private damages, the plaintiff must be injured directly by the antitrust violation. If the defendant is a

---

[42] For a perceptive analysis, see Harrison (1982).

[43] *Arizona v. Maricopa County Medical Society*, 457 US 332 (1982).

[44] 15 USC §15.

[45] *Hanover Shoe, Inc. v. United Shoe Machinery Corporation*, 392 US 481 (1968).

[46] *Illinois Brick Company, v. Illinois*, 431 US 720 (1977).

seller, the plaintiff must have purchased directly from the defendant rather than from an intermediary. If the defendant is a buyer, the plaintiff must have sold directly to the defendant. In short, private suits are limited to those who have been injured directly by an antitrust violation.[47] In *Kamakahi*, the aggrieved parties were past donors who had been underpaid pursuant to the collusive agreement among the fertility clinics. The donors would appear to be the direct victims since the collusion was aimed at limiting the price paid for eggs and the donors were the sellers of those eggs.

Second, the Supreme Court has confined compensable injuries to *antitrust* injuries. In order to have standing to sue under Section 4 of the Clayton Act, the plaintiff(s) must have suffered antitrust injury. In its *Brunswick Corporation* v. *Pueblo Bowl-o-Mat*[48] decision, the Supreme Court defined the concept of antitrust injury:

> Plaintiffs must prove *antitrust* injury, which is to say injury of the type the antitrust laws were intended to prevent and that flows from that which makes defendants' acts unlawful. The injury should reflect the anticompetitive effect either of the violation or of anticompetitive acts made possible by the violation.[49]

In *Kamakahi*, the alleged antitrust violation involved collusion among the fertility clinics, that is, the buyers of the eggs. The purpose of collusive monopsony is to depress the prices buyers pay. Consequently, the underpayment experienced by the donors appears to be antitrust injury since it results from that which makes the collusive conduct unlawful.

Several requirements must be met in order for a price restraint to be successful. First, the members of the collusive agreement must decide on the price to be paid. In this case, the price restraint was accomplished by ASRM and SART through their ethical guidelines

---

[47] The most extensive treatment of antitrust standing is provided by Areeda et al. (2021, at ¶¶335–363).

[48] *Brunswick Corporation* v. *Pueblo Bowl-o-Mat*, 429 US 477 (1977).

[49] *Brunswick Corporation* v. *Pueblo Bowl-o-Mat*, 429 US 477 (1977), at 477–478.

and imposed on all member fertility clinics and donor agencies. Second, the collusive monopsony must be comprised of all or most of the buyers in the market. Otherwise, other buyers could purchase inputs at higher prices and thereby capture most of the market. In this way, nonparticipants act like participants who cheat on a cartel agreement, which undermines the success of the price restraint. Currently, SART has market power; over 90 percent of ART clinics in the United States are participating members.[50] Third, cheating on the collusive agreement needs to be discouraged or prevented. Fertility clinics were required to adhere to both the general and ethical guidelines to maintain membership with SART.[51] Additionally, the collusive agreement extended to independent egg donor agencies. In 2005, SART (with support from two other fertility associations, RESOLVE and AFA) sent letters to egg donor agencies indicating that in order to serve SART clinics, they must also adhere to the ethical guidelines.[52] For complicit donor agencies, SART would maintain their name on the SART website in a list of its approved agencies. Failure to comply with the guidelines would result in removal from the list. These conditions appear to have been satisfied, and the price restraint was effective for years.

Antitrust Damages

The measure of damages in a collusive monopsony case is the underpayment:

$$\Delta = (P_{bf} - P_a)Q_a,$$

where Δ is the damage, P_{bf} is the price that would have been paid but for the antitrust violation, P_a is the actual price paid, and Q_a is the

---

[50] www.sart.org/patients/what-is-sart/.

[51] *Kamakahi* v. *American Society for Reproductive Medicine*, No. 3:11-cv-1781:16 (N.D. Cal. 2011), Order Regarding Motions to Exclude Expert Opinions and Motion for Class Certification, at 6.

[52] Krawiec (2009).

actual quantity purchased. In Figure 15.1, the antitrust damages would be $\Delta = (F_1 - F_2)N_2$, which is equal to the rectangular area F_1gfF_2.

Note that the cognizable damage is less than the total reduction in donor surplus. The difference is the loss in donor surplus suffered by those who were priced out of the market. These would-be donors fall between N_1, the competitive number, and N_2, the restricted number of donors. They are denied recovery largely due to problems of proof. First, if monetary rewards are involved, everyone who did not donate eggs has an incentive to claim that she would have done so at the competitive fee. Second, even if a court could be sure that only those potential donors between N_1 and N_2 made claims, it would be extremely difficult to prove each person's reservation price. Everyone would have an incentive to claim a reservation price of F_2 plus a penny and thereby maximize the damage award.

Unfortunately, it is difficult to identify the damages suffered by egg donors in practice. Ordinary business records will suffice for the actual values. Clinic records can provide hard evidence of P_a and Q_a, which are F_2 and N_2 in Figure 15.1. The hard part is estimating the but-for fee (F_1). It will be a difficult econometric challenge to estimate F_1 in Figure 15.1.

In many cases, analysts employ the so-called before-and-after method. If the requisite data are available, the fees paid before or after the collusion are compared to the fees paid during the collusive period in order to estimate the but-for fee. One must also control for other economic variables that influence the level of fees.

In the case of oocytes, this would be challenging, and in *Kamakahi* it was specifically challenging. The collusive restrictions had been in place for a long time and were so ubiquitous that the plaintiff's expert was only able to identify three fertility clinics that participated in the agreement at one time but withdrew from the agreement at a different time. In a situation like this, it would be important for the expert to demonstrate that these three clinics were similar to, or representative of, all the other participating fertility clinics that allegedly underpaid donors. The plaintiff expert's analysis showed a range of possible underpayments using these three fertility clinics in his damage analysis, which led the court to determine that the underpayment was speculative.[53]

The alleged class in *Kamakahi* was defined as

> All women who sold Donor Services for the purpose of supplying human eggs to be used for assisted fertility and reproductive purposes ("AR Eggs") within the United States and its territories at any time during the time period from April 12, 2007 to the present (the "Class Period") to or through: a. any clinic that was, at the time of the donation, a member of [SART] and thereby agreed to follow the Maximum Price Rules, as set forth by SART and [ASRM]; and/ or b. any AR Egg Agency that was, at the time of the donation, agreeing to follow the Maximum Price Rules.[54]

The problem with this class definition is that it includes women who may not have been injured. Those women would not have standing under Section 4 of the Clayton Act.

In the analysis presented in Figure 15.1, we have assumed that the maximum fee for donor services (F_2) is a binding constraint. This means that everyone who supplied donor services was paid the maximum. There is evidence, however, that many women were offered a smaller fee and accepted it.[55] Arguably, these women were not injured by the collusive agreement or the maximum fee that would be paid. The clinic pays a bargain price due to asymmetric information. Taking advantage of uninformed donors may be unseemly, but it is not an antitrust violation.

---

[53] *Kamakahi* v. *American Society for Reproductive Medicine*, No. 3:11-cv-1781:16 (N.D. Cal. 2011), Order Regarding Motions to Exclude Expert Opinions and Motion for Class Certification, at 15, 32–44.

[54] *Kamakahi* v. *American Society for Reproductive Medicine*, No. 3:11-cv-1781:16 (N.D. Cal. 2011), Order Regarding Motions to Exclude Expert Opinions and Motion for Class Certification, at 10.

[55] There is also suggestive evidence that some women received higher payments in violation of the ethical guidelines (Levine 2012).

There is a counterargument to this claim. All fertility clinics know that they do not face price competition from one another. As a result, the offers made can be quite low and the actual fee paid may well be influenced by the conspiracy.

Although it may be true that the actual fees below the maximum were influenced by the existence of the maximum, it is difficult to estimate the extent of this influence. The plaintiffs must only provide a just and reasonable estimate once liability has been shown. This does not mean, however, that the estimate can be a stab in the dark.[56]

15.7   DISPOSITION OF *KAMAKAHI*

In *Kamakahi*, the court was asked to consider (1) whether the class should be certified and (2) whether the expert reports should be used to aid in the determination of class certification, as the case involved motions to exclude the respective expert reports.[57]

For class certification under Rule 23(a), the class is obligated to meet the following requirements: (1) numerosity, (2) commonality, (3) typicality, and (4) adequacy.[58] Additionally, Rule 23(b) also has four criteria, but only one of them must be satisfied for class certification.[59] The most common antitrust classes are certified under Rule 23 (b)(3), which provides for class certification under a predominance standard.[60] Generally, Rule 23(b)(3) has two requirements. First, "questions of law or fact common to the members of the class predominate over any questions affecting only individual members."[61]

---

[56] The Supreme Court's requirements for precision are summarized in Areeda et al. (2021, ¶392).

[57] *Kamakahi* v. *American Society for Reproductive Medicine*, No. 3:11-cv-1781:16 (N.D. Cal. 2011), Order Regarding Motions to Exclude Expert Opinions and Motion for Class Certification, at 10.

[58] See ¶331. For a more extensive discussion, see ABA Section of Antitrust Law (2017, 820–862.

[59] ABA Section of Antitrust Law (2017, 941).

[60] ABA Section of Antitrust Law (2017, 943).

[61] *Kamakahi* v. *American Society for Reproductive Medicine*, No. 3:11-cv-1781:16 (N.D. Cal. 2011), Order Regarding Motions to Exclude Expert Opinions and Motion for Class Certification, at 19.

Second, a class action must be "superior to other available methods for the fair and efficient adjudication of the controversy."[62]

The expert for the fertility clinics was a bioethicist who was asked to offer opinions about the ethics of compensation for egg donation and the role of the ethical guidelines in that process. In his report, he argued that the guidelines did not actually constitute an agreement to fix prices, but rather provided some helpful language in thinking about compensation and left the ultimate pricing decision to each individual clinic.[63] The expert argued that the guidelines were designed to promote altruism as the motivation for the donation and to protect donors so that "payments to women who provide eggs for fertility treatment must be fair but not so high as to end up harming patients and doctors."[64] The court ruled that the expert's report was not admissible and that these portions of the report addressed merit issues but not class certification questions.

The expert representing the class of egg donors offered opinions on the extent of the underpayment that donors suffered from the price-fixing arrangement. He estimated this antitrust damage by using data from three agencies that switched their participation status. That is, they participated in the agreement for a period of time and then removed themselves from the agreement. The court reviewed the problems with this approach from the perspective of class certification, finding that these three agencies were "neither random nor representative." Not only was there no evidence offered to support the idea that these three agencies were representative of all agencies participating in the agreement, but individual analyses of each clinic

---

[62] *Kamakahi* v. *American Society for Reproductive Medicine*, No. 3:11-cv-1781:16 (N.D. Cal. 2011), Order Regarding Motions to Exclude Expert Opinions and Motion for Class Certification, at 20.

[63] *Kamakahi* v. *American Society for Reproductive Medicine*, No. 3:11-cv-1781:16 (N.D. Cal. 2011), Order Regarding Motions to Exclude Expert Opinions and Motion for Class Certification, at 26.

[64] *Kamakahi* v. *American Society for Reproductive Medicine*, No. 3:11-cv-1781:16 (N.D. Cal. 2011), Order Regarding Motions to Exclude Expert Opinions and Motion for Class Certification, at 30.

yielded different underpayments (ranging from \$300 to \$2,800), indicating that the expert's approach failed to establish a method of proving damages through common proof.[65] Some questions existed as to how each individual clinic adhered to the guidelines, as the evidence suggested that there was little variation in prices paid within clinics and little difference between the actual and posted prices paid by the clinics.[66]

With respect to class certification, the court held that class treatment was appropriate from the perspective of the price-fixing claim, but the court was not convinced that class treatment was appropriate to calculate damages and so reserved this until a finding was made on the antitrust violation itself. In coming to this decision, the judge addressed issues of numerosity, commonality, typicality, and adequacy as described in Rule 23(a). According to the court, the proposed class was sufficiently large (numerosity), an agreement to fix prices through a set of ethical guidelines was common to all class members (commonality), the guidelines outlining compensation limits were common to the class (typicality), and the named plaintiffs adequately represented the class members (adequacy). The court also reviewed ascertainability through objective means, concluding that records existed identifying which clinics participated in the ethical guidelines and compensation agreement and additional records that identified women who donated eggs to specific clinics or agencies.[67]

In 2015, the class was certified, but it was constrained to class members who donated after April 2007 to a SART member clinic or agency that also followed the ethical guidelines. In 2016, the parties

---

[65] *Kamakahi* v. *American Society for Reproductive Medicine*, No. 3:11-cv-1781:16 (N.D. Cal. 2011), Order Regarding Motions to Exclude Expert Opinions and Motion for Class Certification, at 37.

[66] *Kamakahi* v. *American Society for Reproductive Medicine*, No. 3:11-cv-1781:16 (N.D. Cal. 2011), Order Regarding Motions to Exclude Expert Opinions and Motion for Class Certification, at 30, 37–38.

[67] *Kamakahi* v. *American Society for Reproductive Medicine*, No. 3:11-cv-1781:16 (N.D. Cal. 2011), Regarding Motions to Exclude Expert Opinions and Motion for Class Certification, at 53–56.

settled this case, although the defendants denied any wrongdoing. The terms of the egg donor class action settlement required that ASRM eliminate the collusive price-restraint language from the ethical guidelines, thereby removing any suggestion about what reasonable or appropriate prices should be for donated eggs. ASRM agreed to pay $1.5 million for plaintiffs' counsel fees and litigation costs plus $150,000 to cover notices to class members about the settlement.[68,69]

15.8 CONCLUDING REMARKS

Collusion among buyers has become a more prevalent issue in antitrust litigation in recent years. In this chapter, we used *Kamakahi* as a leading example. In this case, the antitrust issues involved an ethical rule promulgated by the American Society for Reproductive Medicine and the Society for Assisted Reproductive Technology that imposed a collusive price ceiling on the fee that could be paid to egg donors. The associations argued that this restraint was reasonable, as compensation must be limited to avoid undue influence. The courts have ruled repeatedly that neither firms nor associations can decide what a reasonable price is; a reasonable price is determined by a competitive market. The restraint in this case was effective in lowering the level of compensation for donated eggs used in assisted reproductive technology procedures.

While donated eggs are not the type of good that courts typically face in price-fixing conspiracy litigation, women who donated eggs under a collusive price ceiling experienced an underpayment and suffered antitrust injury and damages. Such behavior is precisely the type of behavior that the Sherman Act is designed to prevent.

---

[68] *Kamakahi* v. *American Society of Reproductive Medicine*, No. 3:11-cv-1781 (N.D. Cal. 2011), JCS, Plaintiffs' Unopposed Motion for (1) Preliminary Approval of Settlement; (2) Certification of Class for Settlement Purposes; and (3) Approval of Class Notice; Memorandum of Points and Authorities in Support (2016).
[69] Knaub (2016).

If policymakers decide that ethical concerns prevail against market forces in the oocyte market, other steps would be required to address those payment concerns (i.e., public regulation or prohibitions of payments); collusive price restraints that are justified by reasonableness are clearly objectionable under the Sherman Act.

REFERENCES

American Bar Association Section of Antitrust Law. (2017). *Antitrust Law Developments*. 8th ed. Chicago: American Bar Association.

Areeda, Phillip E., and Herbert Hovenkamp (2021). *Antitrust Law*, 5th ed. Vol. VII. New York: Wolters Kluwer.

Areeda, Phillip E., Herbert Hovenkamp, Roger D. Blair, and Christine Piette Durrance. (2021). *Antitrust Law*. 5th ed. Vol. IIA. New York: Wolters Kluwer.

Blair, Roger D. and Christine P. Durrance (2021). "Reducing the Price of Eggs: Collusion in the Oocyte Market," Herbert Hovenkamp, Liber Amicorum in Nicolas Charbit et al, ed.

Centers for Disease Control and Prevention. (2018). 2016 Assisted Reproductive Technology: National Summary Report. www.cdc.gov/art/pdf/2016-report/ART-2016-National-Summary-Report.pdf.

Centers for Disease Control and Prevention. (2020). Assisted Reproductive Technology (ART) Data: National Data. https://nccd.cdc.gov/drh_art/rdPage.aspx?rdReport=DRH_ART.ClinicInfo&rdRequestForward=True&ClinicID=9999&ShowNational=1.

Harrison, Jeffrey L. (1982). Price Fixing, the Professions, and Ancillary Restraints: Coping with Maricopa County. *University of Illinois Law Review* 4: 925–950.

Hsieh, Carina. (2017). *16 Things You Need to Know about Donating Your Eggs*. CCRM Fertility. www.ccrmivf.com/news-events/eggdonation/.

Gelinas, Luke, Emily A. Largent, I. Glenn Cohen, Susan Kornetsky, Barbara Bierer, and Holly Fernandez. (2018). A Framework for Ethical Payments to Research Participants. *New England Journal of Medicine* 378: 766–771.

Knaub, Kelly. (2016). *Egg Donors Get Pay Limits Axed with Antitrust Settlement*. Law360. www.law360.com/articles/753389/egg-donors-get-pay-limits-axed-with-antitrust-settlement.

Krawiec, Kimberley D. (2009). Sunny Samaritans and Egomaniacs: Price-Fixing in the Gamete Market. *Law & Contemporary Problems* 72: 59–90.

Krawiec, Kimberley D. (2014). Egg-Donor Price Fixing and Kamakahi v. American Society for Reproductive Medicine. *Virtual Mentor, American Medical Association Journal of Ethics* 16: 57–62.

Krawiec, Kimberly D. (2015). Markets, Morals, and Limits in the Exchange of Human Eggs. *Georgetown Journal of Law and Public Policy* 13: 349–365.

Levine, Aaron. (2012). Self-Regulation, Compensation, and the Ethical Recruitment of Oocyte Donors. *Hasting Center Report* 40: 25–36.

Williams, Erin P., and Jennifer K. Walter. (2015). When Does the Amount We Pay Research Participants Become "Undue Influence"? *American Journal of Medical Ethics* 17: 1116–1121.

16 No-Poaching Agreements and Antitrust Policy

16.1 INTRODUCTION

Agreements to fix prices by sellers of a good or service have long been considered naked restraints of trade.[1] These agreements violate Section 1 of the Sherman Act and are judged under a per se standard since price fixing is unambiguously harmful to consumers. Collusion on the buying side is similarly impermissible and receives comparable antitrust treatment.[2] In recent years, the exercise of monopsony power has become more prevalent in labor markets, particularly through anticompetitive agreements among firms. *No-poaching agreements* are agreements among rival employers to refrain from hiring one another's employees.[3] No-poaching agreements affect the wage paid for labor through reduced competition in the labor market. In 2016, the antitrust Agencies released guidelines for human resource professionals that outline impermissible agreements that harm employees and reduce their compensation. The guidelines indicate that the Agencies will seek criminal prosecution and penalties for those involved in naked agreements that harm employees, including no-poaching agreements.

No-poaching agreements deprive employees of the competitive benefits that result from outside employer interest. Recent litigation in a variety of industries highlights the competitive concerns with no-poaching agreements. First, collusive no-poaching agreements

[1] *United States* v. *Socony-Vacuum Oil Company*, Inc., 310 US 150 (1940).
[2] *Mandeville Island Farms* v. *American Crystal Sugar Company*, 334 US 219 (1948).
[3] In some cases, these agreements may also include provisions to share information on wages, salary, benefits, and other contractual terms.

received antitrust scrutiny in recent agency investigations, government actions, and private litigation. For example, in the *High-Tech Employees*[4] litigation, a number of high-tech firms were alleged to have conspired through no-poaching agreements for their skilled employees using methods such as agreeing to not actively recruit one another's employees, to provide notification when making an offer to a rival's employee, and to not make counteroffers. Second, franchise agreements have received antitrust scrutiny for contract provisions that prohibit franchisees from hiring another franchisee's employees. Franchise agreements have both vertical (franchisor to franchisee) and horizontal (franchisee to franchisee) elements, and as such, they have received rule-of-reason treatment as some courts have considered no-poaching agreements to be ancillary to the franchise agreement itself. Finally, no-poaching (or anti-tampering) agreements exist in every professional North American sports league (e.g., Major League Baseball, National Football League, and National Basketball Association), where restrictions are intended to prevent teams from soliciting other teams' players, coaches, scouts, and front office personnel.[5]

In this chapter, we explore the role of monopsony and buying power in no-poaching agreements. In Section 16.2, we review some high-profile no-poaching litigation. Then, in Section 16.3, we narrow our focus to no-poaching agreements in health care settings, specifically *Seaman* v. *Duke University*, which involved a no-poaching agreement between the deans of the medical schools of Duke University and the University of North Carolina at Chapel Hill (UNC). In Section 16.4, we provide an economic analysis of no-poaching agreements and a theory of damages. In Section 16.5, we review the recent DOJ–FTC guidelines to human resource professionals and provide concluding thoughts in Section 16.6.

---

[4] *United States* v. *Adobe Systems*, No. 1:10-cv-01629 (D. D.C. 2011).

[5] Blair and Lopatka (2016).

16.2 BACKGROUND

High-Tech Employees and Digital Animators

No-poaching agreements have received recent public and private antitrust scrutiny.[6,7,8] First, the Department of Justice (DOJ) initiated an investigation into several high-tech companies and digital animators, including Adobe Systems, Apple, Google, Intel, Intuit, Pixar,[9] Lucasfilm,[10] and eBay.[11] In these industries, employers demand workers with highly specialized skills. The no-poaching agreements were said to have been in place between 2005 and 2009 and included agreements not to cold-call or solicit each other's employees. In 2010, the DOJ reached an agreement with Adobe Systems, Apple, Google, Intel, Intuit, and Pixar to cease their anticompetitive practices.

---

[6] Lindsay (2019) reviews some of the recent court history in no-poaching litigation.

[7] In *Therapy Source*, the FTC charged two Texas staffing companies, Your Therapy Source and Integrity Home Therapy, with violations of Section 5 of the FTC Act because of allegations of pay rate exchange information and agreements to reduce the pay of therapists employed in their home health agencies. They were also alleged to have attempted to recruit other competitors to join their conspiracy. The companies entered into a consent decree with the FTC to cease the wage information–sharing and wage-setting behavior. Your Therapy Source, LLC, FTC File No. 1710134 (FTC 2018).

[8] Knorr-Bremse, Westinghouse Air Brake, and Faiveley (which was acquired by Westinghouse Air Brake in 2016) each produce rail equipment for passenger and freight rail purposes. The companies compete in the labor market for skilled rail industry employees. Beginning in 2009, all three companies were alleged to have entered into no-poaching agreements with one another, which prohibited the recruiting or hiring of each other's employees. The agreements were said to have "denied employees access to better job opportunities, restricted their mobility, and deprived them of the competitively significant information they could have used to negotiate better terms of employment." The Court found for the government and prohibited the defendants from engaging in future no-poaching agreements. Following the settlement, a class action of employees filed suit against the rail equipment suppliers for damages. *United States* v. *Knorr-Bremse AG and Westinghouse Air Brake*, No. 1:18-cv-00747 (D. D.C. 2018) Complaint.

[9] *United States* v. *Adobe Systems*, No. 1:10-cv-01629-RBW (D. D.C. 2011).

[10] *United States* v. *Lucasfilm*, No. 1:10-cv-02220 (D. D.C. 2010).

[11] *United States* v. *eBay*, No. 5:12-cv-05869-EJD (N.D. Cal. 2012).

Private antitrust class actions were also filed.[12] Defendants were alleged to have conspired and specifically agreed to (1) not recruit each other's employees, (2) provide notification if making an offer to a rival's employee, and (3) limit pay packages offered to prospective employees at the initial offer, thereby not increasing counteroffers.[13] In 2014, Lucasfilm and Pixar agreed to pay $9 million, and Intuit agreed to settle for $11 million. In 2015, Apple, Google, Intel, and Adobe Systems agreed to settle for $415 million. These settlements were paid out to more than 64,000 affected employees. A private class action suit was also filed against the employers of digital animators, including Walt Disney, DreamWorks Animation, Sony Pictures, and Blue Sky Studios.[14] The class settled for a total of $169 million, with $100 million from Disney and its subsidiaries, $50 million from DreamWorks, $13 million from Sony, and $5.95 million from Blue Sky Studios.[15]

Franchise Contracts

In 2018, 11 attorneys general began investigating no-poaching agreements among fast-food franchises.[16] In response, some franchisors immediately removed any language from their contracts that constituted a no-poaching agreement. In addition, there have been myriad private class actions filed in the franchise arena.[17] In some

---

[12] *In re High-Tech Employee Antitrust Litigation*, No. 5:11-cv-02509-LHK (N.D. Cal. 2011).

[13] *In re High-Tech Employee Antitrust Litigation*, No. 5:11-cv-02509-LHK (N.D. Cal. 2011).

[14] *In re Animation Workers Antitrust Litigation*, No. 14-cv-04062-LHK, 123 F. Supp. 3d 1175 (N.D. Cal. 2015).

[15] Amidi (2018).

[16] Young (2019). In 2018, Senators Cory Booker and Elizabeth Warren introduced Senate Bill 2480, the End Employer Collusion Act, which proposed prohibitions for no-poaching agreements in franchise contracts.

[17] Carl's Jr. (*Bautista* v. *Carl Karcher Enterprises*, No. BC 649777 (Sup. Ct. Cal. 2017)); McDonald's (*Deslandes* v. *McDonald's USA, LLC*, No. 17-cv-04857

franchise agreements between the franchisor and the franchisee, there are prohibitions on recruiting or hiring another franchisee's employees. In fact, 58 percent of franchise agreements were found to contain no-poaching language.[18] These agreements are horizontal in nature because they effectively limit competition for employees between franchisees, but also vertical in nature because the agreements are bound between the franchisor and the individual franchisee. Upon the filing of three private cases against Auntie Anne's, Arby's, and Carl's Jr.,[19] the DOJ issued statements of interest to clarify the Agencies' view of no-poaching agreements in the franchise setting. The DOJ took the position that agreements between the franchisees and franchisor should be judged under a rule of reason rather than a per se rule because franchise restrictions may have both procompetitive purposes and anticompetitive effects. They further suggested that it would be important to consider whether the restraint is ancillary to the larger franchise collaboration.[20]

(N.D. Ill. 2017)); Pizza Hut (*Ion* v. *Pizza Hut, LLC*, No. 4:17-cv-00788 (E.D. Tex. 2017)); Jimmy John's (*Butler* v. *Jimmy John's Franchise, LLC*, No. 18-133 (S.D. Ill. 2018)); Arby's (*Richmond* v. *Bergey Pullman, Inc.*, No. 2:18-cv-00246 (E.D. Wa. 2018)); Cinnabon (*Yi* v. *SK Bakeries, LLC*, No. 18-5627 RJB (W.D. Wa. 2018)); Little Caesars (*Ogden* v. *Little Caesars Enterprises, Inc.*, No. 2:18-cv-12792 (E.D. Mi. 2018)); Burger King (*Michel* v. *Restaurant Brands International Inc.*, No. 1:18-cv-24304 (S.D. Fl. 2018)); and Dunkin Donuts (*Avery* v. *Albany Shaker Donuts LLC*, No. 1:18-cv-09885 (S.D. N.Y. 2018)).

[18] Krueger and Ashenfelter (2018) obtained data on US Franchise Disclosure Documents (FDDs). They analyzed franchise agreements from 156 of the largest US franchise chains, finding that 58 percent of franchise agreements in the sample had no-poaching language.

[19] *Stigar* v. *Dough Dough, Inc. (Auntie Anne's)*, No. 2:18-cv-00244 (E.D. Wa. 2019); *Richmond* v. *Bergey Pullman (Arby's)*, No. 2:18-cv-00246 (E.D. Wa. 2019); *Harris* v. *CJ Star, LLC (Carl's Jr., Hardee's)*, No. 2:18-cv-00247 (E.D. Wa. 2019).

[20] Corrected Statement of Interest of the United States of America, *Stigar* v. *Dough Dough, Inc.*, No. 2:18-cv-00244-SAB (E.D. Wa. 2019); *Richmond and Rogers* v. *Bergey Pullman*, No. 2:18-cv-00246-SAB (E.D. Wa. 2018); *Harris* v. *CJ Star, LLC*, No. 2:18-cv-00247-SAB (E.D. Wa. 2018).

16.3   NO-POACHING AGREEMENTS IN HEALTH CARE:
SEAMAN V. *DUKE UNIVERSITY*

No-poaching agreements have received antitrust scrutiny in health care settings.[21,22] This section describes one particular high-profile case involving collusion between two prominent medical schools in North Carolina.

Seaman *v.* Duke University

The Research Triangle of North Carolina houses several major universities, including Duke University, the University of North Carolina at Chapel Hill (UNC), and North Carolina State University, along with Research Triangle Park (RTP). Both Duke and UNC have medical schools and are two of the largest academic medical systems in North Carolina, as well as two of the largest employers of physicians in the area. *Seaman* v. *Duke University*[23] was a private suit that arose because Dr. Danielle Seaman, a Duke faculty physician in radiology, was interested in an open position at the UNC School of Medicine. Despite being a "great fit," Dr. Seaman could not be considered because "lateral moves between Duke and UNC medical schools are

---

[21] There are other examples of no-poaching agreements in health care. For example, a private class of registered nurses filed suit against eight Detroit hospitals, alleging a conspiracy to restrain the compensation of nurses and the exchange of information about compensation. After 10 years of litigation, the class recovered more than $90 million in damages (*Cason-Merenda* v. *VHS of Michigan, Inc.*, No. 06-cv-15061, 862 F. Supp. 2d 603 (E.D. Mich. 2012)). In *United States* v. *Geisinger*, No. 4:20-cv-01383 (M.D. Pa. 2020), the DOJ discovered that Geisinger and Evangelical Community Hospital had a history of engaging in no-poaching agreements with one another. In its Complaint, the DOJ pointed out that Geisinger and Evangelical Community Hospital enjoyed a market share of more than 70 percent. In 2021, nurses filed a class action against Geisinger and Evangelical alleging no-poaching agreements (*Leib* v. *Geisinger Health*, No. 4:21-cv-00196 (M.D. Pa 2021)).

[22] In 2021, the DOJ indicted Surgical Care Associates for no-poaching agreements with other health care companies. Several civil complaints have also been filed as a result of the DOJ allegations (e.g., *Roe* v. *Surgical Care Affiliates, LLC*, No. 1:21-cv-00305 (N.D. Ill. 2021); *Spradling* v. *Surgical Care Affiliates*, No. 1:21-cv-01324 (N.D. Ill. 2021)).

[23] *Danielle Seaman* v. *Duke University*, No. 1:2015-cv-00462 (M.D. N.C. 2018).

not permitted."[24] Dr. Seaman filed suit on behalf of a class of similarly situated hospital faculty employees. The agreement was alleged to have been made between the deans of the medical schools at the respective institutions and effectively prohibited the poaching of employees at the same rank.

Evidence presented in this case included email communication indicating that the recruiter "received confirmation today from the Dean's office that lateral moves of faculty between Duke and UNC are not permitted. There is reasoning for this 'guideline' which was agreed upon between the deans of UNC and Duke a few years back." In later correspondence, UNC's chief of cardiothoracic imaging admitted that "the 'guideline' was generated in response to an attempted recruitment by Duke a couple of years ago of the entire UNC bone marrow transplant team; UNC had to generate a large retention package to keep the team intact." It was further explained that "the only way [Duke and UNC] can hire each other's faculty is if there is an upward move, i.e., a promotion."[25]

The defendants argued that UNC, as a state institution, was immune from antitrust scrutiny under the state action doctrine.[26] A statement of interest in this case filed by the US attorney general[27] took the position that UNC is not a state actor as articulated by the state action doctrine and clearly fails the two-part test that requires (1) a clear state purpose and (2) active supervision. In this case, there was no state articulation of a policy for restraining hiring between employers, nor was there state supervision of this restraint of trade. The defendants also argued that the alleged agreement should be evaluated under the rule of reason rather than a per se standard since the agreement was ancillary to collaboration between UNC and Duke. There was no evidence, however, to support an ancillary restraint.

---

[24] *Danielle Seaman* v. *Duke University*, No. 1:2015-cv-00462 (M.D. N.C. 2018).
[25] *Danielle Seaman* v. *Duke University*, No. 1:2015-cv-00462 (M.D. N.C. 2018).
[26] *Parker* v. *Brown*, 317 US 341 (1943).
[27] *Danielle Seaman* v. *Duke University*, No. 1:2015-cv-00462 (M.D. N.C. 2018). Statement of Interest of the United States (2019).

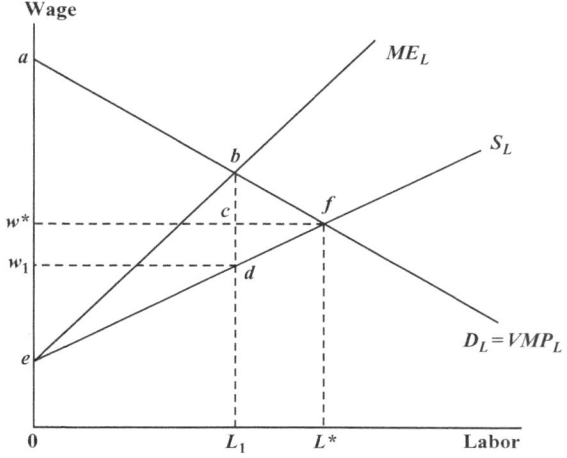

FIGURE 16.1 Competitive and monopsony labor market equilibrium

In February 2018, UNC settled its lawsuit and agreed to never again enter a no-hire agreement. In April 2019, Duke University School of Medicine settled its case and Duke University Health System agreed to pay $54.5 million. In 2020, new allegations emerged that this original conspiracy involved more than the medical schools, encompassing broad no-poaching agreements of non-medical faculty for 40 years from 1978 to 2018.[28] In 2021, a settlement was reached where Duke agreed to pay $19 million to class members employed at either institution in any department between 2001 and 2018.[29]

16.4   DAMAGE THEORY

In a competitive labor market, wages are determined by the interaction of supply and demand, where each firm is a wage taker. In the labor market, firms demand labor (D_L) and employees supply labor (S_L) at different wages (w). In Figure 16.1, the competitive wage and quantity of labor hired are w^* and L^*, respectively. In the competitive

---

[28] *Binotti* v. *Duke University*, No 20-cv-470 (M.D. N.C. 2020).
[29] *Binotti* v. *Duke University*, No. 1:20-cv-470 (M.D. N.C. 2020); Duke UNC Employee Settlement, https://dukeuncemployeesettlement.com/.

model, the sum of consumer surplus and producer surplus is maximized and represented as area *afe*. In this setting, social welfare is maximized.

Now compare the competitive labor market to a monopsonistic labor market, where there is only one employer to hire labor. In Figure 16.1, S_L is the supply of labor while ME_L is the marginal expenditure. The demand for labor (D_L) is also noted as the value of the marginal product of labor (VMP_L).[30] Profit maximization by the monopsonist leads to an employment of L_1 units of labor and a wage of w_1.[31] The monopsonistic buyer is able to depress the wage below w^* and restrict the number of workers hired below L^*. This restriction in the number of workers hired and the wage paid leads to a social welfare loss given by area *bfd*. This is the economic argument against monopsony.

No-poaching agreements are not equivalent to pure monopsony, but they are similar to buyer cartel models where groups of firms collude to create and utilize monopsony power. Consider some economic possibilities that explain the effects of no-poaching agreements. Recall that in *Seaman*, Duke and UNC are both large academic medical centers and large employers in the area.

---

[30] The value of the marginal product of labor (VMP_L) is the increase in output attributable to a small increase in labor times the price of the output (i.e., labor's contribution to the employer's total revenues). Joan Robinson (1933) referred to the VMP–wage gap as "monopsonistic exploitation."

[31] The monopsonist has buying power; as a result, the wage paid by the monopsonist is a function of the number of people it hires, $w(L)$. The monopsonist's profit function is given by $\pi = pQ - w(L)L - r\bar{M}$, where p is the output price of the product, Q is the output, w is the wage, L is the labor input, M is the fixed capital input, and r is the rental rate of the fixed input. Profit maximization leads to $\frac{\partial \pi}{\partial L} = p\frac{\partial Q}{\partial L} - [w(L) + L\frac{dw}{dL}] = 0$. Because $\frac{\partial Q}{\partial L}$ is the marginal product of labor, or MP_L, which indicates the contribution to total product from a small increase in labor input, the first term, $p\frac{\partial Q}{\partial L}$, represents the value of the marginal product of labor (VMP_L). The second term, $w(L) + L\frac{dw}{dL}$, represents the marginal expenditure (ME_L), which is made up of two complementary effects. When the monopsonist hires an additional worker, it must pay that new worker the higher wage $(w(L))$, and it also must increase the pay of all the previously employed workers to the higher wage $(L\frac{dw}{dL})$. The sum of these two effects is the ME_L. Profit maximization for the monopsonist requires employing the quantity of labor where VMP_L is equal to ME_L. This profit maximization results in paying a wage of w_1 and hiring L_1 workers.

Employers like UNC and Duke, therefore, already have some power to depress wages below the competitive level. It is costly for employers to identify and recruit employees with desirable skills and qualifications. As such, employers want to retain these employees at the lowest cost, avoid competitive bidding wars for employees with rivals, and minimize turnover. Employers could make their positions more attractive through retention methods such as offers with higher compensation, more attractive benefits, and flexible working conditions. This type of retention activity is procompetitive and could preempt departures. If employers jointly decide to not solicit a rival's employees, retention is preserved at a lower cost, but in violation of the antitrust laws. No-poaching agreements can lead to competitive harm in several ways.

First, consider a market with a small number of employers, such as the high-tech or digital animator market. Assume these firms collude to fix the wages paid to their employees. Wage setting was not alleged in *Seaman*, but it has been alleged elsewhere.[32] The economic effects of price-fixing or wage-setting agreements are well known and receive per se treatment under the antitrust laws. In its simplest form, a wage-fixing agreement emulates the monopsony solution in Figure 16.1, leading to the same wage reduction, labor input reduction, and resulting deadweight social welfare loss. Such behavior is a per se violation of Section 1 of the Sherman Act, which forbids conspiracies that restrain trade. No-poaching agreements, however, are not equivalent to wage-setting agreements.

Second, firms that agree to participate in no-poaching agreements conspire to not compete on certain dimensions, even if not explicitly agreeing to set wages. In this way, no-poaching agreements may be more similar to employee allocation, which is the equivalent of market division or customer allocation on the selling side, where firms agree to divide the market for employees, to hire only from its own market for employees, or not to hire from a rival's market for employees. In this setting, each firm would have a monopsony in its

---

[32] *Danielle Seaman* v. *Duke University*, No. 1:2015-cv-00462 (M.D. N.C. 2018).

own labor market. In this way, firms could offer different wages in their respective market but not directly compete for workers. In *Seaman*, the damage theory was based on UNC and Duke implementing an employee allocation agreement, given that UNC and Duke are unique employers in the area. In this agreement, wages were not set directly, but the agreement required the rivals not to compete on the recruiting and hiring dimension, which reduced competition in the faculty physician labor market.

Third, no-poaching agreements affect buying power, or the degree to which an employer can depress the wage paid below the competitive wage.[33] Consider the Lerner index as adapted to monopsony power.[34] Let λ be the measure of buying power, which is given by the deviation from the competitive outcome, or

$$\lambda = \frac{(VMP_L - w)}{w},$$

which is equal to the inverse of the elasticity of supply (ε_s),[35] or

$$\lambda = \frac{1}{\varepsilon_s}.$$

The elasticity of supply measures the responsiveness of the supply of labor to changes in the wage. In other words, the more responsive (elastic) workers are to changes in wage, the less monopsony power the employer has. Mathematically, this makes sense since the larger the denominator, ε_s, the smaller the overall buying power (λ). Put simply, the gap between the VMP_L and wage narrows as buying power is reduced. Now consider the implementation of a no-poaching agreement. The agreement effectively reduces ε_s because it reduces the likelihood that a worker can leave one employer for another.

[33] Naidu, Posner, and Weyl (2018) discuss the role of the elasticity of supply in labor market power. Additionally, Sullivan (1989) adapted the Lerner Index to the nurse labor market.

[34] The Lerner index for monopoly power was developed by Abba Lerner (1934).

[35] Recall that under profit maximization, $VMP_L = ME_L$ and that $ME_L = w(L) + L\frac{dw}{dL}$. Therefore, the buying power index is given by: $\lambda = \left[w + L\frac{dw}{dL} - w\right]/w$ or $\lambda = \frac{L}{w}\frac{dw}{dL}$ or $1/\varepsilon_s$. See, for example, Blair and Harrison (2010).

This, in turn, increases the buying power (λ), which exacerbates the gap between the wage and VMP_L.

If no-poaching agreements do not require specific agreements on price, then how do they affect workers' wages? No-poaching agreements effectively restrict the information available to all employees about their marketability or value in the labor market through the prohibition of recruiting. Moreover, there are fewer (or no) employers competing for employees, which reduces competition. Information asymmetries work against the party with less information, that is, the employee. Without outside offers from a rival employer, an employee is foreclosed from upward mobility both with the current employer and a rival employer. In the absence of a no-poaching agreement, if a faculty physician at UNC were recruited by Duke, UNC could respond in two ways if they wanted to retain the employee. UNC could either make a preemptive retention offer with a higher salary to discourage the faculty physician's interest in the Duke position or, alternatively, make a (presumably higher) counteroffer if the faculty physician received a competing offer from Duke. The faculty physician would need to decide between staying at UNC or leaving for Duke.[36] In either case, the faculty physician's salary will increase. Under the no-poaching agreement, neither of these scenarios is possible and salary increases of this type are not attainable. In addition, the employer also avoids paying higher salaries to faculty physicians who are not being recruited. Information exchange and employee movement between employers would impact both the employees involved in recruiting, as well as other employees not currently being recruited.

In response to a faculty physician departure, a hospital may increase wages for its remaining employees to improve the likelihood

---

[36] Of course, there are other academic medical centers outside the Research Triangle of North Carolina. But locally, the two provide alternative employment options with the lowest switching costs. A faculty physician could, of course, choose to move outside of North Carolina, but the switching costs (e.g., relocating, purchasing a new residence, relocating research projects or grant funding) are much larger.

of retention. In other words, rising tides lift all boats. If an employer wants to retain its employees, it must incentivize them to stay in their positions. By using no-poaching agreements, the hospitals avoid paying higher salaries necessary to retain employees who would otherwise be recruited. In addition, employers also avoid the increased cost of the remaining faculty physicians' salaries. No-poaching agreements will necessarily have effects on all employees under the agreement given existing salary structures. Duke and UNC, like other academic institutions, have some salary structure both at baseline and within rank (e.g., assistant, associate, and full professor), where promotions between some ranks are further complicated by tenure procedures. When no-poaching agreements eliminate lateral hiring, they affect all employees because the pressure on employers to raise compensation through preemptive or reactive retentions is removed, information about competitive salaries is blunted, and worker mobility is restricted.

A Theory of Damages

When firms make no-poaching agreements, resulting employee wages are depressed. This reduction in the actual wage relative to the but-for wage (i.e., the wage that should have been paid but for the no-poaching agreement) constitutes antitrust injury and is compensable in the form of antitrust damages. Antitrust damages resulting from an underpayment would be sustained by all employees of the colluding employers. The underpayment for each worker is given by

$$Damage = (w_{bf} - w_a)L,$$

where w_a represents the actual wage paid, w_{bf} represents the but-for wage, and L is the number of units of labor employed.

Estimating damages involves identifying the wages that employees actually received (w_a), using administrative business records. Additionally, it requires identifying the wages that employees would have received in the absence of the no-poaching agreement (the but-for wage, or w_{bf}). With data available during the no-poaching agreement period as well as data available outside of the no-poaching agreement (either before or after or both), it would be possible to estimate the underpayment using regression analysis. This approach would involve estimating a wage equation, where the dependent variable is the individual worker wage. The key independent variable is an indicator for the time period during the no-poaching agreement (relative to outside of the no-poaching agreement). Other independent variables must include control variables for other important factors that would necessarily affect the wage of the employee, such as years of experience, highest degree attained, other specific skills, geographic location, and rank. Using this approach, the estimated harm to all employees under a no-poaching agreement could be credibly estimated.[37]

16.5 GOVERNMENT REGULATION

DOJ–FTC Guidance

The Antitrust Division of the Department of Justice and the Federal Trade Commission issued joint guidance in 2016 for human resource professionals[38] on the competitive processes of hiring and retaining workers. In response to concerns about no-poaching and other anticompetitive hiring agreements, the Agencies have put human resource professionals on notice and specifically stated,

> An agreement among competing employers to limit or fix the terms of employment for potential hires may violate the antitrust laws if the agreement constrains individual firm decision-making with regard to wages, salaries, or benefits; terms of employment; or even job opportunities.[39]

---

[37] An approach of this type was taken by the economic expert Dr. Edward Leamer, in *High Tech Employees Antitrust Litigation*, submitted October 1, 2012.

[38] Department of Justice and Federal Trade Commission (2016).

[39] Department of Justice and Federal Trade Commission (2016, 1).

Firms may unilaterally set their own hiring and recruiting policies, but firms are not permitted to make agreements with other firms about those hiring policies or to agree not to compete on any terms of employment. Any agreement among firms to set wages or to implement no-poaching agreements could be subject to a per se rule if these agreements are *naked* restraints of trade. As such, the per se standard would not require investigation of any procompetitive aspects of the agreement; rather, only proof of an agreement would be necessary. The Agencies have said such an agreement could be "informal or formal, written or unwritten, spoken or unspoken."[40] The Agencies assert in their guidelines that the DOJ intends to prosecute such naked restraints in criminal proceedings.[41] Any no-poaching agreement, therefore, could be a violation of the antitrust laws. Such a violation could result in criminal prosecution by the DOJ against the individual and/or company, civil prosecution by the DOJ or FTC, and/or private suits that are eligible for treble damages if successful. Even information sharing without an overt agreement can reduce competition in the labor market. Specifically, the Agencies caution against sharing wage and benefit information with other employers, as this information sharing could be used to negatively affect compensation for employees. This kind of information sharing can also be offensive to the antitrust laws and lead to scrutiny by the Agencies or private claims.

Federal and State Laws

Recently, state laws have been passed that would prohibit no-poaching agreements or severely restrict them. For example, the Massachusetts Noncompetition Agreement Act, passed in 2018, banned no-poaching agreements for certain medical professions, including physicians, nurses, psychologists, and a few other

---

[40] Department of Justice and Federal Trade Commission (2016, 3).
[41] Department of Justice and Federal Trade Commission (2016, 4).

non-health-care-related professions.[42] Florida also passed a similar law in 2019 that banned no-poaching agreements between medical specialists and their employers.[43] Other states, such as California, Washington, North Dakota, Oklahoma, Maine, and New Hampshire, also have no-poaching agreement legislation.[44]

In keeping with his tough stance on antitrust issues, President Biden seeks to ban most no-poaching agreements, except for those that are necessary to protect trade secrets. In July 2021, he signed the Executive Order on Promoting Competition in the American Economy that would do just that. The hope is that harmful no-poaching agreements will be limited.

16.6 CONCLUDING REMARKS

The Agencies have made very clear statements to employers and their human resource representatives about how no-poaching agreements will be perceived and subsequently treated under the antitrust laws. It is clear that no-poaching agreements are harmful to the competitive process, to employees and their compensation, and to social welfare. Collusive no-poaching agreements result in the depression of wages through reductions in recruiting and information available to employees. Employees affected by no-poaching agreements have suffered antitrust injury in the form of undercompensation and should be able to collect antitrust damages.

REFERENCES

Amidi, Amid. (2018). *Animation Workers Set to Receive $170 Million Payout from Wage-Theft Lawsuit*. Cartoonbrew. www.cartoonbrew.com/artist-rights/animation-workers-set-to-receive-170-million-payout-from-wage-theft-lawsuit-161482.html.

Blair, Roger D., and Jeffrey L. Harrison. (2010). *Monopsony in Law and Economics*. New York: Cambridge University Press.

---

[42] Massachusetts Noncompetition Agreement Act, MGL c.149, Section 24L (2018).
[43] Pazanowski (2019).   [44] Milizio (2021).

Blair, Roger D., and John E. Lopatka. (2016). The Economic Effects of Anti-Tampering Rules in Professional Sports Leagues. *Managerial and Decision Economics* 38:704–713.

Department of Justice and Federal Trade Commission. (2016). Antitrust Guidance for Human Resource Professionals. www.justice.gov/atr/file/903511/download.

Krueger, Alan B., and Orley Ashenfelter. (2018). *Theory and Evidence on Employer Collusion in the Franchise Sector*. NBER Working Paper No. 24831.

Lerner, Abba. (1934). The Concept of Monopoly and Measurement of Monopoly Power. *Review of Economic Studies* 1: 157–175.

Lindsay, Michael A. (2019). McDonald's and Medicine: Developments in the Law of No-Poaching and Wage-Fixing Agreements. *Antitrust* 33: 18–28.

Milizio, Joseph G. (2021). *Biden Pushes for National Ban of Non-Compete Agreements*. Vmm Legal. www.vmmlegal.com/publications/2021/july/biden-pushes-for-national-ban-of-non-compete-agr/.

Naidu, Suresh, Eric A. Posner, and Glen Weyl. (2018). Antitrust Remedies for Labor Market Power. *Harvard Law Review* 132: 537–601.

Pazanowski, Mary Anne. (2019). *Florida Can Enforce Law Outlawing Doctors' Noncompete Contracts*. Bloomberg Law. https://news.bloomberglaw.com/health-law-and-business/florida-can-enforce-law-outlawing-doctors-noncompete-contracts.

Robinson, Joan. (1933). *The Economics of Imperfect Competition*, London: Macmillan.

Sullivan, Daniel. (1989). Monopsony Power in the Market for Nurses. *Journal of Law and Economics* 32: 135–178.

Young, A. Christopher. (2019). *Legal Challenges to No-Poach Provisions in Franchise Agreements*. Pepper Hamilton LLP. www.pepperlaw.com/publications/legal-challenges-to-no-poach-provisions-in-franchise-agreements-2019-01-07/.

PART V **Mergers and Acquisitions**

In this final section of the book, we focus on mergers, both horizontal and vertical. The health care sector has been marked by ever-increasing merger activity in the past 20 years.[1] The total annual number of health care mergers grew from under 800 health care transactions in 2000 to 1,588 health care transactions in 2019. Scholars in part attribute rising health care costs to horizontal mergers, which have rapidly increased concentration in many sectors. Other mergers in health care are vertical, whose effects may be pro-competitive, competitively neutral, or anticompetitive.

HORIZONTAL MERGERS

In Chapter 17, we outline the theory of horizontal mergers. When merging firms have been competing with one another in the same market, the merger is considered horizontal. By definition, horizontal mergers increase concentration in an industry, which can lead to the exercise of monopoly or monopsony power. Yet, horizontal mergers can also introduce efficiencies that benefit consumers.

In Chapter 18, we chronicle how Sutter Health, a hospital system in Northern California, strategically consolidated with other hospitals and physician groups, which allowed it to increase its prices by 113 percent over a decade. By increasing concentration and thereby increasing market power, such mergers can harm consumers. Horizontal mergers, however, can also introduce efficiencies, such as achieving economies of scale in production and administration.[2]

---

[1] We consider mergers to encompass mergers, acquisitions, and affiliations.
[2] When the average cost of a product decreases with increased production, firms should expand production or merge to take advantage of the increased efficiency of the lowered average cost of production. This is known as economies of scale.

Often, merged firms can take advantage of economies of scale and offer a greater number of products at a lower average cost, which benefits consumers. For example, some hospitals merge in order to consolidate capital, which would allow them to invest in advanced IT systems, data analytics, and population health initiatives.[3] By consolidating, the average cost of these investments is lower than if each hospital needed to purchase these goods on its own. Consumers then receive higher-quality care at a lower price than if the firms had not merged.

VERTICAL MERGERS

In Chapter 19, we examine vertical mergers. When the firms that operate at different levels of a supply chain merge, the merger is vertical. If an acute care hospital merges with a rehabilitation facility, that merger is vertical. If a drug store chain acquires a pharmacy benefit manager, that merger is also vertical. In general, vertical mergers pose fewer anticompetitive challenges than horizontal mergers since the merging firms were not competing with each other. Vertical mergers often lead to substantial efficiencies that benefit consumers, but the Agencies should be careful to consider the possibilities of market foreclosure and raising rivals' costs. In a successive monopoly case, where there is a monopoly at two or more levels of the supply chain, double marginalization arises as each firm individually maximizes its profit by charging a significant markup. Vertical integration allows the integrated firm to maximize joint profits and thereby eliminate double marginalization, which benefits consumers. Vertical mergers can also lead to reductions in transaction costs, which make firms more efficient.

Although two vertically integrated firms were not directly competing before the merger, the integration leads to a change in profit incentives. Now, instead of each firm trying to maximize its own profits, joint profits are maximized. This can be a problem when an

---

[3] Herschman et al. (2020).

integrated firm can leverage its market power at one level of the supply chain and impose it at a different level. The integrated firm may find it profitable to stop selling inputs (market foreclosure) or raise the price of those inputs (raising rivals' costs) to other downstream firms in order to increase its downstream profits.

The antitrust Agencies, the DOJ and the FTC, review mergers and are tasked with ensuring that only mergers that are procompetitive or competitively neutral on balance are allowed to proceed. Using economic theory, prior experience, and professional judgment, as well as certain tools, such as measures of market concentration, the Agencies determine the likely effects that a merger will have after its consummation. The Agencies can be quite effective at stemming the tide of anticompetitive mergers. Not only have they blocked a number of anticompetitive mergers, but moreover, increased enforcement activity leads to a reduction in proposed mergers, especially those that are more likely to be anticompetitive. In Chapters 18 and 20, we discuss the methodology that the Agencies use to evaluate horizontal mergers and vertical mergers, respectively. We illustrate their processes using specific health care examples.

REFERENCE

Herschman, Gary W., Anjana D. Patel, Larry Kocot, and Hector M. Torres. (2020). *INSIGHT: Health-Care Consolidation Strong in 2019: Expect Even Stronger 2020*. Bloomberg Law. https://news.bloomberglaw.com/health-law-and-business/insight-health-care-consolidation-strong-in-2019-expect-even-stronger-2020.

17 The Economics of Horizontal Mergers

17.1 INTRODUCTION

Mergers are ubiquitous in various health care markets,[1] including pharmaceutical manufacturers, acute care hospitals, health insurers, medical device manufacturers, and physician groups. In most instances, mergers are horizontal, which means that two or more competitors join forces. In other instances, mergers are vertical, which means that a supplier buys its customer or an end user buys one of its suppliers. This chapter and Chapter 18 focus on horizontal mergers while Chapters 19 and 20 examine vertical mergers.

There are two key reasons a merger increases concentration in a market, which could increase monopoly power and be anticompetitive. First, a merger could alter the market structure such that the newly merged entity would have the ability to exercise unilateral market power. Second, the merger might alter the market structure such that overt or tacit collusion is more likely. The economic concerns surrounding either unilateral or coordinated effects are familiar: higher prices, lower quantity and/or lower quality, and reduced consumer and social welfare.[2]

At the same time, however, mergers can also lead to substantial efficiencies that would not be realized otherwise. These efficiencies increase social welfare by freeing up resources for other socially beneficial pursuits. Gains in efficiency improve profits by reducing costs,

---

[1] In some technical respects, mergers, acquisitions, consolidations, and joint ventures are legally distinct. For our purposes, however, we refer to all of them simply as "mergers." If any distinctions are important in specific instances, we will note that at the time.

[2] See Part I and Part II for more information about the harms of unilateral and coordinated effects in output markets.

whereas gains in quality improve profits by making the merged firm's output more attractive to consumers.

Merger policy in the United States is governed by Section 7 of the Clayton Act, which forbids mergers that are apt to impair competition or tend to create a monopoly. Since Section 7 is a preventive – rather than a remedial – provision, the DOJ or FTC need not demonstrate actual harm. The Agencies need only prove that adverse effects are likely to accompany that merger. A careful review of the change in the market structure following the proposed merger is often employed to determine the likelihood of an adverse effect.[3]

In Section 17.2, we discuss the economic incentives for and consequences of horizontal mergers for the merging firms. In Section 17.3, we then examine the trade-off between welfare-enhancing efficiencies and increases in monopoly power that result from a merger between sellers. The section also covers the Williamson welfare trade-off. We adapt this analysis to mergers between buyers in Section 17.4. In Section 17.5, we review the trade-offs for mergers that result in higher quality. We provide concluding remarks in Section 17.6.

17.2   MERGERS TO MONOPOLY

For antitrust purposes, we are primarily concerned with mergers that are likely to result in noncompetitive prices and outputs. Although cartels may accomplish the same end, a merger that combines all the firms in an industry, which would result in complete monopolization, is far superior for a firm than forming a cartel. After a merger, no cheating and disputes over prices, territories, customers, or market shares exist because a single-firm monopoly has resulted. Moreover, there will be no non-price competition threatening to dissipate the economic profits. The only remaining difficulty for the firm is controlling entry, which, of course, may prove to be difficult in the

---

[3] We discuss how the Department of Justice and Federal Trade Commission evaluate horizontal mergers in Chapter 18.

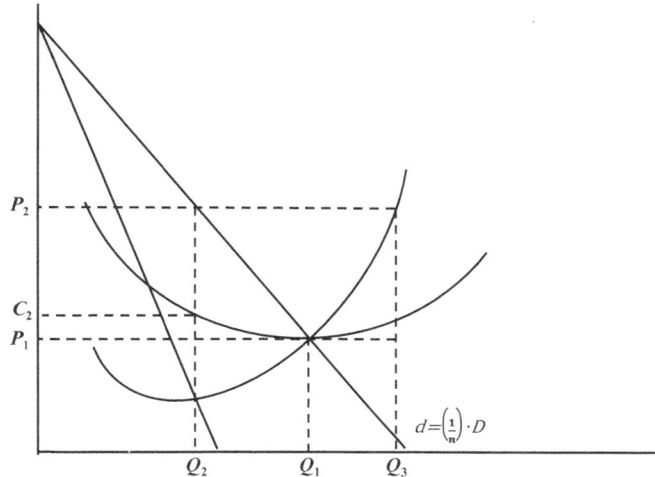

FIGURE 17.1 The problem of merging to monopoly

presence of positive economic profits. Merging to a complete monopoly, however, will seldom succeed due to the profit incentive for non-merged firms to remain outside the consolidation.

In attempting to merge to monopoly, it will become increasingly expensive for a dominant firm to acquire the remaining independent firms. This increasing cost of additional acquisitions can be seen in Figure 17.1, where a representative firm's average and marginal cost curves are labeled AC and MC, respectively, and the proportional demand function and the associated marginal revenue are d and mr.[4] Before the merger, each firm would have produced the competitive output of Q_1 and sold it at the competitive price of P_1. In the short run, the goal of a merger to monopoly in this industry is to have each firm reduce its output to Q_2, which is its share of the total

---

[4] At each price, the quantity on the proportional demand curve is $(1/n) \cdot Q$, where n is the number of firms and Q is the corresponding quantity on the market demand curve.

monopoly output. As a result of the reduced production, the price would rise to P_2 and excess profits per firm would be $(P_2 - C_2)Q_2$, which is the monopoly equilibrium price and profit, where C_2 represents the average cost at Q_2.

The value to the independent firm of refusing to merge, however, will be much larger. If the firm depicted in Figure 17.1 were to remain independent, it could act as a price taker and view P_2 as its marginal revenue function.[5] The optimal output for this firm would then be Q_3 where its marginal cost equals P_2. Its profit in this case is much larger than $(P_2 - C_2)Q_2$. Thus, it is more profitable for a single firm to remain outside the consolidation. Consequently, to convince a reluctant firm that merger is in its best interest, the merging firm may have to resort to some sort of predatory, or economically coercive, conduct designed to lower the independent firm's profits.[6]

Another alternative would be to simply ignore the firms that refuse to merge. In that case, the optimal price and output would follow the dominant firm model. Because the dominant firm model yields a price and profit that are above competitive equilibrium levels, however, mergers that fall short of complete monopolization of the industry can, nonetheless, prove to be profitable and welfare-reducing. Such mergers increase the degree of monopoly power held by the combined organization, even though a pure monopoly may not result.

Rather than coercing all industry members to merge, the willing partners will simply maximize their profits subject to the presence of independent firms. If the newly merged firm is dominant, it will exercise unilateral market power. To the extent that the resulting price and output are at noncompetitive levels, there will be losses in both consumer welfare and social welfare.

---

[5] The increase of quantity sold by the independent firm will decrease the price to some extent. However, if the number of firms in the industry is large, one firm's deviation will negligibly affect the price.

[6] In the Gilded Age (1870s to around 1900), the robber barons, such as Standard Oil, used predatory practices to force smaller rivals to sell their holdings to the larger firm. If it were profitable to merge, the smaller firms would have willingly given up their businesses without need for predatory practices.

In spite of the independent rivals, the dominant firm may still be able to price above the competitive level and thereby reduce both social welfare and consumer welfare. Beyond the risk of anticompetitive pricing from either a pure monopoly or a dominant firm, some mergers may create a market environment wherein collusion – either tacit or overt – among the remaining firms becomes more likely.

17.3   MERGERS OF PRODUCERS TO REALIZE EFFICIENCIES

Mergers may evoke competitive concerns regarding either unilateral monopoly power or collusive monopoly power. In some instances, the merging parties will experience efficiencies that cannot be realized in the absence of the merger, increasing social welfare.[7] These *merger-specific* efficiencies may offset the competitive concerns in some cases, but not in others. We revisit the welfare analysis introduced by Williamson[8] to clarify a possibly misunderstood aspect of the cost savings.

When formerly competing sellers merge, concentration in the relevant market necessarily increases. The magnitude of the change in concentration depends on the relative sizes of the merging firms. If the merger yields merger-specific efficiencies, one of three things is apt to happen. First, if the market is unconcentrated before and after the merger, this merger poses no antitrust concerns since the price will remain competitive. Given the premerger and postmerger market structure, this merger would not attract much attention from the Agencies.

Second, the merger could alter the market structure in such a way that noncompetitive pricing occurs, but the postmerger actual price is still below the premerger price due to substantial cost savings. If these efficiencies are merger specific, this merger should still be applauded because consumers benefit from lower prices and greater output. The fact that actual prices are above the postmerger

---

[7] Here, we provide an example of such an efficiency. There are two firms that produce the same product but have excess capacity at their plants. By merging, the firms can concentrate production of the product at one plant and direct resources invested in the second plant to other pursuits.

[8] Williamson (1968).

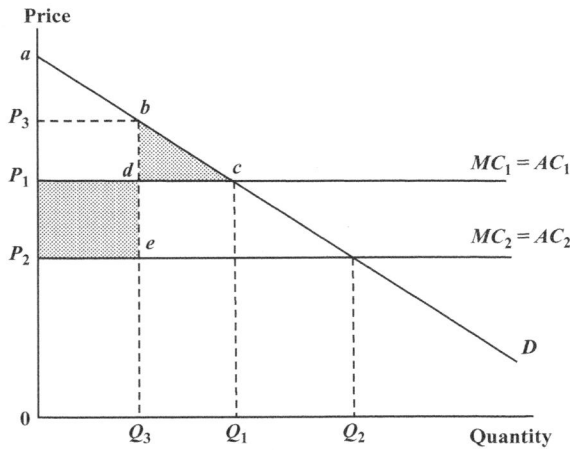

FIGURE 17.2 The Williamson welfare trade-off

competitive level may seem anticompetitive, but consumers are still better off on balance. Moreover, this type of merger satisfies the standards set forth in the 2010 Merger Guidelines: "[T]he Agency considers whether cognizable efficiencies likely would be sufficient to reverse the merger's potential to harm consumers in the relevant market, e.g., by preventing price increases in that market."[9] This is the pass-through requirement: The cost savings are large enough to result in lower prices for consumers in spite of the increase in monopoly power.

The third and most interesting possibility involves the Williamson trade-off.[10] In this case, merger-specific efficiencies reduce the per unit cost of production and/or distribution, but the increase in market concentration is sufficient to produce a price above the pre-merger level. Thus, the pass-through requirement is not met and such a merger is apt to be prohibited. In some instances, this is the correct outcome, but in others it is not. This case is illustrated in Figure 17.2.

---

[9] Yde and Vita (1996, 2006). DOJ/ FTC Horizontal Merger Guidelines, §4 (2010). This pass-through effect and its relationship to market power has been discussed at length by Paul Yde and Michael Vita.

[10] Williamson (1968). See Bet and Blair (2019) for an overview of the Williamson welfare trade-off.

The premerger price and quantity, P_1 and Q_1, respectively, are determined by the equality of demand (D) and the competitive supply, which is shown as $MC_1 = AC_1$. The merger increases efficiency as reflected in the decrease in costs to $MC_2 = AC_2$. If market power does not increase as a result of the merger, the merger raises no apparent antitrust policy concerns. Competition leads to a price reduction from P_1 to P_2 as the cost savings are passed on to consumers.

Complications arise when market power increases due to the efficiency-enhancing merger. Consider Figure 17.2. Suppose that the merger leads to the indicated cost savings, but the exercise of the resulting market power leads to an increase in price from P_1 to P_3 with a corresponding decrease in quantity from Q_1 to Q_3. The evaluation of this merger is somewhat complicated. From the social welfare perspective, the desirability of our efficiency-enhancing merger depends on the relative magnitudes of the allocative inefficiency caused by the price increase and the cost savings.

Reviewing mergers from a social welfare perspective requires the Williamson (1968) welfare trade-off. Whether social welfare rises or falls depends on the relative magnitudes of the allocative inefficiency and the cost savings. In Figure 17.2, the allocative inefficiency is given by the triangular area bcd. The cost savings are given by the rectangle $P_1 de P_2$. As Figure 17.2 is drawn, the cost savings appear to be larger than the allocative inefficiency. In that event, the merger should not be barred because the social benefits of the cost savings outweigh the allocative inefficiency and social welfare increases. The merger is Kaldor-Hicks efficient because the winners (the producers) *could* compensate the losers (the consumers) and still be better off.[11] But this result need not always be the case. When the allocative inefficiency outweighs the cost savings, the merger reduces both consumer welfare and social welfare. The merger is inefficient on the Kaldor-Hicks criterion because the winners cannot compensate

[11] Hicks (1939); Kaldor (1939); Miceli (2009); Just, Hueth, and Schmitz (2004).

the losers. The DOJ and FTC should prevent such a merger. Since we cannot presume that the net effect of an efficiency-enhancing merger of rival sellers will inevitably be positive or negative, we need reliable estimates of the cost savings as well as the allocative inefficiency. This is particularly daunting because both estimates are needed before the merger is actually consummated.[12] This is even more complicated when the merger stops short of monopoly. In that event, the merged firm experiences cost savings while the rivals do not, but all firms realize price increases and higher profits.[13]

The Merger Guidelines demand large – even extraordinary – efficiencies if a structural analysis predicts a substantial anticompetitive effect. But this may be too demanding. To see this, suppose that demand is given by $P = 100 - 0.001Q$ and marginal cost is 20. The competitive solution is, of course, $P = 20$ and $Q = 80,000$. Now suppose a merger-specific efficiency would decrease marginal cost by 10 percent to 18. The price would have to increase by more than two times the per unit cost reduction for the merger to be socially inefficient. If the price rose from 20 to 24.21, the allocative inefficiency would be precisely equal to the cost savings.[14]

Since the Merger Guidelines adopt consumer welfare, rather than social welfare, as the appropriate standard of analysis, it is important to analyze this merger on that restricted basis. From the consumer's perspective, the merger appears to be clearly undesirable. The price paid rises, the quantity consumed falls, and the consumer does not appear to enjoy any of the benefits of the cost reduction. The allocative inefficiency flowing from the exercise of market power causes consumer surplus to fall from area acP_1 to area abP_3. If the

---

[12] Mergers that have already been consummated can, of course, be challenged after the fact. In that event, proof of the cost savings will be possible – at least in principle – but estimating the allocative inefficiency will be no easy task.

[13] The other firms would appear to have an incentive to merge to realize similar cost savings. This could result in further increases in price and further antitrust enforcement issues.

[14] Finding P_3 involves equating the area of P_1deP_2, which is $(P_1 - P_2)Q_3$ and bde, which is $\frac{1}{2}(P_3 - P_1)(Q_1 - Q_3)$ and solving for P_3.

lawfulness of the merger is determined solely on the basis of consumer welfare in this market, then this merger would be unlawful.

This result depends on confining the cognizable consumer benefits to the relevant antitrust market. But this is too narrow because even if the focus is solely on *consumer* welfare, the cost savings benefit consumers generally. These cost savings do, of course, improve the profits of the sellers in this market.[15] But it would be a mistake to dismiss these cost savings as of no consequence to consumers.[16] The sellers' costs fall because fewer scarce resources are needed to produce any given quantity of output. In Figure 17.2, the cost savings of $(AC_1 - AC_2)Q_3$ represent resources that are not needed to produce Q_3. These resources are then available to produce goods and services in other markets. The consumer benefits flowing from these cost savings may be diffused throughout the economy, but they exist nonetheless.[17]

17.4   MERGERS OF BUYERS TO REALIZE EFFICIENCIES

At times, buyers of the same input merge in order to realize efficiencies. Such mergers may arouse antitrust concerns. On the one hand, mergers among buyers may raise competitive concerns when they result in monopsony power, which is the power to depress price below the competitive level by curtailing purchases.[18] On the other hand, these mergers may foster efficiencies that can offset the competitive

---

[15] The profits flowing from the merger are equal to $(P_3 - P_2)Q_3$. Part of this profit is due to market power and part is due to the cost savings.

[16] We are not counting the cost savings twice. We could dismiss those savings as beneficial to the sellers, but we should consider them benefits to consumers.

[17] Williamson alludes to this type of effect in his qualifications of a partial equilibrium approach. He stated, "Whereas partial equilibrium analysis indicates that an increase in the monopoly price in any one sector invariably yields a loss, viewed more generally such an isolated price increase may actually lead to a desirable reallocation of resources. Conceivably, therefore, a merger that has monopoly power and cost-saving consequences could yield benefits in both respects although it is probably rare that operational content can be supplied" (Williamson 1968).

[18] Blair and Harrison (1992).

concerns in whole, in part, or not at all. Here, we extend the welfare trade-off presented by Williamson to the case of monopsony.

When formerly competing buyers merge, concentration on the buying side of the relevant market necessarily increases. Whether the merger is objectionable, however, depends on the change in market structure after the merger. If both the premerger and postmerger market structures are competitive or nearly so, a merger will have little negative impact on the welfare of input suppliers. The merger most likely yields efficiencies that will wholly offset the entire harm to the suppliers. This merger would not attract much attention from the Agencies since (1) it would have no discernible effect on the price the newly merged firm pays and (2) the merger could alter the market structure in such a way that noncompetitive pricing would occur, but the postmerger price paid would still be above the premerger price due to substantial efficiencies. There are two factors at play. First, the merger-specific efficiencies would cause derived demand to shift upward, which would increase the price paid to the suppliers. Second, the postmerger market structure is more concentrated, which leads to monopsony power and lower prices paid. As long as the benefit from the efficiencies compensates the input suppliers for the increased concentration, this merger would not be objectionable.

Another scenario involves the Williamson welfare trade-off as adapted to monopsony. In this case, merger-specific efficiencies reduce the transaction costs of the buyers, but the increase in market concentration is sufficient to produce a price and quantity below the premerger level. Even though social welfare increases, the wins and losses are distributed unevenly. The buyers realize increased surplus at the expense of the input suppliers.

More specifically, we consider the situation in which the buyers purchase an intermediate good that is used to produce a final good. The demand for the intermediate good is derived from consumer demand for the final good. If the cost of transforming the intermediate good into a final good falls, then the derived demand will shift to the right and the intermediate good becomes more valuable to the buyers.

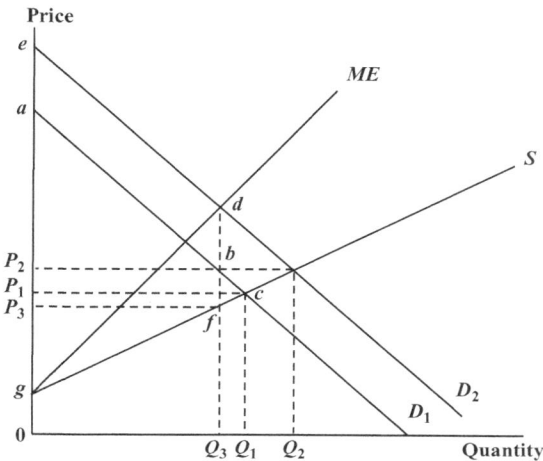

FIGURE 17.3 Merger-specific efficiencies and monopsony: The welfare trade-off

In this case, transactional efficiencies lead to a shift in the derived demand for the intermediate good in question. The economic effects are illustrated in Figure 17.3.

The premerger price (P_1) and quantity (Q_1) are determined by the equality of derived demand (D_1) and supply (S). The efficiencies resulting from the merger of buyers lead to a shift in the derived demand from D_1 to D_2. If the merger of formerly competing buyers confers no monopsony power, then the quantity will expand to Q_2 due to the increased value of the intermediate good. Due to the positively sloped supply, the price received by the suppliers rises from P_1 to P_2. In this case, everyone is a winner as buyer surplus and producer surplus both increase.[19] As a result, social welfare rises. The DOJ and FTC should permit such mergers because they pose no competitive threats.

If, however, the efficiency-enhancing merger results in monopsony power, the quantity purchased will be determined by the equality of the marginal expenditure (ME) and the derived demand (D_2).

---

[19] We refer to buyer surplus rather than consumer surplus because the buyers of the intermediate good are firms. The concept is the same.

In Figure 17.3, the profit-maximizing quantity falls from Q_1 to Q_3 and the price falls from P_1 to P_3. As a result, there is a welfare loss due to allocative inefficiency as well as enhanced buyer surplus that flows from the efficiency.[20] To be sure, there will be an increase in buyer surplus that is simply a transfer from producers due to the monopsony power employed. But there is additional buyer surplus that results from the efficiency. It is only the latter that should be compared to the allocative inefficiency in evaluating the impact on social welfare.

If the lawfulness of this merger depends solely on its impact on the competitive suppliers, then the merger would be unlawful due to the reduction in producer surplus from the premerger area P_1cg to the post-merger area P_3fg. On social welfare grounds, however, the allo-cative inefficiency captured by the triangular area bcf must be com-pared to the reduction in cost captured by the area between the two derived demand curves, that is, area $abde$. If the cost savings outweigh the allocative inefficiency, then the merger should be allowed; other-wise, it should not be allowed.

In the event that the reduction in transaction costs outweighs the allocative inefficiency, the DOJ and FTC should not bar the merger since it would be Kaldor-Hicks efficient. The buyers could compensate the input suppliers and still be better off, which indicates an overall increase in social welfare. But when the allocative ineffi-ciency outweighs the cost savings, the merger reduces both producer welfare and social welfare. The merger is inefficient on the Kaldor-Hicks criterion because the winners cannot profitably compensate the losers and, therefore, the merger should be forbidden.

The problems associated with providing a sound evidentiary basis for drawing inferences regarding the welfare effects of a merger of buyers is the same as those for a merger of sellers.

---

[20] It is possible for the derived demand to shift enough for the postmerger quantity to increase in spite of the monopsony power. In this event, producer surplus would increase even though there would be some allocative inefficiency. This is the second possible outcome of a merger that was described earlier in Section 17.3.

From an economic perspective, social welfare is the correct standard for evaluating the economic effects of a merger among buyers. The Supreme Court, however, is not clear on this. At times, the Court refers to social welfare, but at other times it refers to consumer welfare. Since an argument can therefore be made that the appropriate standard of analysis is input supplier welfare rather than social welfare, it is important to analyze this merger on that restricted basis.[21] From the supplier's perspective, the merger appears to be clearly undesirable. The price the suppliers receive falls, the quantity sold falls, and the suppliers do not appear to enjoy any benefits from the cost reduction. This conclusion depends, however, on confining the cognizable supplier benefits to the relevant antitrust market. But this is too narrow because even if our focus is solely on *supplier* welfare, the cost savings benefit suppliers generally. It would be a mistake to dismiss these cost savings as having no consequence for the suppliers. The buyers' costs fall because fewer scarce resources are needed to produce the output being sold. These resources are then available to produce goods and services in other markets. The benefits to the input supplier flowing from these cost savings may be diffused throughout the economy, but they exist nonetheless.

17.5 MERGER EFFICIENCIES RESULTING IN INCREASED QUALITY

Consider a merger that leads to a better product. All consumers prefer the improved product over the old, lower-quality product and are willing to pay more for it.[22] In short, demand for the improved product lies above demand for the old product. The result of a merger that improves quality may well be an increase in price, but that does not

---

[21] The 2010 Merger Guidelines are designed to deal with merging sellers and seek to protect customers. As applied to merging buyers, the concern shifts to protecting suppliers.

[22] *Quality* is a general term that acquires meaning from the context. Quality may refer to fit, finish, durability, colorfastness, taste, appearance, and functionality, among other attributes. More of any attribute is usually desirable and, therefore, enhances the product's value to the consumer.

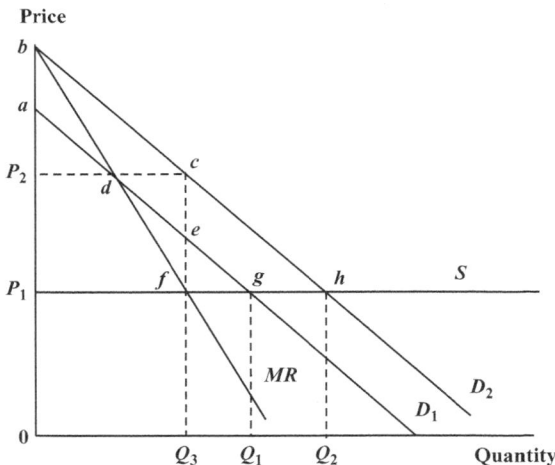

FIGURE 17.4 The welfare trade-off of a quality-enhancing merger

necessarily mean that the merger is anticompetitive. The effect on consumer welfare is ambiguous. In fact, consumer surplus may rise, fall, or stay the same depending on what happens to the price of the product.

In Figure 17.4, D_1 represents the demand for the product in question before the quality-improving merger and S is the perfectly elastic supply.[23] The premerger price and quantity are P_1 and Q_1, respectively. Now suppose that a merger enables the newly merged firm to improve the quality of the product. For ease of exposition, we assume that the efficiencies permit the product improvement without an increase in cost.[24] This means that the supply curve of the improved product is identical to the supply of the old, lower-quality product. The improved quality causes the demand to shift. Assuming that all consumers value the improved quality equally, there will be a parallel shift in demand from D_1 to D_2 and social welfare will

---

[23] The welfare results are more complicated when the supply is positively sloped.
[24] This assumption can be relaxed, but doing so adds some complications that are not relevant to the present analysis.

increase.[25] If the market remains competitive, then the price will remain at P_1 but the quantity will expand to Q_2. The effect of the improved quality is an unambiguous increase in consumer (and social) welfare. The premerger consumer surplus is equal to area agP_1, whereas the postmerger consumer surplus is equal to area bhP_1. Presumably, this merger would not arouse any antitrust concerns because it does not alter the market structure in a competitively significant way.

Suppose, however, that the quality-improving merger resulted in substantial market power. The enhanced market power leads, say, to an increase in price from P_1 to P_2 and a decline in quantity from Q_1 to Q_3. In that event, the welfare trade-off would be analogous to the one developed by Williamson. In this case, the allocative inefficiency of merging is equal to the triangular area egf, whereas the gain in consumer and producer surplus due to the quality improvement is equal to area $abce$. The relative magnitudes of these two areas cannot be determined on an a priori basis. If the gain due to the quality improvement exceeds the loss in allocative efficiency, the merger is desirable in spite of the increase in market power. This merger improves social welfare and, therefore, should be permitted on that basis. Conversely, if the allocative inefficiency swamps the gain in consumer surplus, then the merger is undesirable on social welfare grounds.

The Merger Guidelines focus on consumer welfare rather than social welfare. On this more restricted basis, the relevant comparison is (1) area $abcd$, which is the increase in consumer surplus due to the quality improvement; and (2) area P_2dgP_1, which is the allocative inefficiency plus the conversion of premerger consumer surplus into profit. Obviously, if the former exceeds the latter, then the merger is pro-consumer and would be desirable on that basis.

---

[25] The assumption that all consumers value the quality improvement equally is unimportant to the generality of the welfare results when the supply is perfectly elastic.

17.6   CONCLUDING REMARKS

Firms merge to improve their profits. The incentive to merge flows from enhanced efficiencies that are made possible by the merger. When the improved efficiencies are unaccompanied by increased market power, the merger should be applauded. When increased efficiency is accompanied by increased market power, there are conflicting welfare effects that should be weighed in determining the legality of the merger. This weighing is complicated by the fact that mergers are usually evaluated on an ex ante basis.

In any event, if a merger's cost savings exceed the anticipated loss in social welfare, the merger is beneficial on Kaldor-Hicks reckoning. If a merger simply increases market power, it should be banned. Whether the goal of antitrust policy is to promote and preserve consumer welfare or social welfare, mergers that increase market power without any offsetting welfare gains should be proscribed.

REFERENCES

Bet, German, and Roger D. Blair. (2019). Williamson's Welfare Trade-off around the World. *Review of Industrial Organization* 55: 515–533.

Blair, Roger D., and Jeffrey L. Harrison. (1992). The Measurement of Monopsony Power. *The Antitrust Bulletin* 37: 133–150.

Hicks, John. (1939). The Foundations of Welfare Economics. *The Economic Journal* 49: 696–712.

Just, Richard E., Darrel L. Hueth, and Andrew Schmitz. (2004). *The Welfare Economics of Public Policy*. Northampton, UK: Edward Elgar.

Kaldor, Nicholas. (1939). Welfare Propositions in Economics and Interpersonal Comparisons of Utility. *Economic Journal* 49: 549–552.

Miceli, Thomas J. (2009). *The Economic Approach to Law*. 2nd ed. Redwood City, CA: Stanford University Press.

Williamson, Oliver E. (1968). Economies as an Antitrust Defense: The Welfare Tradeoffs. *American Economic Review* 58: 18–36.

Yde, Paul, and Michael Vita. (1996). Merger Efficiencies: Reconsidering the "Passing-On" Requirement. *Antitrust Law Journal* 64: 735–747.

Yde, Paul, and Michael Vita. (2006). Merger Efficiencies: The "Passing-On" Fallacy. *Antitrust* 20: 59–65.

18 Horizontal Merger Policy

18.1 INTRODUCTION

In Chapter 17, we defined horizontal mergers and discussed their possible anticompetitive and procompetitive effects. In this chapter, we review the tools and tactics that the antitrust Agencies use to distinguish anticompetitive from procompetitive mergers and illustrate them with various examples. Effective merger policy is more important than ever due to increased merger and acquisition activity in health care markets.

There are numerous examples of horizontal mergers in every health care market. For instance, two or more physician groups may join forces. Or one acute care hospital may acquire another hospital in the same geographic market. A large pharmaceutical producer may acquire a smaller rival. These mergers may be procompetitive or anticompetitive depending on the structure of the market in which the merger takes place.

A horizontal merger necessarily reduces competition. After all, where once there were two rivals, now there is a single firm. The economic significance of this change in the competitive landscape depends on the number and size distribution of the firms in the market as well as the position of the merging firms in the market. If the merging firms are large enough, they will be required to notify the antitrust Agencies before consummating the merger. In doing so, they will provide a good deal of information about themselves and the market, which will help the antitrust Agencies decide whether to challenge the proposed merger. If the government has decided that the proposed merger poses a competitive threat, the parties can often settle their differences by divesting some assets, which thereby reduces the risk of anticompetitive behavior.

Existing Supreme Court precedent for horizontal mergers does not provide much guidance since the decisions are quite old and were based on outdated economic reasoning. In fact, the precedents laid down in the 1960s may simply reflect unbridled animosity toward big business. In any case, there is little doubt that these cases would be decided differently today.

In this chapter, we begin in Section 18.2 with an examination of Section 7 of the Clayton Act, which is the statutory foundation for merger policy by the Department of Justice (DOJ) and the Federal Trade Commission (FTC). We also examine the role of the DOJ and FTC Horizontal Merger Guidelines, which set out the enforcement policies of the antitrust Agencies. In Section 18.3, we turn our attention to the administration of US merger policy. In Section 18.4, we examine the economic inferences that one may draw from structural conditions. In Section 18.5, we examine *Sutter Health* and showcase the anticompetitive harms that can arise from too much consolidation. We also explore some of the most common tools and tactics used by the Agencies to evaluate horizontal mergers by discussing examples among health insurers, physician groups, and pharmaceutical manufacturers in Section 18.6. We close with some concluding remarks in Section 18.7.

18.2   HORIZONTAL MERGER POLICY

Antitrust policy regarding horizontal mergers resides in Section 7 of the Clayton Act. The language of Section 7 makes it clear that this is a preventive, rather than remedial, measure. More specifically, Section 7 provides that

> No person engaged in commerce . . . shall acquire, directly or
> indirectly, the whole or any part of the stock or other share
> capital . . . or any part of the assets of another person engaged also
> in commerce. . ., where in any line of commerce . . . in any section of

the country, the effect of such acquisition may be substantially to lessen competition, or to tend to create a monopoly.[1]

There are several things worth noting about this provision. First, it is intended to be a preventive measure. When either the DOJ or the FTC challenges a merger, it need not prove actual competitive harm. In fact, neither Agency could prove actual harm since their merger review takes place before the proposed merger is consummated. Consequently, the Agency only has to show that the merger will lead to a change in market structure that *may* substantially lessen competition or tend to create a monopoly. As we will see below, inferences of harm are based primarily on market structure and the presence of entry barriers for new firms. Second, the potential adverse economic effects must occur in an antitrust market in which the forces of supply and demand determine price, quantity, quality, service, and so on. For antitrust purposes, a market has a product dimension and a geographic dimension.

As it turns out, defining an antitrust market is not a trivial exercise. For the most part, market definition is determined by reasonable substitutability. This is often complicated. For example, are all acute care hospitals in the same product market? Or are hospitals with different characteristics (e.g., university teaching hospitals, for-profit hospitals, not-for-profit hospitals, and those with religious affiliations) in separate markets? The answer cannot be found with a priori reasoning. Instead, the answer is an empirical matter.

The DOJ and FTC share the responsibility for public enforcement of Section 7 and are motivated – at least in part – by efficiency considerations. For example, the FTC has developed some expertise in analyzing hospital mergers. Consequently, it is less costly for the FTC to handle new merger proposals by formerly competing hospitals than it would be for the DOJ, so the FTC usually takes the hospital cases.

For decades, both the DOJ and the FTC faced a serious problem in enforcing Section 7 of the Clayton Act. Although it was easier to

---

[1] 15 USC §18.

recognize the competitive harm after a merger had been consummated, it was much more difficult to break up a merger and return to a market structure that lacked the competitive harm. Two firms would merge and one management team would survive. Production facilities would be altered. Some brands would disappear and some products would be abandoned. Channels of distribution would change to reflect the business model of the newly merged firm. There could be significant personnel changes and plant relocations. If either the DOJ or the FTC challenged the merger after its consummation and were successful, restoring the premerger market structure would prove to be extremely complicated, as all of the postmerger changes would have to be undone. Congress recognized this problem and passed the Hart-Scott-Rodino Antitrust Improvements Act of 1976.

Hart-Scott-Rodino Act

Under the Hart-Scott-Rodino (HSR) Act, any proposed merger that exceeds a specific dollar value threshold is subject to the HSR premerger notification requirement. As of 2021, mergers with a combined valuation of assets above $92 million were subject to review.[2] The parties must complete an extensive disclosure and submit it to the DOJ and FTC. The Agencies then decide which of them will evaluate the merger. That Agency has 30 days to decide whether (1) to allow the merger to proceed, (2) to challenge the merger as being anticompetitive, or (3) to make a second request. If the Agency makes a second request, the parties are asked to provide a wealth of additional information. Presumably, the information is necessary for the Agency to make a final assessment of the proposed merger's competitive effects.

In many instances, the merging parties and the Agency settle their differences. This settlement could require divestiture of certain assets or a firewall to restrict the flow of information between the two firms. Once a settlement has been reached, the parties are free to

---

[2] The dollar threshold is adjusted every year.

consummate the merger. For example, the FTC first condemned UnitedHealth's 2019 acquisition of DaVita, a deal worth \$4.3 billion, due to its concern that the merger would significantly harm competition in two Nevada counties. The FTC required that UnitedHealth "divest DaVita's health care provider organization in the Las Vegas Area to Intermountain Health."[3] Once agreed upon, the merger was allowed to proceed.

If the parties do not settle and the Agency still objects to the merger, the Agency will go to court to seek an injunction that prohibits consummation. If the merging parties do not abandon the merger, they will be headed to trial. Generally, if the merging firms cannot resolve the Agency's competitive concerns, the proposed merger will be abandoned. The prospect of a lengthy and costly legal battle may convince the firms that the delay will undermine the economic advantages of the merger.

Horizontal Merger Guidelines

In 2010, the DOJ and the FTC jointly published the 2010 Horizontal Merger Guidelines, which describe how the Agencies evaluate mergers that meet the HSR threshold.[4] These guidelines recognize that mergers have both procompetitive effects, through the merger-specific efficiencies they create, and anticompetitive effects, due to increased market power, which can lead to unilateral or coordinated effects to raise prices for consumers or depress prices for suppliers. When the procompetitive effects outweigh the anticompetitive effects, the merger should be allowed. A merger that is anticompetitive on balance will be condemned. In order to determine whether a proposed merger is anticompetitive or competitively neutral or procompetitive, the Agencies compare the premerger market structure to the postmerger market structure. In the next sections, we describe the

---

[3] Federal Trade Commission and Department of Justice (2019).
[4] Department of Justice and Federal Trade Commission (2010).

Agencies' methods of doing this. The first step in this process is to define the relevant antitrust market.

18.3 DEFINING THE RELEVANT ANTITRUST MARKET

To explain how the DOJ or FTC defines relevant antitrust markets, we use the example of X-rays, which are used for radiological imaging. Suppose that the Agencies are concerned about the effect a merger of two physician clinics may have on the X-ray market in the town of Radio Lodge. The Agencies' first step would be to define a relevant market.[5] First, the Agencies would need to define which products are in the relevant market. This includes X-rays and any reasonable substitutes, such as CT scans.

One conventional measure of substitutability is the cross-elasticity of demand (θ), which is defined as

$$\theta_{xc} = \frac{\partial Q_x}{\partial P_c} \frac{P_c}{Q_x},$$

where Q_x is the quantity of X-rays, P_c is the price of CT scans, and $\frac{\partial Q_x}{\partial P_c}$ is the change in Q_x resulting from a small change in P_c.

If θ_{xc} is positive, then X-rays and CT scans are substitutes. This methodology makes intuitive sense. If the price of CT scans goes up, consumers will switch to using X-rays since they are comparatively cheaper. The term $\frac{\partial Q_x}{\partial P_c}$ is positive since a small increase in the price of CT scans would lead to an increase in the quantity of X-rays purchased, which makes θ_{xc} positive. It does not mean, however, that they are perfect substitutes. Two products may be substitutes without being completely interchangeable.

Second, the DOJ or FTC must define the geographic market for X-rays. The market for X-ray devices and technology is national or even global. The physician clinics in Radio Lodge would likely buy their X-ray machines from manufacturers that also have plenty of

---

[5] An extensive discussion of market definition can be found in chapter 6 of Blair and Kaserman (2009).

other customers nationally. This would indicate that a merger would not significantly increase monopsony power. The market for patient X-rays, however, is more concentrated in Radio Lodge. A patient will usually get an X-ray in a very localized market. It could be in a physician's office or in a nearby imaging center. The cross-elasticity of demand can also be used to describe the geographic market. Essentially, it determines to what extent patients will substitute an X-ray at their doctor's office for an X-ray at another practice if the price of X-rays at their doctor's office goes up.

There are two problems associated with using θ_{xc} to define the relevant market. First, θ_{xc} must be empirically estimated, which is difficult to do in practice. It would be difficult to conduct experiments to determine how many consumers would switch to using X-rays if the price of CT scans increased or how many consumers would move their business to a different practice if the price of X-rays went up. Without a price change, it can be difficult to determine what would happen.

Second, there is no threshold that separates reasonable substitutes from remote substitutes. Ordinarily, we are only concerned with reasonably close substitutes. If, for example, $\theta_{xc} = 0.10$, X-rays and CT scans are substitutes. But are they close enough substitutes for antitrust purposes? If θ_{xc} equals 0.10, a 20 percent increase in the price of CT scans will lead to a 2 percent increase in the use of X-rays. In contrast, if θ_{xc} equals 0.01, a similar 20 percent hike in the price of CT scans will lead to only a 0.2 percent increase in the use of X-rays.

In both cases, the data show that CT scans and X-rays are substitutes. For antitrust purposes, the question is whether they are close enough substitutes to provide competitive discipline. In this example, one might readily infer that a quantity shift from CT scans to X-rays amounting to about 0.2 percent would be insufficient. Whether 2 percent would be enough is open to debate. The same difficulty of using the cross-elasticity of demand is also evident in defining the geographic market.

As a result of these difficulties, the Agencies developed the so-called SSNIP test to find the smallest relevant market in which a hypothetical monopolist or cartel could profitably raise prices by a "small but significant, non-transitory increase in price" (SSNIP). In practice, "small but significant" means 5 percent and "non-transitory" means one year. First, the Agencies would look at a hypothetical market where a monopolist controls all patient X-rays in Radio Lodge. If the monopolist could profitably raise its price by 5 percent, the relevant antitrust market would be X-rays in Radio Lodge. If, however, the price increase would lead to so many defections that the price rise would be unprofitable, the market must be expanded. Suppose the price of X-rays rises, and consumers either travel within a 50-mile radius of Radio Lodge for a better deal on X-rays or switch to CT scans. The SSNIP test would be conducted again, supposing that a monopolist controlled the market for X-rays and CT scans within a 50-mile radius of Radio Lodge. The test is repeated until the supposed monopolist can profitably raise its price.

Determining substitutability on the basis of the SSNIP test has one serious weakness: It is purely hypothetical. The Agencies rely on past data of customer purchasing habits and surveys as well as the conduct of industry participants, among other things, to inform their analysis. Nonetheless, the exercise is hypothetical.

18.4   ECONOMIC EVIDENCE OF COMPETITIVE EFFECTS

Once the DOJ or the FTC has defined the relevant antitrust market, the inquiry turns to market structure. If the health care market in question is highly competitive, with many buyers and sellers of a substantially homogenous product and reasonably easy entry, the Agencies will usually permit mergers without much difficulty. In contrast, when there are few sellers and many buyers or few buyers and many sellers, a proposed merger is apt to receive a careful look because an increase in market concentration may impair competition. In evaluating the likely competitive effects of the proposed merger, the Agency will be interested in premerger and postmerger market structure and the barriers to entry – if any.

Measuring Market Concentration

Once an antitrust market has been defined, the task is to assess the degree of competition that exists in that market. The most relied-upon summary statistic that captures the essence of market structure is the Herfindahl-Hirschman Index (HHI).[6] The HHI is the sum of the squared market shares,

$$HHI = \sum_{i=1}^{n} S_i^2,$$

where n is the number of firms in the market and S_i is the market share of firm i. In order to make computations simpler, one can treat the shares as whole numbers, that is, use 15 in place of 0.15.

As market shares fall and the number of firms increase, the HHI will decline. The lower bound of the HHI is 0. As market shares rise and the number of firms falls, the HHI will rise. The upper bound is 10,000 (for a single-firm monopoly).

The HHI can be used to calculate the "numbers equivalent," which is the number of equal-sized firms that will generate the observed value of the HHI. For example, suppose that there are 20 firms of varying sizes in the market and the HHI is 1,250. The numbers equivalent (N) is

$$N = \frac{10,000}{HHI} = 8.$$

That is, eight firms of equal size will also generate an HHI of 1,250.

Merger Guidelines Thresholds

The Merger Guidelines characterize concentration in three categories: highly concentrated, moderately concentrated, and unconcentrated.

---

[6] This is the statistic that has been incorporated in the DOJ/FTC Horizontal Merger Guidelines.

Table 18.1. *Calculating the HHI*

Hospital	Share	S^2 in decimals	S^2
1	0.1	0.01	100
2	0.05	0.0025	25
3	0.15	0.0225	225
4	0.25	0.0625	625
5	0.12	0.0144	144
6	0.03	0.0009	9
7	0.03	0.0009	9
8	0.09	0.0081	81
9	0.07	0.0049	49
10	0.04	0.0016	16
11	0.05	0.0025	25
12	0.02	0.0004	4
Total	1	0.1312	1312

Note: The third column shows the share squared; the fourth column removes the decimals by multiplying by 10,000.

If the HHI exceeds 2,500, the industry is characterized as highly concentrated. In that event, the number of firms with equal market share must be less than $\frac{10,000}{2,500} = 4$. A market is said to be moderately concentrated if the HHI falls between 1,500 and 2,500. The corresponding firm number equivalent is in the 4–6.67 range. Finally, the market is considered unconcentrated if the HHI is below 1,500, which would correspond to any market that has more than 6.67 firms with equivalent market shares.

Sample Calculation

Suppose that there are 12 hospitals in a metropolitan area. The market shares and the HHI calculations are displayed in Table 18.1. Based on these hypothetical values, the HHI is 0.1312. To avoid decimals, the Guidelines recommend multiplying by 10,000, which converts the HHI to 1,312. This market would be deemed unconcentrated by the standards set forth in the Horizontal Merger Guidelines.

Calculating Delta (Δ)

When two firms merge, the HHI necessarily increases.[7] For purposes of antitrust policy, the question is whether the increase or change in the HHI, which is usually referred to as Δ, is economically significant. As a matter of arithmetic, Δ will always be positive, but any change in price, quantity, and quality may be imperceptible. In theory, some effect will exist, but its economic significance may be extremely small.

The Agencies generally allow mergers that would cause a small change in concentration that corresponds to a change of less than 100 in the HHI, especially in an already unconcentrated market. If the merger would increase the HHI by more than 100 points in a moderately concentrated market, it would often warrant scrutiny. In highly concentrated markets, a change in HHI of between 100 to 200 points would raise significant competitive concerns. If the HHI were to increase more than 200 points, the Agencies would presume that the merger would enhance market power. Only a convincing argument that the merger would not enhance market power would be enough to save this merger.[8]

18.5 MERGERS AND THEIR ANTICOMPETITIVE EFFECTS: *SUTTER HEALTH*

The Agencies are charged with the responsibility of ensuring that anticompetitive mergers do not proceed. But sometimes the Agencies get it wrong or fail to review mergers that ultimately prove to be anticompetitive. Those mergers may lead to increased prices, decreased quantities, and decreased quality of health care services.

---

[7] Prior to the merger, the firms A and B contribute S_A^2 plus S_B^2 to the HHI. Following the merger, the new firm contributes $(S_A + S_B)^2 = S_A^2 + S_B^2 + 2S_A S_B$. Thus, the HHI increases by twice the product of the premerger market shares of the merging firms.

[8] In theory, the merging firms could also make a claim that the substantial efficiencies created by the merger would offset the anticompetitive harms. In reality, a condemned merger has never been approved on the sole basis of an efficiency argument.

This may happen more often than one might expect. First, a number of small mergers may miss the $92 million HSR threshold and cause anticompetitive harm, especially in small local markets.[9] But anticompetitive mergers with a transaction size below the threshold may avoid scrutiny. Indeed, this almost occurred with Otto Bock Healthcare's merger with Freedom Innovations.[10] Second, the Agencies have budget constraints that limit their ability to closely inspect all mergers. By focusing on mergers that are most likely to yield anticompetitive harm, a harmful merger may slip past them, especially since the number of mergers is on the rise.

Sutter Health (Sutter) is a hospital system in Northern California that strategically acquired other hospitals and physician groups in order to increase its market power and thereby increase its profits by raising prices.[11] Sutter now owns hospitals in 24 locations, 36 ambulatory surgery centers, nine cancer centers, seven cardiac centers, and nine major physician organizations. It employs more than 12,000 doctors and serves millions of patients annually.[12] The strategy of market consolidation was profitable, as hospital charges rose by 113 percent from 2004 to 2013 for Sutter and Dignity Health, the two largest hospital systems in California, in comparison to only a 70 percent increase for other hospitals in California.[13]

Hospital rates are generally kept in check by insurance companies that bargain on behalf of their policyholders.[14] Thus, prices are determined based on the relative bargaining power of insurance

[9] Premerger Notification Office Staff (2021).

[10] *In re Otto Bock HealthCare North America, Inc.*, FTC Docket No. 9378 (Federal Trade Commission 2017). Otto Bock was the leading manufacturer of mechanical prosthetic knees, and Freedom Innovations was its main competitor. Although this merger did not fall under the purview of the Hart-Scott-Rodino Act, the FTC discovered this merger and dismantled it soon after it was consummated.

[11] *People of the State of California* v. *Sutter Health*, No. CGC-18-565398 (Sup. C. Cal. 2018). We will discuss mergers between hospitals and physician groups in Chapter 20.

[12] Sutter Health (2021).   [13] Melnick and Maerki (2020).

[14] Due to being small in number, uninsured patients have little power as individuals to influence hospital prices.

companies and hospital networks. In the 1990s, employers moved to large managed care plans. At the same time, there was a rise in merger activity in the hospital sector. A second wave of mergers commenced after the passage of the Affordable Care Act in 2010. According to a 2020 study, 44 percent of all privately insured health care spending can be attributed to short-term hospital costs, and hospital costs can explain a sizable share of the increase in health care spending.[15] Hospital mergers may be contributing to these increases.

Sutter Hospital was first established in Sacramento in 1923, and Sutter Maternity Hospital opened in 1937. Beginning in 1986, Sutter began merging with a number of hospital systems, which allowed it to increase its market share in strategic areas. Notably, in 1996 it merged with the California Healthcare System, which was composed of five large hospitals and gave Sutter a dominant position in San Francisco.[16] By the time it was first challenged for its merger with Summit Health in 1999, Sutter was affiliated with 26 hospitals in Northern California.

The proposed merger was between Sutter's Alta Bates Medical Center and Summit Medical Center, two of the largest hospitals in the Bay Area that were located only three miles apart. The merger was challenged by California Attorney General Bill Lockyer, but Sutter successfully pleaded its case by pointing to travel costs that were allegedly low enough so that other hospitals in the area could success-fully compete with it.[17] Additionally, Sutter pointed to the fact that insurers can steer their patients to lower-cost centers and thereby provide competition.[18] The court ignored a number of internal memos indicating that Sutter was following a strategy of consolidation so that it could leverage its bargaining power over health insurers to increase its prices.[19]

---

[15] Berenson et al. (2020).   [16] Spetz, Seago, and Mitchell (1999).   [17] Tenn (2008).
[18] *People of the State of California* v. *Sutter Health*, No. CGC-18-565398 (Sup. C. Cal. 2018), Complaint for Violations of the Cartwright Act.
[19] Waters (2020).

Allowing this merger to be consummated was a mistake. A retrospective report on this merger conducted by the FTC showed that prices rose after the merger. Specifically, the prices at Summit were estimated to have increased between 23.2 to 50.4 percent due to the merger when controlling for other factors.[20] Additionally, there were other indicators that Sutter would use its market power to its own advantage. Before this case, Sutter had already leveraged its market power in the Sacramento markets in 1998. Sutter threatened to foreclose Blue Cross policyholders from its hospitals unless Blue Cross increased the prices it paid for claims.[21] Blue Cross took these threats seriously. A 2004 report showed that Blue Cross paid 73 percent more for claims at Sutter hospitals than at other hospitals for the same services.[22] In turn, this led to an increase in the prices consumers paid for health insurance.

Sutter used all-or-nothing offers to extract surplus from health insurers. Essentially, it threatened to foreclose policyholders from all its hospitals unless the health insurer agreed to pay higher prices and put Sutter in a more favorable tier. Since Sutter controlled a dominant share of the market, health insurers complied with Sutter's demands. For example, because Sutter dominated maternity care in the Bay Area, any health insurer who wanted to offer maternity care to its policyholders would have to include Sutter in its network. Additionally, Sutter required health insurers to sign contracts that prohibited their sharing any price data with other parties. This limited the ability of government officials or other interested parties to recognize Sutter's anticompetitive actions.[23]

Through consolidation and strategic dominance, Sutter was able to earn higher profits for its hospital services to the detriment of health insurers and consumers. Northern California had a 110 percent higher HHI than Southern California. Hospital prices were also 70 percent higher in Northern California as demonstrated by the

[20] Tenn (2008).   [21] Spetz, Seago, and Mitchell (1999).
[22] California Healthline (2004).   [23] Waters (2020).

median inpatient procedure rate, which was $223,278 in Northern California and only $131,586 in Southern California.[24] This difference can be attributed in part to the higher levels of consolidation seen in Northern California.

In 2018, the State of California brought Sutter Health to court alleging that Sutter had illegally used its market power to increase hospital rates. In the end, Sutter settled for $575 million and was prohibited from using all-or-nothing offers and forcing health insurers to place it in favorable tiers.[25] They also faced a federal suit that went to trial in February 2022, which was decided in Sutter Health's favor.[26] This case clearly shows the dangers of allowing too much consolidation in a market.[27] The number of mergers in the US health care sector, however, continues to rise. The antitrust Agencies have their work cut out for them to ensure that markets do not become too consolidated. In the next section, we discuss how the Agencies review various horizontal mergers.

18.6 AGENCY ANALYSIS OF MERGERS IN HEALTH CARE MARKETS

We turn our attention to some examples of mergers involving health insurers, physician groups, and pharmaceutical companies. We show how the courts analyze merger-specific efficiencies, how the courts have used market share to predict anticompetitive harm, and finally how divestiture may be able to save an otherwise objectionable merger.

Health Insurer Merger: Anthem–Cigna

In 2015, Anthem and Cigna agreed to merge in a $54 billion deal.[28] At the time, Anthem and Cigna were the second and third largest health

---

[24] Nicholas C. Petris Center (2018).   [25] Waters (2020).

[26] *Sidibe* v. *Sutter Health*, No. 3:12-cv-04854 (N.D. Cal. 2021).

[27] In 2021, HCA Healthcare in eastern North Carolina was sued for similar behavior (Bulusu 2021).

[28] *United States* v. *Anthem, Inc., and Cigna Corporation*, No. 1:16-cv-01493 (D. D.C. 2016).

insurers in the United States and competed on a regular basis.[29] Anthem was the largest of 36 insurers in the Blue Cross Blue Shield Association, owned an exclusive license in 14 states to do business under the Blue Cross brand, and had about 39 million members. In certain local markets, Anthem's market share was even larger due to reduced competition. Although Cigna was the third largest health insurer, it was considerably smaller than Anthem, with some 13 million policyholders in the United States. It competed with Anthem, which leveraged its size to negotiate steep discounts with its in-network providers, through innovative health care plans and better customer service. Cigna's plans included value-based alternatives that would incentivize hospitals and doctors to focus on good patient outcomes. Cigna's revenue grew on average by 13 percent in the six years before 2015.[30] Anthem and Cigna competed for national and individual accounts as well as access to health care providers on the basis of price, customer service, care management, wellness programs, and reputation.

National accounts are deals made with large employers with more than 5,000 employees. These employers generally enter into "administrative services only" contracts where the employer takes on the risk of its employees' medical costs but relies on the insurer for administering claims processing and for access to their in-network providers (i.e., a self-insurance plan).[31] Anthem and Cigna were both major players in this market, especially in the 14 states where Anthem was the Blue Cross Blue Shield licensee. A combined merger in the 14 states would have led to a combined 40 percent market share for national accounts. The combined market share for the entire

---

[29] At about the same time, Humana and Aetna, two other dominant health insurance companies, had also agreed to merge. If both of the mergers had been consummated, there would have been only three major health insurers rather than five.

[30] *United States* v. *Anthem, Inc., and Cigna Corporation*, No. 1:16-cv-01493 (D. D.C. 2016), Complaint.

[31] *United States* v. *Anthem, Inc., and Cigna Corporation*, No. 1:16-cv-01493 (D. D.C. 2016), Plaintiffs' Proposed Findings of Fact: Phase 1.

United States would have been 30 percent.[32] Cigna was not affiliated with the Blue Cross Blue Shield brand. Merging with Anthem, however, would have reduced its incentives to compete with other Blue Cross Blue Shield health insurers due to its affiliation with Anthem. The Blue Cross Blue Shield network of health insurers often shared responsibilities for national accounts and thus did not vigorously compete with one another to gain clients. Competition generally came from firms such as Cigna, who were not affiliated with the Blue brand. If, however, Anthem and Cigna had merged, Cigna would have had little incentive to compete for business with other Blue Cross Blue Shield health insurers. Consequently, the negative effects of such a merger, although concentrated in areas where Anthem and Cigna would have had a large combined market share, would also have had far-reaching effects in other areas of the country.

A merger between Anthem and Cigna would also have had deleterious effects on large local employers who purchase health insurance plans from the two parties. The DOJ complaint in this litigation identified at least 35 metropolitan areas, including New York, Los Angeles, San Francisco, Atlanta, and Indianapolis, where Anthem and Cigna would have a large combined market share. Anthem often cited Cigna as its main competitor in these markets, so a merger would drastically reduce competition in these areas. A merger to monopoly would make a bad situation much worse for many local firms, especially since Cigna and Anthem were fierce competitors.

In addition, Cigna and Anthem also compete for individual exchanges, which are plans offered to individuals and families. These exchanges are only sold at county levels, which makes the exchanges market especially prone to high levels of concentration. In many counties, Cigna and Anthem were the only providers of insurance and a merger would reduce other options for individuals

---

[32] *United States* v. *Anthem, Inc., and Cigna Corporation*, No. 1:16-cv-01493 (D. D.C. 2016), Complaint.

and families, who already had little bargaining power. Additionally, a merger would eliminate competition since Cigna had actively been growing in these markets primarily due to diverting market share from Anthem. This competition had led to better-quality plans, better customer service, and other benefits. A merger would have reduced incentives for such innovation.

Finally, a merger could significantly reduce the bargaining power of hospitals and health care providers to receive competitive rates for their services. Insurers compete for doctors, hospitals, and other health care providers in their networks. If health care providers have other options, they can negotiate better rates by threatening to move to a different network. A merger, however, can reduce their options and can lead to substantial monopsony power, which would reduce reimbursement rates to doctors and reduce the quantity of medical services provided.

Such a merger between two of the largest health insurers would have led to a substantial increase in monopoly and monopsony power in many insurance markets across the United States, leading to reductions in the quantity and quality of medical care. Robust competition, however, usually leads to quality insurance plans, better customer service, and innovative value-based contracts. Even though some mergers may increase efficiencies, in this case, a merger would have led to substantial harm to healthcare providers and patients. For this reason, the merger was challenged by the DOJ. Anthem and Cigna countered by indicating that substantial merger-specific efficiencies would outweigh the anticompetitive harm.

The district court rejected this argument, since the proposed efficiencies were neither merger specific nor attainable, and ruled in favor of the DOJ. The decision was appealed to the D.C. Circuit Court of Appeals.[33] On appeal, the main issue was not whether the proposed merger was likely to lessen competition in violation of Section 7 of

---

[33] *United States* v. *Anthem, Inc., and Cigna Corporation*, No. 1:16-cv-01493 (D.C. Court of Appeals 2017).

the Clayton Act, but rather whether the claimed efficiencies created by the merger were both merger specific and large enough to offset any adverse competitive effects. Anthem and Cigna imagined a merged entity that would combine Cigna's innovative insurance plans with Anthem's lower reimbursement rates.

Anthem and Cigna claimed that the merger would lead to savings of $2.4 billion, 98 percent of which would be passed on directly to consumers. These efficiencies would mostly arise due to increased bargaining power that would allow the joint firm to negotiate even steeper discounts with health care providers. Their economic expert determined that this savings would completely offset any anticompetitive harm that could result from the merger. The D.C. Circuit observed, however, that the merger would result in an increase in market power in the health insurance market. As for the claimed efficiencies, the court found that the parties had not proven that the efficiencies were achievable.

Moreover, the alleged cost savings were not the product of true efficiencies resulting from more efficient production. Instead, the reduced expenditure would be driven by the increased exercise of monopsony power, a fact ignored by both the district and appellate courts.[34] Ignoring the adverse welfare effects due to monopsony was unfortunate. The exercise of monopsony leads to a reduction in quantity and perhaps in quality as well.[35] Thus, the exercise of monopsony in the input markets results in consumer welfare losses in the output market.

Next, Anthem claimed that it could incorporate Cigna's innovative plans into its service line, which would benefit consumers. The goal was to offer Cigna's plans at Anthem's lower rates. The appellate court, however, claimed that this efficiency was not merger specific since Anthem could have developed similar plans on its own. Anthem

[34] The district court did not address the government's monopsony concern because it had already deemed the efficiencies to be not merger specific. The appellate court followed the district court's actions in this matter, although the approach was criticized by Justice Brett Kavanaugh, who dissented.

[35] For a thorough treatment of monopsony, see Chapter 11.

claimed that they had had difficulty in developing their own wellness program, but they offered few details that would prove their failure in the past had originated from impossible challenges rather than a lack of effort and a commitment of resources. Thus, the efficiency was not merger specific. Additionally, the alleged efficiencies were found to be both speculative and uncertain. Indeed, the merger may have led to an inferior Cigna product being offered since lower rates would require lower quality and thereby harm consumers.

Both the district and appellate courts enjoined the merger between Anthem and Cigna with good reason. A merger would have significantly reduced competition that had led to innovative health care plans beneficial to consumers. Additionally, it would have led to increases in monopsony power, which would have allowed the firms to depress the rates paid to their in-network health care providers. Although Anthem and Cigna claimed that significant efficiencies could offset this harm, they failed to prove that the efficiencies were attainable and merger specific.

Merger of Physician Groups: Sanford Health–Mid-Dakota Clinic

Physician groups conduct their medical practices, which are businesses, in localized markets. A horizontal merger of two or more physician groups reduces competition in the local market. The economic effect, therefore, could be a significant increase in physician charges, reduced access to care, and even a reduction in quality. In spite of these potential harmful effects, such mergers may be missed by the Agencies because they do not hit the $92 million HSR threshold. But some mergers of physician groups do attract Agency attention. The Sanford Health–Mid-Dakota deal was one such merger.[36]

Sanford Health and Mid-Dakota Clinic agreed to join forces by merging. The FTC contended that the merger would violate Section 7 of the Clayton Act. The FTC identified four relevant service

---

[36] *Federal Trade Commission* v. *Sanford Health*, 926 F. 3d 959 (8th Cir. 2019).

Table 18.2. *Combined shares of the merging physician groups in the Bismarck-Mandan area*

Product market	Combined share in Bismarck-Mandan area (%)
Adult primary care	77
Pediatric care	83
Obstetrics/gynecology	88
General surgery	100

Source: *Federal Trade Commission* v. *Sanford Health*, 926 F. 3d 959 (8th Cir. 2019), Complaint.

markets: adult primary care, pediatric care, obstetrics and gynecology, and general surgery physician services. The FTC identified the geographic market as the four-county Bismarck-Mandan, North Dakota area. We show the relevant combined market shares of Sanford and Mid-Dakota, as estimated by the FTC, in Table 18.2. It was clear that patients would have few options following the proposed merger.

The FTC alleged that the proposed merger would have several adverse competitive effects: "healthcare costs will rise and the incentives to increase service offerings and improve the quality of healthcare will diminish."[37] The FTC pointed out that Sanford and Mid-Dakota are each other's closest competitors. Sanford and Mid-Dakota compete with one another by "purchasing new equipment, updating technology, expanding services, recruiting high quality physicians and providing patients with convenient and accessible physician and surgical services."[38] Since Sanford and Mid-Dakota compete with one another, health insurers benefit in negotiating reimbursement rates. If they stopped competing, reimbursement rates were apt to rise. Consequently, the health insurer would have to raise premiums charged to employers and individuals. Moreover, the postmerger firm would have reduced incentives to improve its quality of care.

[37] *Federal Trade Commission* v. *Sanford Health*, 926 F. 3d 959 (8th Cir. 2019), Complaint at 2.
[38] *Federal Trade Commission* v. *Sanford Health*, 926 F. 3d 959 (8th Cir. 2019).

Table 18.3. *Service market concentration*

Service market	Premerger HHI	Postmerger HHI	Difference
Adult primary care	3220	6013	2793
Pediatric care	3750	7083	3333
Obstetrics/gynecology	4464	7855	3391
General surgery	5200	10000	4800

Source: *Federal Trade Commission* v. *Sanford Health*, 926 F. 3d 959 (8th Cir. 2019), Complaint.

The FTC argued that any merger resulting in an HHI increase of 200 where the postmerger HHI is greater than or equal to 2,500 is presumptively unlawful. In the case at hand, the FTC found that the postmerger HHI was well above the threshold of 2,500. All four service markets were already above 2,500 premerger, but the proposed merger would have made matters much worse. As shown in Table 18.3, the postmerger HHIs increased significantly and the changes in HHI were well above 200. Thus, the proposed merger would make a highly concentrated market even more concentrated.

The FTC identified the anticompetitive consequences of a merger of the two provider groups. First, adverse consequences for health insurers and their policyholders were considered. A health insurance plan must assemble a network of health care providers. The plan's negotiating power is reduced when the number of attractive sources of supply is reduced. The result is higher reimbursement rates to the providers, which translates into higher costs for employers and higher premiums, copayment rates, and deductibles for consumers.

There is a second adverse effect. As in-network providers of a health plan, Sanford and Mid-Dakota were bound by the contract to charge the same fees for the services performed. Without the ability to compete on price, they competed for patients on nonprice terms such as better quality of care, better amenities, better services, and efforts to improve overall patient satisfaction. The merger of Sanford and Mid-Dakota would have eliminated the pressure to compete on non-price terms that would benefit patients.

In spite of the presumptively unlawful consequences of the proposed Sanford–Mid-Dakota merger, efficiencies – if they are merger specific and substantial – could save the merger. In fact, the FTC analyzed the efficiency claims of the parties and found them lacking. The FTC found the cost savings claimed by the parties to be speculative, unsubstantiated, and not merger specific. Moreover, even if they were cognizable, they would not offset the adverse consequences of losing the benefits of competition between Sanford and Mid-Dakota. Sanford decided to drop its proposed acquisition of Mid-Dakota, and the FTC dropped its charges.

Mergers of Pharmaceutical Manufacturers: Amneal–Impax

Pharmaceutical firms manufacture and sell a variety of pharmaceutical drugs. When analyzing a pharmaceutical firm merger, the Agencies may be concerned that the merger will reduce competition in the markets for a few of the pharmaceutical drugs, even though the vast majority of the drug markets in which the firms operate will not be affected. In this scenario, the Agencies may require a divestiture of the problem drugs. In other words, the Agencies may require the firm to sell intellectual property rights, manufacturing plants, equipment, or other assets related to the drug. In this way, the Agencies ensure that competition is not compromised in a few drug markets, while allowing an efficiency-enhancing merger to proceed. We review the acquisition of Impax Laboratories, Inc. (Impax) by Amneal Pharmaceuticals, LLC (Amneal).[39]

Amneal is one of the largest and fastest-growing generic drug companies in the United States. The company was founded in 2002 by

---

[39] *In re Amneal Holdings, LLC, Amneal Pharmaceuticals, LLC, Impax Laboratories, Inc., Impax Laboratories, LLC*, Docket No. C-4650 (Federal Trade Commission 2018).

brothers Chirag and Chintu Patel, who have grown the company through merger and acquisition. The company has numerous manufacturing facilities around the world, many of which are located in India. The company boasts a wide range of generic drugs and injectable drugs.[40]

Impax was a pharmaceutical firm that produced generic drugs as well as a few branded drugs that treated central nervous system diseases. Before the merger, it had a pipeline of 126 generic drugs that had FDA-approved ANDAs. In addition, Impax was developing or in the application process for a number of other generic drugs. Its specialty was controlled-release products.[41]

The merger with Impax made Amneal Pharmaceuticals the fifth largest generic drug manufacturer in the United States, with one of the broadest generic pipelines. It boasted an offering of over 200 generic product families with a variety of dosage forms and delivery systems along with another 220 drugs in the application or development process. For many of these drugs, the company was the first to file or first to market, indicating it could capture a large market share in the generic drug market. Before merging with Impax, Amneal offered no branded drugs.[42]

The merger led to a number of efficiencies that could be considered procompetitive. The merger allowed the firms to consolidate administrative offices and manufacturing and distribution plants. A number of duplicative employment positions could be eliminated, leading to lower salary costs.[43] Additionally, a number of Impax's drugs could be produced by Amneal manufacturing plants, reducing Impax's reliance on contract manufacturers. Finally, the merger increased the countervailing power of Amneal, which allowed it to negotiate better deals with a consolidated retail and wholesale sector.

---

[40] Amneal Pharmaceuticals (2021).   [41] Impax Laboratories (2016).
[42] Amneal Pharmaceuticals (2018).
[43] Note that employees are being let go not because of monopsony power, but because consolidation led to the possibility for a more efficient labor allocation.

The company estimated that they would see $200 million in annual cost savings after three years.

The FTC, who reviewed this merger, was concerned that the merger would decrease current or future competition in the markets for 10 generic drugs. Amneal and Impax were both current producers of 3 of the 10 drugs. The other seven drugs were produced by one of the two generic firms. The FTC was concerned that future competition could be constrained for these drugs since either Amneal or Impax was one of a few firms that could provide entry into the concentrated generic drug market. The FTC recognized the procompetitive aspects of the merger but required the divestment of assets associated with these 10 drugs to mitigate anticompetitive concerns. We review two of these drugs, felbamate and aspirin/dipyridamole.

Amneal and Impax were two of four companies that sold generic felbamate tablets, which are used to treat epilepsy, in the United States at the time. The merger would have led to a reduction from four to three suppliers. At the time of the merger, Amneal had a monopoly on generic aspirin and dipyridamole ER capsules, which are used to mitigate the risk of stroke. The FTC deemed Impax as one of a limited number of firms that was capable of entering this market and competing with Amneal. The FTC reasoned that the merger would reduce the probability of future entry.[44] For this reason, the FTC required divestment of assets. Seven of the drugs were acquired by ANI Pharmaceuticals, Incorporated. The rights to two drugs were acquired by Perrigo Company, plc. Finally, G&W Laboratories acquired the marketing rights for the last drug.[45]

The purpose of a divestiture is to maintain competition in the relevant market. The main idea is that a divestiture will lead to the status quo. The same number of firms will operate in the market and the same number of firms with higher entry probability will exist.

[44] *In re Amneal Holdings, LLC, Amneal Pharmaceuticals, LLC, Impax Laboratories, Inc., Impax Laboratories, LLC*, Docket No. C-4650 (Federal Trade Commission 2018).

[45] Federal Trade Commission (2018).

Using divestiture to resolve merger cases is simple since it requires the Agencies to make the fewest assumptions about the market and has the lowest risk. The key to any divestment agreement is that the company sells a business unit that can operate autonomously after its sale. The FTC generally requires a buyer up front and requires the merging firms to divest within six months to mitigate depreciation of the divested assets. The divestment may include manufacturing facilities, access to key inputs, access to markets for ancillary supply, research and development capabilities, intellectual property, technology, access to personnel, marketing and distribution capabilities, supply, service and customer relationships, capital, and anything else the acquiring firm may need to operate the business effectively.[46]

In the case of felbamate, the merged firm would have had to divest one of its felbamate business units, either Amneal or Impax.[47] The firms could have also offered a "mix and match" divestment that would have allowed them to propose a divestment package including assets from both companies. These packages are more difficult to get approved since it requires more analysis to ensure that the combined asset package will allow a buyer to operate the business autonomously. Because of this divestment, four firms still produce felbamate: Amneal, the two original firms, and a new entrant who bought Amneal's felbamate business unit. Thus, competition is maintained.

Amneal would have divested its aspirin and dipyridamole business unit to another firm according to the settlement. Although Amneal divested its business units, the merged firm would be a prime entrant into the market. According to their online product catalog, Amneal does produce aspirin and ER dipyridamole. Presumably, concentration has decreased in this generic drug market due to Amneal's divestment and eventual reentry.

---

[46] Feinstein (2012).
[47] Note that due to the private nature of the settlement, it is unclear which assets were divested.

Divestment is a simple method the Agencies can use to mitigate the anticompetitive effects a merger may have in certain problem drug markets. Although Amneal needed to divest the business units for 10 generic drugs, its acquisition of Impax proceeded and yielded substantial efficiencies.

18.7 CONCLUDING REMARKS

There have been myriad horizontal mergers in various health care markets. Too much consolidation in local health care markets can lead to decreases in quantity and increases in prices for consumers, leading to a reduction in social welfare. As the *Sutter Health* case shows, effects on price can be quite severe. The Agencies employ various methods, such as a market definition approach, to determine whether a proposed merger would be anticompetitive or whether it would introduce substantial efficiencies and be procompetitive. Sometimes, divestiture can save an otherwise anticompetitive merger. On behalf of consumers, it is important that the Agencies only allow mergers that are procompetitive or competitively neutral to be consummated.

REFERENCES

Amneal Pharmaceuticals. (2018). United States Securities and Exchange Commission Form 10-K. https://s22.q4cdn.com/186279204/files/doc_finan cials/annual/2018/Annual-Report-on-Form-10-K-for-the-Year-Ended-December-31-2018.pdf.

Amneal Pharmaceuticals. (2021). www.amneal.com/about/our-story/.

Berenson, Robert A., Jaime S. King, Katherine L. Gudiksen, Roslyn Murray, and Adele Shartzer (2020). *Addressing Health Care Market Consolidation and High Prices.* Urban Institute. www.urban.org/research/publication/addressing-health-care-market-consolidation-and-high-prices.

Bulusu, Siri. (2021). *HCA Faces Antitrust Claims After North Carolina Hospital Deal.* Bloomberg Law. https://news.bloomberglaw.com/health-law-and-busi ness/hca-faces-antitrust-claims-after-north-carolina-hospital-deal.

Blair, Roger D., and David L. Kaserman. (2009). *Antitrust Economics.* 2nd ed. New York: Oxford University Press.

California Healthline. (2004). *CalPERS Considers Plan to Eliminate Coverage at 45 Hospitals*. https://californiahealthline.org/morning-breakout/calpers-considers-plan-to-eliminate-coverage-at-45-hospitals/.

Department of Justice and Federal Trade Commission. (2010). Horizontal Merger Guidelines. www.justice.gov/sites/default/files/atr/legacy/2010/08/19/hmg-2010.pdf.

Federal Trade Commission. (2018). FTC Approves Final Order Imposing Conditions on Merger of Generic Drug Marketers Amneal Pharmaceuticals LLC and Impax Laboratories Inc. www.ftc.gov/news-events/press-releases/2018/07/ftc-approves-final-order-imposing-conditions-merger-generic-drug.

Federal Trade Commission and Department of Justice. (2019). Hart-Scott-Rodino Annual Report: Fiscal Year 2019. www.ftc.gov/system/files/documents/reports/federal-trade-commission-bureau-competition-department-justice-antitrust-division-hart-scott-rodino/p110014hsrannualreportfy2019_0.pdf.

Feinstein, Richard. (2012). *Negotiating Merger Remedies*. Federal Trade Commission. www.ftc.gov/tips-advice/competition-guidance/merger-remedies.

Impax Laboratories. (2016). United States Securities and Exchange Commission Form 10-K. https://s22.q4cdn.com/186279204/files/doc_financials/2016/annual/Impax-Labs-2016-10K.pdf.

Melnick, Glenn, and Susan Maerki. (2020). *Commissioning Change: How Four States Use Advisory Boards to Contain Health Spending*. California Health Care Foundation. www.chcf.org/wp-content/uploads/2020/01/Commissioning ChangeFourStatesAdvisoryBoards.pdf.

Nicholas C. Petris Center on Health Care Markets and Consumer Welfare. (2018). Consolidation in California's Health Care Market 2010–2016: Impact on Prices and ACA Premiums. https://petris.org/wp-content/uploads/2018/03/CA-Consolidation-Full-Report_03.26.18.pdf.

Premerger Notification Office Staff. (2021). *HSR Threshold Adjustments and Reportability for 2021*. Federal Trade Commission. www.ftc.gov/news-events/blogs/competition-matters/2021/02/hsr-threshold-adjustments-reportability-2021.

Spetz, Joanne, Jean Ann Seago, and Shannon Mitchell. (1999). *Changes in Hospital Ownership in California*. Public Policy Institute of California. www.ppic.org/content/pubs/report/R_1099JSR.pdf.

Sutter Health. (2021). What Is Sutter Health? www.sutterhealth.org/about/what-is-sutter-health.

Tenn, Steven. (2008). *The Price Effects of Hospital Mergers: A Case Study of the Sutter-Summit Transaction*. Federal Trade Commission Working Paper

No. 293. www.ftc.gov/sites/default/files/documents/reports/price-effects-hos
pital-mergers%C2%A0-case-study-sutter-summit-transaction/wp293_0.pdf.

Waters, Rob. (2020). *California's Sutter Health Settlement: What States Can Learn about Protecting Residents from the Effects of Health Care Consolidation.* Milbank Memorial Fund. www.milbank.org/wp-content/uploads/2020/09/ Sutter-History-Report_v3.pdf.

19 The Economic Theory of Vertical Integration

19.1 INTRODUCTION

Health care providers, hospitals, health insurance companies, pharmaceutical manufacturers, and suppliers of medical devices and equipment all use inputs to produce goods and services.[1] To the extent that they produce some of the needed inputs themselves, they are said to be vertically integrated.

In his pathbreaking work, Ronald Coase[2] explained that the extent of vertical integration within a firm is driven by considerations of profit maximization. In particular, Coase emphasized the role of transaction costs that are incurred in market exchange. Through vertical integration, these costs may be reduced or eliminated altogether. In this chapter, we apply Coase's teaching to participants in health care markets.

In Section 19.2, we examine transaction costs and the ways in which they can be reduced through vertical integration. In Section 19.3, we analyze how vertical integration by a monopolist into a competitive downstream market affects prices and profits. Given this market structure, vertical integration is either competitively neutral or procompetitive. In Section 19.4, we address the successive monopoly problem. Here, both the upstream and the downstream firms are monopolists. Given this market structure, we show that vertical integration is both profitable and welfare enhancing. In Section 19.5, we discuss some of the anticompetitive effects that may arise with vertical mergers, including foreclosure and raising rivals' costs. Next,

---

[1] This chapter relies extensively on Blair and Kaserman (1983) and Blair and Kaserman (2009). Our debt to Ronald Coase (1937) will be obvious.

[2] Coase (1937).

we review recent empirical evidence of vertical mergers in Section 19.6, which provides context for the theories we discuss. In Section 19.7, we turn our attention to mergers of complementary input suppliers, which are common in health care markets. We close with some concluding remarks in Section 19.8.

19.2   VERTICAL INTEGRATION

When a hospital buys beds, hires nurses, or employs a billing service, it engages in market transactions and thereby incurs transaction costs.[3] Searching for those inputs and contracting for their exchange require the hospital to use scarce resources. If the hospital were vertically integrated, it would produce its own beds and bypass the market. In that event, managers would allocate resources that may result in cost savings and higher profit.

Transaction Costs

Transaction costs refer to any expenditure of resources associated with using the market mechanism in transferring a good or service from one party to another. Coase described three categories of costs that are associated with the use of the market mechanism.

First, there are search costs that the parties must bear in order to discover the relevant prices. Because it is in the buyer's interest to pay the lowest price possible and in the seller's interest to charge the highest price possible, both parties involved in a given transaction must carry out some search activity to ensure that he or she is not being taken advantage of by the other party. Second, using the market mechanism often requires the parties to negotiate (and, later, enforce) contracts that stipulate precisely what the buyer and seller are agreeing to do. These contracts usually specify not only the price and quantity of the product to be traded, but also such details as product quality, warranties, delivery dates, buyback agreements, and escalator

---

[3] For the seminal work, see Coase (1937). For extensions and application to antitrust policy, see Williamson (1983).

clauses. Such detailed specification of the items affecting the purchase and sale is necessary to ensure that both parties will live up to the terms of the agreement because performance incentives may change drastically after the initial contract is signed. Generally, the longer the term of such contracts, the greater the costs of negotiation and enforcement since specifying future contingencies becomes increasingly problematic as the time horizon is extended. Moreover, the more complex the product or trading environment becomes, the more difficult it is to specify all future contingencies and the parties' contractual obligations should those contingencies arise. And any contingencies that are not covered by the terms of the contract leave one or both firms vulnerable to opportunistic behavior by the other party. Consequently, each party must monitor and enforce performance under the contract.

Finally, in addition to negotiation and enforcement costs, there are costs of reduced flexibility associated with market transactions that use long-term contracts. If the market price of the input falls during the term of the contract, the buyer will bear an opportunity cost in being unable to take advantage of the lower, spot market price because of its obligation to purchase the input at the higher price specified in the contract. The seller of the input bears a similar opportunity cost if the market price increases unexpectedly during the term of the contract. Changes in market conditions involving aspects other than price (e.g., the introduction of a superior intermediate product) can impose analogous costs on either party. The basic point is that by entering into the contractual agreement, each party locks itself into a predetermined pattern of behavior in order to assure the other party that it has not misrepresented its future intentions. An unexpected change in market conditions often makes this behavior suboptimal and, therefore, costly *ex post*.

By replacing the system of market exchanges with internal transfers, vertical integration may substantially reduce these transaction costs. Instead of buyers and sellers negotiating the sale of an intermediate product, managers organize the production and transfer of this product from the upstream division to the downstream division of the integrated firm. Replacing market transactions with administrative decisions can reduce transaction costs for two fundamental reasons.

First, internalizing the transfer alters the relationship between the affected parties (buyer and seller) from an adversarial relationship to a partnership. Without vertical integration, one firm often stands to gain profits at the expense of the other firm. If firm A can increase its profits by $1 by pursuing a certain course of action, it may be expected to do so even if such an action reduces firm B's profits by $100 (thereby reducing the combined profits of the two firms by $99). By combining the profit functions of the two firms, vertical integration brings about a convergence of goals and thereby eliminates (or greatly reduces) the incentive for this sort of counterproductive behavior. Such convergence, in turn, reduces the costs of completing the given transaction because the parties involved will no longer find it necessary to expend resources designing and negotiating contracts to protect themselves from the anticipated opportunism of the other party.

Second, vertical integration reduces transaction costs because the incentive and control options available to the firm are much more extensive for intrafirm as opposed to interfirm transfers. It is far easier for the manager of a firm to discover and, as necessary, reward or penalize the behavior of employees than it is to exercise similar controls over the behavior of another firm. In the absence of vertical integration, discovery of opportunistic behavior is relatively costly, and haggling or litigation may be the only means available for encouraging more desirable performance. Failure to elicit such performance can lead to a termination of the contractual relationship, which, in turn, requires a search for a new supplier or customer and negotiation of a new contract, all of which entail additional costs.

By combining the profit streams of the buyer and seller, vertical integration increases the amount of information available to the parties for the transaction and sharpens the incentives of all parties to behave in a manner that promotes the profitability of the overall operation.

In addition, vertical integration would substantially mitigate transaction costs in situations involving *transaction-specific assets*. Such assets arise from investments that are undertaken to support some particular set of market transactions. For example, computer software used to coordinate sales of medical products from a group purchasing organization to a hospital could be considered a transaction-specific asset, especially if the computer software could not be used in other applications.

The problem with transaction-specific investments is that once these assets are put in place, the firm that owns them becomes vulnerable to the *hold-up problem*. Specifically, the firm's contracting partner will recognize that the investing firm's trading options become severely limited *ex post* and, consequently, may attempt to capture a portion of the returns for itself when the contract comes up for renewal. Or, in the extreme, the firm may simply renege on the contract and insist upon negotiation. The potential for such opportunistic behavior may prevent the first firm from undertaking these sorts of investments, despite the potential cost reductions that can be reaped from them.

An obvious solution to the hold-up problem is vertical integration. If both parties to the transactions for which the assets are specifically designed are owned by the same firm, incentives for hold-up are eliminated entirely. Thus, vertical integration may be motivated by the desire to avoid hold-up problems stemming from transaction-specific investments.

Because transaction costs are associated with all real-world markets, the incentive for firms to vertically integrate is pervasive. Yet, firms do continue to use some intermediate product markets. No company manufactures all of its inputs. The reason for this lack of complete integration is that vertical integration itself tends to increase the firm's costs. Expanding the firm's operations to an additional stage of production increases the problems of coordinating all the firm's activities. As more and more intermediate products are brought within the firm's control, efficient management of the total operation becomes increasingly difficult due to managerial diseconomies. Eventually, the additional costs of trying to coordinate one more stage of production will exceed the transaction cost savings that result from internalizing this additional stage. At that point, the firm will refrain from further vertical integration and will use the intermediate product market for the allocation of the input.

Although transaction costs provide firms with a major incentive to vertically integrate, managerial diseconomies place a limit on the extent to which such integration will occur. Consequently, the extent of vertical integration is determined where the incremental cost of internalization equals or exceeds the incremental cost of market exchange. By expanding the firm's breadth of operations to this point, the overall costs of producing and delivering the final product to the consumer are minimized. The optimal mix of internal and market exchanges is selected, and the range of firm activities is determined.

19.3   VERTICAL INTEGRATION AND COMPETITIVE DISTRIBUTION

In this section, we use an example to exhibit the economic effects of vertical integration. Initially, we assume that there are no transaction costs in order to focus on the consequences of market structure and vertical control. Suppose, a hypothetical firm, Medical Devices International (MDI), has a valid patent on a specific device for which there is no reasonable substitute. MDI is a monopolist and sells its device to a competitively structured distribution sector.

In Figure 19.1, D represents the demand by health care providers for MDI's devices. This is the demand that the distributors face. MDI faces a wholesale demand d, which is derived from the final demand, D.

Since the health care sector is competitive, the firm knows that market forces will drive the price of the device in the output market down to marginal (and average) cost, that is, the wholesale price plus

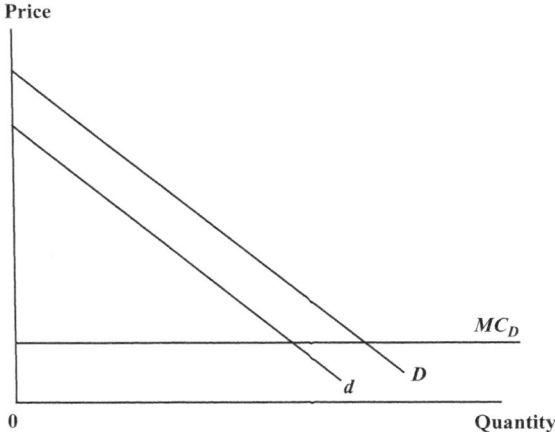

FIGURE 19.1 Derived demand in a competitive market

the marginal cost of distribution (MC_D). This economic principle helps the firm to find the derived demand. Given the final good demand, the maximum wholesale price for any given quantity is found by

$$w = P - MC_D,$$

where w is the wholesale price, P is the final good price, and MC_D is the constant marginal (and average) cost of performing the distribution function. This becomes our derived demand, d. The MC_D does not include the distributor's cost of acquiring the devices. It only includes the cost of distribution, such as sales personnel, rent, and utilities. Since the distribution market is competitive, the price of the medical device must equal the cost to the distributor, which includes the wholesale price charged by MDI, and the distribution cost. The marginal cost of a device at retail, therefore, is equal to the wholesale price plus the marginal cost of distribution.

In Figure 19.2, D and MR correspond to the demand for the device in the output market and marginal revenue, respectively. We have constructed the marginal revenue curve (mr) that corresponds to the derived demand for the input (d). We have also included MDI's

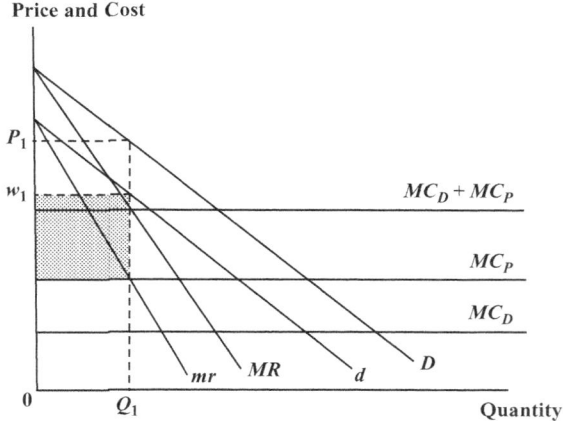

FIGURE 19.2 Monopoly profits of an upstream supplier facing a competitive downstream market

marginal cost of producing devices, which is shown as MC_P. In order to maximize profits, MDI must produce where mr equals MC_P. At this point, the quantity produced will be Q_1. The wholesale price is w_1, which is the height of the derived demand at that quantity. Competition will force the final price to equal w_1 plus MC_D at Q_1, so the retail price will be P_1. The distributors will earn a normal return but enjoy no economic profit. MDI, however, will earn a handsome economic profit,

$$\Pi = (w_1 - MC_P)Q_1,$$

which is represented by the shaded area in Figure 19.2.

MDI has a monopoly on its extraordinarily popular devices. The company is earning economic profits by simply producing the devices and letting others distribute them. Can profits be increased through vertical integration? Put differently, if MDI monopolized both production and distribution of its devices, would profits rise? Our intuition suggests that the answer is yes. After all, monopolizing the production sector and the distribution sector would seem to be more profitable than having a monopoly only in production. But as we will show, this is not the case.

If MDI vertically integrates, it will both produce and distribute its devices. It will sell to consumers, so the retail demand is now relevant for all managerial decisions. Profit maximization requires producing and distributing the quantity of devices where marginal revenue at the final good stage is equal to the sum of the marginal costs of production and distribution:

$$MR = MC_D + MC_P.$$

This profit maximization occurs again at Q_1 with a corresponding price of P_1. Profits are now

$$\Pi = (P_1 - MC_D - MC_P)Q_1.$$

These profits are precisely the same as those MDI earned by only producing the medical devices and distributing them to competing distributors. Our earlier analysis revealed that P_1 was equal to w_1 plus MC_D, so by substitution, we get the same profit function as before the monopolist vertically integrated. Consequently, it is clear that, given this market structure, vertical integration does not improve profits – nor does it harm consumers since price does not rise.

A Numerical Example

Suppose that the demand for MDI's devices is $P = 100 - 2Q$, where Q is measured in millions of units. The marginal cost of distribution (MC_D) is constant and equal to \$10. The marginal cost of production (MC_P) is constant and equal to \$50.

If the distribution sector is competitive, the derived demand for MDI will be $w = P - MC_D = 100 - 2Q - 10 = 90 - 2Q$ and the associated marginal revenue will be $mr = 90 - 4Q$. Profit maximization will yield the quantity found by equating mr to MC_P, so $Q = 10$ with a corresponding wholesale price of $w = 70$ and a consumer price of $P = 80$. The distributors earn a normal return on their investment but no economic profits. MDI, however, earns profits of $\Pi = (w - MC_P)Q = \$200$, which is in millions.

If MDI vertically integrates, then it will produce and distribute its own devices. Profit maximization requires marginal revenue (MR) to equal the combined marginal costs of production and distribution. In this case, $MR = 100 - 4Q = 60 = MC_P + MC_D$. Therefore, profit maximization leads MDI to produce a quantity, $Q = 10$, with a corresponding price, $P = \$80$. Finally, MDI's profits are $\Pi = (P - MC_P - MC_D)Q = \$200$, which is the same profit as before vertical integration.

As we can see, when the distribution stage is organized competitively, the manufacturer's profits are the same whether the firm is vertically integrated or not. If vertical integration confers no efficiencies, it will not improve profits, but it will cause no competitive harm either. Consequently, a vertical merger under these economic conditions must be motivated by the prospect of cost-saving efficiencies.

Backward Integration

Suppose that a hospital has local monopoly power and buys its plastic cups in a competitive market. In the absence of efficiencies, the hospital has no incentive for vertical integration into the production of plastic cups. Since plastic cups are sold at a competitive price, they are sold at marginal cost. Assuming that the hospital could produce plastic cups with the same efficiency as the current plastic cup manufacturers, it would be indifferent between buying or producing plastic cups. If the cost of producing plastic cups is higher for the hospital, the hospital would earn more profit if it bought plastic cups on the competitive market. This is easy to show. The hospital's profit function can be written as

$$P(Q) = Q(x_1, \ldots, x_n),$$

$$\Pi = P(Q) \cdot Q - \sum_{i=1}^{n} w_i x_i,$$

where $P(Q)$ is the inverse demand function for acute care hospital services, which gives us our price (P), and $Q(x_1, \ldots, x_n)$ is the production function, which yields the quantity (Q) of those services that will be produced. Additionally, w_i is the competitive price of the ith input, and x_i is its quantity. The first-order condition for maximizing profit requires employing x_i such that

$$\frac{\partial \Pi}{\partial x_i} = MRP_i - w_i = 0,$$

where $MRP_i = \left(P + Q\frac{dP}{dQ}\right)\left(\frac{\partial Q}{\partial x_i}\right)$.

If the hospital were vertically integrated, it would produce and employ x_i such that

$$\frac{\partial \Pi}{\partial x_i} = MRP_i - MC_{Pi} = 0,$$

where MC_{P_i} is the marginal cost of producing x_i. Assuming that the hospital is as efficient as other producers of x_i, w_i will equal MC_{P_i}. Thus, the hospital would gain nothing by vertically integrating, and it would not begin producing plastic cups.

With this market structure, vertical integration will be profitable only if production costs and/or transaction costs fall as a result. As mentioned in Section 19.2, the firm will vertically integrate to the point where the incremental cost of internalization equals the incremental cost of buying the good in the market. If there are extensive cost savings from vertically integrating that do not exceed the cost of managerial diseconomies, it would make sense for the hospital to vertically integrate. Since we seldom see hospitals merging with plastic cup producers, it is safe to conclude that the cost of internalization may exceed the transaction cost of buying plastic cups in the competitive market.

19.4   SUCCESSIVE MONOPOLIES IN PRODUCTION AND DISTRIBUTION

We now turn to a different market structure: Successive monopoly occurs when there exists a monopoly upstream and a separately owned and operated monopoly downstream.[4] To illustrate the economic effects of vertical integration in the presence of successive monopoly,

---

[4] Again, initially, we assume an absence of transaction costs.

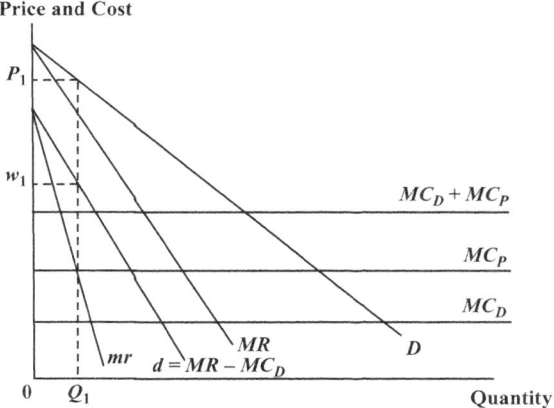

FIGURE 19.3 The dreaded double marginalization with successive monopoly

we can modify our medical device example. MDI still has monopoly power in the medical device market. Instead of selling its devices to a competitive distribution sector, however, it sells them to Dynamic Device Distributors, Inc. (DDD), which is a distribution monopolist.

MDI and DDD are separately owned and independently operated firms. Consequently, each will have an independent incentive to maximize its own profits. The effect of these independent efforts is to reduce total output, raise the price of the good to final consumers, and reduce the combined profits of the two firms below that of a vertically integrated firm.

We use Figure 19.3 to illustrate our findings. The key to analyzing the successive monopoly structure is finding the derived demand, which measures DDD's demand for devices from MDI. The derived demand for MDI is determined by the retail demand, which is shown as D in Figure 19.3, and the profit-maximizing behavior of DDD. To maximize its profits, DDD will operate where marginal revenue (MR) is equal to its marginal cost, which is the sum of the wholesale price (w) and the marginal cost of distribution (MC_D):

$$MR = w + MC_D.$$

The derived demand for MDI is found by rearranging the above expression. We get

$$w = MR - MC_D.$$

In Figure 19.3, the derived demand is shown as the line parallel to MR, which is $d = MR - MC_D$. The marginal revenue associated with the derived demand is mr. MDI's manager will maximize profits by operating where mr is equal to the marginal cost of production (MC_P). This output is Q_1, and the corresponding wholesale price will be w_1.

For DDD, the marginal cost will be the sum of the wholesale price and the marginal cost of distribution. Thus, we have that $MR = MC = w_1 + MC_D$ at the profit-maximizing level. The profit-maximizing quantity will be Q_1, and the retail price will be P_1.
Both firms earn economic profits. MDI earns a profit of

$$\Pi = (w_1 - MC_P)Q_1$$

while DDD earns a profit of

$$\Pi = (P_1 - w_1 - MC_D)Q_1.$$

The effect of vertical integration in this market structure is profound, as Figure 19.4 shows. If MDI vertically integrates, it will operate where MR is equal to the marginal cost of the integrated firm, which is $MC_P + MC_D$. Since $MC_P + MC_D$ is less than $w_1 + MC_D$, the marginal cost of the integrated firm is less than the marginal cost of the nonintegrated firms. The key is recognizing that the marginal revenue of the integrated firm (MR) will be equated to the sum of the marginal cost ($MC_P + MC_D$) rather than the sum of w_1 and MC_D, which exceeds the sum of MC_P and MC_D. The result is an increase in total sales from Q_1 to Q_2 and a reduction in the price paid by consumers from P_1 to P_2, making consumers better off. Total industry profits earned soar from $(w_1 - MC_P)Q_1 + (P_1 - w_1 - MC_D)Q_1$ or $(P_1 - MC_P - MC_D)Q_1$ to $(P_2 - MC_P - MC_D)Q_2$.

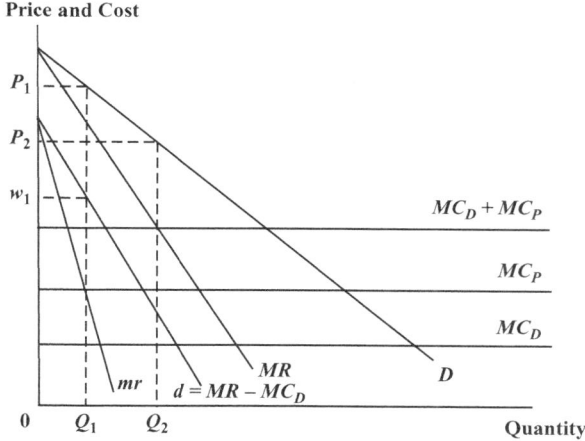

FIGURE 19.4 Vertical integration eliminates double marginalization

A Numerical Example: Successive Monopoly

We return to the previous numerical example but now assume that DDD monopolizes the distribution sector. As a monopolist, the manager of DDD will maximize profits by operating where marginal revenue is equal to marginal cost. Now, the derived demand for MDI is $w = 90 - 4Q$. The corresponding marginal revenue will then be $mr = 90 - 8Q$.

Profit maximization leads MDI to produce where mr equals MC_P: $90 - 8Q = 50$ or $Q = 5$. The optimal wholesale price, w, is then 70, and the profit for MDI will be $\Pi = (w - MC_P)Q = \$100$ million.

DDD will operate where MR equals $w + MC_D$, which gives us $100 - 4Q = 80$ or $Q = 5$. DDD will charge final consumers a price of $P = 100 - 2Q = 90$. Profit for DDD is then $\Pi = (P - w - MC_D)Q = \$50$ million.

With vertical integration, the firm produces and distributes its output. Accordingly, the profit function becomes

$$\Pi = (100 - 2Q)Q - 50Q - 10Q.$$

The firm will produce where its marginal revenue, $100 - 4Q$, is equal to its marginal cost, which is $MC_P + MC_D = \$60$. Thus, $Q = 10$, $P = 80$, and $\Pi = \$200$ million.

With successive monopoly, the total profits will be equal to $150 million, in contrast to the profit of $200 million when the firm is vertically integrated. Successive monopoly is an unstable market structure because total profits can be improved through vertical integration. The manufacturer can improve its profit through forward integration. Similarly, the distributor can improve its profits by backward integration.

As has been shown, vertical integration is a superior market structure to successive monopoly. By vertically integrating, firms can improve their profits by eliminating double marginalization. Additionally, consumers benefit since output expands and price will be reduced. Thus, vertical integration in a successive monopoly situation is procompetitive and should be encouraged by the antitrust Agencies.

19.5 COMPETITIVE CONCERNS WITH VERTICAL MERGERS

In Sections 19.3 and 19.4, we found vertical integration to be either procompetitive or competitively neutral. These findings suggest that antitrust policy should treat vertical mergers with benign neglect. But not all vertical mergers are competitively innocuous. In some instances, a vertical merger may create an opportunity for the vertically integrated firm to raise its rivals' costs and thereby gain a competitive advantage. In those instances, rivals may be entirely foreclosed from the market. To further the goals of antitrust policy, the DOJ and the FTC must consider these anticompetitive possibilities when reviewing a proposed vertical merger.[5]

If an integrated firm forecloses its downstream rivals by restricting their access to vital input supplies, this is known as input (or downstream) foreclosure. When the integrated firm has market power upstream, this conduct may disadvantage rivals such that new firms do not enter, existing firms may exit, or rivals' costs may rise. In such

---

[5] See Salop and Scheffman (1983) and Krattenmaker and Salop (1986) for more details on raising rivals' costs.

cases, quantity decreases and output prices rise, leading to a loss in social welfare and harm to consumers.

We demonstrate the incentives of foreclosure and raising rivals' costs by discussing the case of input foreclosure. By vertically integrating, a firm with sufficient market share in the upstream market may reduce the supply of inputs available by refusing to supply its downstream rivals. Usually, a decrease in supply translates to an increase in price. Hence, the vertically integrated firm hopes that by decreasing the supply of inputs, input prices will rise for other downstream firms, which will disadvantage them. Due to the increase in input prices, the rival distributors may reduce the quantity of output that they sell with a consequent increase in output price. Then the vertically integrated firm may capture market share and would earn higher profits due to the higher margins on the downstream product.

The success of such a strategy relies on whether the vertically integrated firm can maintain the supply shortage for its rivals and whether the raised costs will lead to stable price increases in the downstream market.[6] Competitive forces may undermine this strategy. The input strategy provides an incentive for upstream entry. In this event, new upstream firms will sell inputs to the independent downstream firms at lower prices, and, therefore, output prices may not remain above the premerger level.

In some cases involving vertical integration or vertical mergers, the total effects of vertical integration can be ambiguous because there are both procompetitive and anticompetitive effects. In many cases, a vertical merger is likely to produce efficiencies that can be passed on to consumers. But the vertically integrated firm may also act anticompetitively by foreclosing its rivals. It is up to the Agencies to determine whether the vertical merger will be procompetitive. Some limited empirical surveys show that, on balance, vertical mergers can be procompetitive, anticompetitive, or neutral.[7]

---

[6] For more details, see the seminal work by Krattenmaker and Salop (1986).

[7] See Lafontaine and Slade (2007, 2021) and Beck and Scott Morton (2021).

19.6 EMPIRICAL EVIDENCE ON VERTICAL MERGERS

Due to the ambiguous effects of vertical mergers, empirical evidence is vital to understanding how vertical integration affects consumers. Unfortunately, the current empirical evidence is itself ambiguous.[8] An overview of the most recent empirical studies finds that some vertical mergers are procompetitive, some are anticompetitive, and others have ambiguous effects.

In 2007, Lafontaine and Slade published an overview of the empirical literature on vertical mergers. They concluded that vertical mergers were generally procompetitive, with procompetitive efficiencies overwhelming any anticompetitive harms.[9] But in later work, Lafontaine and Slade (2021) identify more recent studies with mixed effects of vertical integration. The authors concluded that not enough evidence existed to develop presumptions about vertical mergers.[10]

Beck and Scott Morton (2021) reviewed 29 empirical studies of vertical mergers. Fourteen mergers had anticompetitive effects and 14 mergers had procompetitive effects, leading the authors to conclude that no legal presumption could be made for vertical mergers.[11] In these studies, the authors found evidence of both the elimination of double marginalization and instances of foreclosure, which corroborates the theories we have introduced above. Unfortunately, many of the studies that Beck and Scott Morton (2021) reviewed did not provide an analysis of both procompetitive and anticompetitive effects, leaving the total effect unclear. Beck and Scott Morton (2021) reference two empirical studies of vertical mergers in health care markets, which we introduce below.[12]

First, Cuesta, Noton, and Vatter (2019) examined hospital–insurer mergers in Chile from 2013 to 2016. After controlling for

---

[8] See Beck and Scott Morton (2021) for a discussion of the limitations and biases that plague empirical studies.

[9] Lafontaine and Slade (2007).   [10] Lafontaine and Slade (2021).

[11] Some mergers had both anticompetitive and procompetitive effects.

[12] We do not look at the hospital and physician merger examples that the authors point to since acute care hospital services and physician services are complements in providing complete health care. Therefore, these mergers are not vertical.

confounding variables, the authors found that insurance premiums were higher, but hospital billings and patient copayments were lower for patients who bought insurance and services from integrated hospitals. The authors found that although the elimination of double marginalization occurred, the anticompetitive effect of foreclosure overwhelmed the procompetitive benefits. The integrated hospitals raised their rivals' costs by negotiating higher prices with rival insurers. These insurers would then have to raise their premiums for patients, who may have switched to the integrated firm. Quantities decreased and prices rose. The authors suggest that these types of mergers should be banned in Chile. It is unknown whether hospital–insurer mergers in the United States would lead to similar negative effects.

Second, Malik (2011) studied innovation in the pharmaceutical industry during 1994–2005. Controlling for confounding variables, firms that engaged in more joint ventures and acquisitions generally saw higher levels of new product development. Malik, therefore, suggests that vertical integration may be beneficial since it leads to more innovation.[13]

The limited empirical evidence that exists suggests that vertical mergers are not invariably procompetitive or invariably anticompetitive. The vast majority of vertical mergers pass muster with the Agencies, and therefore, must appear to be procompetitive or competitively neutral. Public policy would benefit from further empirical research on the economic effects of vertical mergers.

19.7 MERGERS OF COMPLEMENTARY INPUT SUPPLIERS

Not all health care mergers are clearly horizontal or vertical mergers. For example, a merger between a hospital and a physician group is

---

[13] Beck and Scott Morton (2021) find various faults with this study that may bring the results into question. Malik (2011) may have ignored omitted variable bias of a firm's innovation strategy and also did not observe the timing of the innovation. Additionally, Malik (2011) did not test whether total innovation increased in the pharmaceutical industry.

neither horizontal nor vertical. It is not horizontal since physician services are generally not substitutes for hospital services. The merger is not vertical because neither firm buys inputs from the other firm. Instead, the merger is one that involves suppliers of complementary goods.[14]

Complements are goods that are more valuable when consumed together rather than separately. An injectable vaccine cannot effectively enter the bloodstream unless it is paired with a hypodermic needle. Rotator cuff surgery is generally followed by physical therapy. A visit to the nephrologist is usually paired with visits to a dialysis center for those with kidney failure. These products and services work best when they are administered together. The demand for a good or service therefore relies, in part, on the price of its complementary good or service. For example, if the price of physical therapy increased, a patient who required rotator cuff surgery may decide to delay the surgery since he or she would consider the whole cost of the operation and physical therapy.

When two firms that offer complementary goods are separate, they unilaterally make decisions that will maximize their profits irrespective of the effects on the other firm. This can lead to a negative externality, which occurs when the actions of one firm negatively affect another firm. One commonly cited externality is the Cournot effect that concerns price. A price drop for rotator cuff surgery would have a positive effect on the demand for physical therapy. But the surgeon will not drop his or her price if he or she will lose profit by doing so, even if the lost profits are less than the profits that the physical therapist would gain due to the increase in demand. A merger internalizes this externality and leads to efficiencies. By merging, the firm may have an incentive to lower its margins on the

[14] Most commentators view hospital acquisition of physician practices as vertical. In our view, these mergers really combine complements. Acute care hospital services are combined with physician services to produce health care for an unwell patient. There is no obvious supply chain issue since the hospital does not buy the physician services in the absence of the merger.

rotator cuff surgery to increase demand for physical therapy, which can benefit consumers.[15]

Merging can also lead to efficiencies from coordinating decision making, especially in terms of quality control and investments. A firm will shy away from quality improvements or investments if its realization of the benefits is not sufficient to cover its costs. Yet, some of these investments may be socially beneficial if the benefit to both firms is greater than the cost. Investments that increase the compatibility of the two products may also be undersupplied if the two firms have not merged.

Additionally, conglomerate mergers[16] may lead to economies of scale and economies of scope. Economies of scale may occur if the firms share inputs, skills, knowledge, and efficient management. With economies of scope, it may be more efficient to produce both complementary products together rather than separately. For example, a merger between a surgeon and a physical therapist may make the transfer of paperwork easier and may facilitate communication between the surgeon and physical therapist, increasing the quality of care that the patient receives.

Potential Anticompetitive Effects

Few mergers of complementary goods will raise red flags. But in some cases where a merged firm has sufficient market power in at least one complementary market, it may implement tying, bundling, and other seemingly exclusionary practices that may be anticompetitive.

---

[15] Spulber (2016) argues that the benefits may not be merger specific. He explores a bargaining model with two monopolies of complementary goods and shows that the efficient price is achieved when the firms use supply contracts. Therefore, benefits can be realized without a merger. But in health care markets where health care consumers often have little bargaining power and do not use supply contracts to buy health care services, Spulber's model does not apply.

[16] If a merger is neither horizontal nor vertical, we usually call it a conglomerate merger. For an examination of conglomerate mergers, see Blair and Kaserman (2009).

Tying occurs when a firm sells one good (the tying good) on the condition that the buyer also buy a second good (the tied good). For example, if a pharmaceutical firm has a patent monopoly on a vaccine, it could sell the vaccine on the condition that the buyer also purchase its hypodermic needles. In that event, the needles would be tied to the vaccine. Bundling, which is a close cousin of tying, occurs when a firm sells products as a bundle in fixed proportions. The vaccine monopolist could bundle together its vaccine and needles. In this way, the customer would have to buy the bundle at a single price. The competitive concern is that rival suppliers of hypodermic needles will be foreclosed from selling to the vaccine monopolist's customers. But this concern may be misplaced. If the vaccine monopolist is a more efficient producer of needles, its rivals cannot compete. They are foreclosed by their relative inefficiency. If the rivals are equally efficient, it is immaterial who supplies the needles from a social welfare perspective. If the rivals are more efficient, it is in the vaccine monopolist's interest to buy needles rather than produce needles. The rivals will compete with one another to be the favored supplier. The winner of the competitive battle will not be foreclosed. The others are foreclosed not because of tying or bundling, but because they were underbid by the winner.

Finally, a merged firm may have an incentive to unnecessarily increase demand in the complementary good market. For example, a surgeon may encourage patients to get physical therapy even when it is unnecessary. If patients had perfect information, they could easily see through this ruse, but asymmetric information is rife in the real world, especially in health care markets. Although patients may decide to go to other physical therapists, the merged firm would still benefit from the increased demand from patients who decide to buy its physical therapy services.

There is very little empirical evidence on the economic effects of mergers between complementary input suppliers. A few empirical studies look at the effects of hospital and physician practice mergers on price and output. In one article, the authors found that a significant number of in-office visits were transferred to the acquiring hospital.[17] As a result, patients were billed for the use of hospital facilities as well as the physician's services. The cost to the patient and his or her health insurer would rise. Prices were higher, but at least health outcomes were no worse than before.[18] One study found no significant health differences in patients with diabetes and hypertension after a merger. More research is needed to understand the net effects of these mergers.

19.8 CONCLUDING REMARKS

The economic analysis of vertical integration reveals that vertical mergers can be procompetitive or anticompetitive. When vertical integration is motivated by reductions in transaction costs or by distributional efficiencies, scarce resources are saved, costs fall, and prices fall as well. When vertical integration is motivated by successive monopoly, output expands and prices fall. But a vertical merger may lead to potential anticompetitive effects in the form of raising rivals' costs and market foreclosure. We also reviewed mergers of complementary suppliers, finding that their effect on consumers is ambiguous. In Chapter 20, we discuss various examples that illustrate both the benefits and disadvantages of vertical integration as well as mergers of complementary suppliers.

REFERENCES

Beck, Marissa, and Fiona Scott Morton. (2021). Evaluating the Evidence on Vertical Mergers. *Review of Industrial Organization* 57: 273–302.

Blair, Roger D., and David L. Kaserman. (1983). *Law and Economics of Vertical Integration and Control*. New York: Academic Press.

Blair, Roger D., and David L. Kaserman. (2009). *Antitrust Economics*. 2nd ed. New York: Oxford University Press.

---

[17] Koch, Wendling, and Wilson (2017).
[18] Koch, Wendling, and Wilson (2021) and Capps, Dranove, and Ody (2018).

Capps, Cory, David Dranove, and Christopher Ody. (2018). The Effect of Hospital Acquisitions of Physician Practices on Prices and Spending. *Journal of Health Economics* 59: 139–152.

Cuesta, Jose Ignacio, Carlos Noton, and Benjamin Vatter. (2019). *Vertical Integration between Hospitals and Insurers*. SSRN. https://papers.ssrn.com/sol3/papers.cfm?abstract_id=3309218.

Coase, Ronald H. (1937). *The Nature of the Firm*. Economica 4: 386–405.

Koch, Thomas G., Brett W. Wendling, and Nathan E. Wilson. (2017). How Vertical Integration Affects the Quantity and Cost of Care for Medicare Beneficiaries. *Journal of Health Economics* 52: 19–32.

Koch, Thomas G., Brett W. Wendling, and Nathan E. Wilson. (2021). The Effects of Physician and Hospital Integration on Medicare Beneficiaries' Health Outcomes. *Review of Economics and Statistics* 103: 725–739.

Krattenmaker, Thomas G., and Steven C. Salop. (1986). Anticompetitive Exclusion: Raising Rivals' Costs to Achieve Power over Price. *Yale Law Journal* 96: 209–293.

Lafontaine, Francine, and Margaret Slade. (2007). Vertical Integration and Firm Boundaries: The Evidence. *Journal of Economic Literature* 45: 629–685.

Lafontaine, Francine, and Margaret Slade. (2021). Presumptions in Vertical Mergers: The Role of Evidence. *Review of Industrial Organization* 59: 255–272.

Malik, Tariq. (2011). Vertical Alliance and Vertical Integration for the Inflow of Technology and New Product Development in the Pharmaceutical Industry. *Technology Analysis and Strategic Management* 23: 851–864.

Normann, Hans Theo. (2011). Vertical Mergers, Foreclosure and Raising Rivals' Costs: Experimental Evidence. *Journal of Industrial Economics* 59: 506–527.

Salop, Steven C., and David T. Scheffman. (1983). Raising Rivals' Costs. *American Economic Review* 73: 267–271.

Spulber, Daniel. (2016). *Complementary Monopolies and Bargaining*. Northwestern University School of Law, Law and Economics Series No. 16–10.

Williamson, Oliver E. (1983). *Markets and Hierarchies: Analysis and Antitrust Implications*. New York: Free Press.

20 Vertical Merger Policy

20.1 INTRODUCTION

In Chapter 19, we reviewed the economic theories of vertical integration and mergers of complementary input suppliers. When the supplier of a good acquires its distributor, the merger is said to be vertical. Similarly, if a distributor acquires the supplier of a good that it distributes, the merger is also vertical. A merger of complements occurs when a supplier merges with a supplier of a complementary good. None of these mergers alter the structure of either the upstream or downstream market. As a result, assessing their competitive significance is more complicated and more subtle than assessing the competitive significance of a horizontal merger. In this chapter, we will tease out the competitive concerns that have shaped vertical merger policy.

In the next section, we explore the legal foundation that governs vertical mergers and mergers of complementary input producers. We also review the minimal guidance provided by the Supreme Court in its *Brown Shoe*[1] and *Ford (Autolite)*[2] decisions. In Section 20.3, we turn our attention to enforcement policy. Our analysis relies on the 2020 Vertical Merger Guidelines. These Guidelines recognize the benefits of eliminating double marginalization as well as the competitive concerns associated with raising rivals' costs and market foreclosure. We note, however, that in September 2021, the FTC withdrew and is revising the 2020 Vertical Merger Guidelines. The DOJ has not yet followed suit but plans to carefully review the Guidelines and cooperate with the FTC. In Sections 20.4, 20.5, and 20.6, we review

---

[1] *Brown Shoe Company, Inc.* v. *United States*, 370 US 294 (1962).
[2] *Ford Motor Compoany* v. *United States*, 405 US 562 (1972).

examples of vertical mergers and mergers of complementary input producers. First, we examine Illumina Inc.'s proposed acquisition of GRAIL in the biotechnology industry, in which an upstream input supplier of DNA sequencing instruments wanted to purchase a downstream firm that produces cancer tests. Next, we illustrate some of the procompetitive benefits and anticompetitive harms when insurers acquire providers of health care services, as was the case when UnitedHealth Group Inc. acquired the DaVita Medical Group. Finally, we examine the practice of hospitals acquiring physician groups and observe how these mergers can lead to anticompetitive harm if left unchecked. We close with some concluding observations in Section 20.7.

20.2   LEGAL FOUNDATION

While vertical mergers have always been subject to rule of reason treatment, the aggressiveness of the antitrust Agencies in challenging these mergers and the level of hostility exhibited by the courts have changed considerably as newer economic theories have been incorporated into enforcement decisions. In the beginning of the twentieth century, enforcement actions were limited to the Sherman Act since Section 7 of the Clayton Act only applied to horizontal mergers until a 1950 amendment. Although some vertical merger cases were brought under the more demanding Sherman Act standard, enforcement did not appear to be overly aggressive during this period.[3]

In 1950, the Celler-Kefauver amendment to the Clayton Act expanded that legislation's antimerger provisions to vertical mergers. The legality of all mergers is dictated by Section 7 of the Clayton Act, which holds that

> No person engaged in commerce or in any activity
> affecting commerce shall acquire ... the whole or any part of the
> assets of another person engaged also in commerce or in any activity

---

[3] Blair and Kaserman (2009).

affecting commerce, where in any line of commerce ... in any section of the country, the effect of such acquisition may be substantially to lessen competition, or to tend to create a monopoly.[4]

A vertical merger is therefore forbidden if it substantially lessens competition or tends to create a monopoly. But economic theory has not always been clear on the conditions that would make a vertical merger anticompetitive.

The expansion of the Clayton Act, along with widespread acceptance by the judiciary of an early version of foreclosure theory, led to 20 years of extreme administrative and judicial hostility toward vertical integration. During this period, a number of vertical mergers were blocked that, in retrospect, did not appear to have presented any substantial anticompetitive threats. In our view, the legal precedence from these cases provides no useful guidance for current vertical merger policy. We discuss two examples below.

First, in *Brown Shoe*,[5] the Supreme Court objected to a shoe producer acquiring a retail distributor. The Brown Shoe Company (Brown Shoe) was the fourth largest manufacturer of shoes in the United States, and the G.R. Kinney Company, Inc. (Kinney) operated the largest family-style shoe chain.[6] However, the US shoe market was quite unconcentrated. Brown Shoe only manufactured shoes for about 4 percent of the domestic market. Kinney's sales, meanwhile, accounted for only 1.2 percent of all retail shoes by dollar amount. These market shares are not large enough to generate substantial anticompetitive effects.

The Court, however, proscribed the merger because the justices wanted to halt what they perceived to be a worrying trend toward vertical integration in the shoe industry. Additionally, the Court believed the merger would allow Brown Shoe to force its shoes into

---

[4] 15 USC § 18.   [5] *Brown Shoe Company, Inc.* v. *United States*, 370 US 294 (1962).
[6] There were some horizontal aspects to this case since Brown Shoe operated some retail outlets and Kinney manufactured its own shoes.

Kinney's stores and thereby allow Brown Shoe to gain a competitive advantage over its rivals. These complaints lack merit.

First, although vertical integration was rife in the shoe industry, entry was relatively easy and a number of alternatives existed. It would have been difficult for Brown Shoe to foreclose its rivals, especially since the market shares involved were very small.

Second, the Court claimed that "by eliminating wholesalers and by increasing the volume of purchases from the manufacturing division of the enterprise, [retail outlets of integrated companies] can market their own brands at prices below those of competing independent retailers."[7] Essentially, by creating efficiencies through the merger, Brown Shoe would supposedly disadvantage its rivals. Condemning procompetitive efficiencies in largely unconcentrated markets is seriously misguided.

In *Ford (Autolite)*,[8] the Court condemned Ford's acquisition of a spark plug producer on potential competition grounds. Before the proposed merger, Ford bought the spark plugs that it installed in all of its new vehicles from Champion. Ford decided to enter the spark plug business but determined that internal expansion would be too costly and time-consuming. Ford therefore purchased Champion's main competitor, Autolite. Consequently, Champion lost the Ford account and instead began supplying spark plugs to Chrysler, which had previously been supplied by Autolite. Due to this realignment, Champion's market share of the domestic spark plug market fell from 50 to 33 percent.

The Court proscribed this merger since the justices saw Ford as the most likely *de novo* entrant. Additionally, they believed Ford would foreclose its rivals and thereby limit the pricing discretion of the independent spark plug manufacturers.[9] But the Court did not

---

[7] *Brown Shoe Company, Inc.* v. *United States* 370 US 294 (1962), at 345.

[8] *Ford Motor Company* v. *United States*, 405 US 562 (1972).

[9] At the time, General Motors already produced its own spark plugs. It was reasonable to believe that Ford would make the investment to produce its own spark plugs in the future.

consider the efficiencies that may have arisen due to the merger. Specifically, Ford made a calculated decision to buy a spark plug manufacturer rather than expand internally, which indicates that purchasing may have been more efficient.

These decisions led to new interest in vertical integration theories in the 1970s and substantial pushback from various economists, especially those at the University of Chicago. The Chicago school criticized the early foreclosure doctrine and developed newer theories of vertical integration that emphasized the procompetitive impacts. In response, vertical merger policy retreated to a decade or so of relative inactivity as the Reagan and Bush administrations backed away from the previous period's stringent enforcement activities. The Agencies challenged very few vertical mergers during this time.

As new foreclosure theories have become widely accepted, a second turnaround has emerged. Although we had hoped that the excessively stringent doctrine of the 1960s and 1970s would not return, antitrust policy under the Biden administration seems to be heading in this direction. The antitrust Agencies have shown a much more hostile attitude toward vertical mergers and big business. In the next section, we review the most recent policy guidelines, the 2020 Vertical Merger Guidelines. Although they have been withdrawn by the FTC, no new guidelines have been published at the time of this writing. Thus, we discuss the policy procedures on vertical mergers and mergers of suppliers of complementary products as put forth by the 2020 Vertical Merger Guidelines.

20.3   THE 2020 VERTICAL MERGER GUIDELINES

For decades, the DOJ and the FTC were often surprised to discover a *Wall Street Journal* article about a consummated merger. If one of the Agencies had concerns about the merger's competitive effects, it faced the daunting task of "unscrambling the eggs." This is no longer the case. In 1976, Congress passed the Hart-Scott-Rodino (HSR) Act, which requires premerger notification if the value of the acquired firm exceeds a specific threshold. In 2021, that threshold was $92 million.[10] The Act includes a provision for an initial notification, which requires the parties to provide information that one of the Agencies will review to form a judgment about the competitive consequences of the merger. The initial review period is only 30 days, which may be insufficient. If the Agency is troubled by the proposed merger but not ready to challenge it, the Agency can request more information on specific issues, such as pricing, perceived competitive threats, product development, and expansion plans.

To inform the business community and lawyers of its enforcement policies and actual procedures, the DOJ and the FTC published their Vertical Merger Guidelines (VMGs) in 2020, which replaced the 1984 Merger Guidelines.[11] The Guidelines also provided guidance on mergers of complements. In 2021, the Merger Guidelines were rescinded by the Federal Trade Commission. We anticipate more stringent guidelines will be published by the antitrust Agencies in the near future.

Analyzing the likely effects of a vertical merger is not easy since both procompetitive and anticompetitive effects may be present. A vertical merger may reduce transaction costs and/or eliminate double marginalization. In either event, the result will be expanded output and lower prices for consumers. Alternatively, a vertical merger may permit the firm to raise its rivals' costs or even foreclose them from the market. Such a vertical merger would reduce consumer welfare. Balancing these procompetitive benefits and anticompetitive harms may not be too difficult in theory but may be quite elusive in practice.

The Agencies have developed various strategies to uncover the effects of mergers on balance. When evaluating a merger, the Agencies "consider any reasonably available and reliable evidence" that is relevant to determine the likely effects of a merger.[12] They rely on

---

[10] Premerger Notification Office Staff (2021). The threshold is adjusted on an annual basis.

[11] Department of Justice and Federal Trade Commission (2020, 2).

[12] Department of Justice and Federal Trade Commission (2020, 3).

the documents and statements provided by the merging firms, but documents from customers and other interested parties may be used as well. The Agencies also use their experience with similar mergers or merger simulations along with evaluations of market share and concentration to get a better idea of the likely effects of the proposed merger. These tools assist the Agencies in assessing the likelihood of anticompetitive and procompetitive effects.

First, the Agencies define a relevant market with a specific product, which "could be an input, a means of distribution, access to a set of customers, or a complement."[13] Second, the Agencies calculate the market share of the merging firms and the concentration levels of that market. Higher concentration may indicate a greater likelihood of anticompetitive conduct and would warrant more scrutiny.

When assessing anticompetitive effects, the Agencies look at ability and incentives. First, the Agencies determine whether a merger would allow a firm to act anticompetitively. For example, in the case of foreclosure, if rivals had various substitutes they could easily switch to, the integrated firm would not have the ability to raise its rivals' costs. Now suppose the firm had the ability to foreclose its rivals. The Agencies would assess whether the integrated firm had the incentive to do so, that is, whether the firm could profit from its anticompetitive behavior. This thought experiment allows the Agencies to determine the likelihood of anticompetitive conduct.

The VMGs recognize that vertical mergers may result in efficiencies, or real cost savings. These cost savings must flow from a reduction in the use of scarce resources. Examples of real cost savings include streamlined production, inventory management, or distribution. For these efficiencies to be cognizable, they must be merger specific. In other words, the efficiencies cannot be realized in the absence of the merger.

---

[13] Department of Justice and Federal Trade Commission (2020, 3).

The elimination of double marginalization (EDM) is not an efficiency in the sense that fewer resources are needed to produce, purchase, and distribute the product. EDM is beneficial because it alters the market structure from one of successive monopoly to a single integrated monopoly. As we saw in Chapter 19, EDM results in greater output at reduced prices, which improves consumer welfare.

EDM is not necessarily merger specific since a number of vertical contracts exist that provide the same welfare-enhancing benefits as a merger without the potential anticompetitive harm.[14] But the Agencies do not discount this efficiency. For example, the Agencies will review the past contractual history of the firm to determine the ease with which a welfare-enhancing vertical contract could be created. If no such contract exists in the history of the firm, it may be the case that such contracts have substantial transaction costs that could be eliminated with vertical integration.

Comparing the likelihood of the anticompetitive and procompetitive effects allows the Agencies to determine whether the merger will be anticompetitive, procompetitive, or competitively neutral. In some cases, it will be clear that a merger has no anticompetitive effects. If the reviewing Agency is unsure of the economic effects of a proposed merger based on the HSR filing, it can request more information. The time available for further analysis and evaluation is not severely constrained. This permits the Agency to reach a more considered judgment regarding the proposed merger's competitive significance. Sometimes, the Agencies determine the merger will cause no harm. But in some cases, the Agencies deem the merger to be anticompetitive on balance.

When the Agencies determine that a vertical merger is anticompetitive, they may first look for a satisfactory solution amenable to both the merging firms and the antitrust authorities. This may include divestiture of certain assets that would have increased the

---

[14] See Angerhofer and Blair (2021) for a discussion of various contracts.

likelihood of anticompetitive effects. If an agreement cannot be reached, the Agencies will sue the merging firm and ask for a court's injunction on the proposed merger. Most often, firms settle with the Agencies or abandon a merger before going to court in order to avoid expensive litigation costs. Now we will examine several specific vertical and conglomerate mergers in health care markets to see how the Agencies apply antitrust policy in real situations.

20.4 A MERGER IN BIOTECHNOLOGY: ILLUMINA/GRAIL

Illumina is a biotechnology company with $3.2 billion in annual revenues that specializes in products used to analyze genetic variation and biological function.[15] It is the world leader of next-generation sequencing (NGS) equipment and consumables and provides about 90 percent of the world's DNA sequencing data.

In September 2020, Illumina, Inc., announced its plan to acquire GRAIL for $7.1 billion.[16] GRAIL was founded in 2015 as a unit of Illumina but was divested in 2016.[17] Through its research, Illumina discovered that sequencing DNA in the blood allowed tests to pick up pieces of DNA that were shed by cancerous cells. GRAIL was tasked with developing a multi-cancer early detection (MCED) test. MCED tests will be a game changer for the health care industry, with billions of dollars in annual sales at stake. The Galleri test that GRAIL developed may detect up to 50 types of cancers before patients have symptoms, thereby significantly increasing the chances of cancer survival through early detection.

Since GRAIL uses Illumina's data-sequencing equipment for its MCED test, the acquisition is considered vertical. In addition, Illumina has a virtual monopoly on sequencing equipment since no

---

[15] Illumina (2020).

[16] *In re Illumina, Inc. and GRAIL, Inc.*, No. 9401 (Federal Trade Commission 2021), Complaint, Redacted Public Version.

[17] In 2016, Illumina divested the company but held on to a minority share. At this stage, expensive clinical trials were looming, and Illumina feared the trials could drive up its operating expenses, which could reduce its stock price (Herper 2017).

other firm can match the cost, accuracy, and throughput of its sequencing instruments in this market.[18] The Galleri test, meanwhile, is now available for consumer purchase and will be more widely marketed once it receives FDA approval.[19] The Galleri test is poised to be the first to enter the market and therefore is expected to have a significant market share.

In March 2021, the FTC moved to block the vertical merger, believing that Illumina could use its market power in the DNA sequencing market to foreclose rival MCED test makers.

Antitrust Analysis

When analyzing the Illumina/GRAIL merger, the FTC looked at both potential procompetitive and anticompetitive aspects.[20] As outlined in the 2020 VMGs, the Agencies determined whether the merging firm would have the *ability* and *incentive* to foreclose its rival MCED test makers after the merger and found that Illumina would have both. Illumina is the dominant player in the short-read NGS platform market, which is a critical component of MCED tests.[21] If Illumina refused to provide NGS platform equipment and consumables to other MCED test makers, it is safe to assume that those test makers would be forced to exit the market. The Agencies determined that no substantial procompetitive benefits would arise from the merger that could offset the anticompetitive harm.

---

[18] *In re Illumina, Inc. and GRAIL, Inc.*, No. 9401 (Federal Trade Commission 2021), Complaint, Redacted Public Version.

[19] Before FDA testing is complete, the MCED test can be launched as a laboratory-developed test (LDT) from the developer's own proprietary lab. Without FDA testing, however, commercial opportunity is limited since insurers may not pay for tests that do not have FDA approval.

[20] Most of the following analysis comes from *In re Illumina, Inc. and GRAIL, Inc.*, No. 9401 (Federal Trade Commission 2021), Complaint, Redacted Public Version.

[21] Thermo Fisher Scientific, Inc., also provides a short-read NGS platform, but it is not a viable alternative. Beijing Genomics Institute cannot sell its NGS platform in the US market due to a patent infringement lawsuit that Illumina filed. *In re Illumina, Inc. and GRAIL, Inc.*, No. 9401 (Federal Trade Commission 2021), Complaint, Redacted Public Version.

The possibility of an NGS platform substitute is unlikely to provide a useful check on Illumina's ability to foreclose. First, launching a new NGS platform faces substantial legal and commercial barriers. Besides technological challenges, various patents protect Illumina's monopoly. Even if an entrant were to bypass these barriers and enter the market, MCED test makers would need to invest substantial capital and time to ensure compatibility and would need to repeat expensive clinical trials, making it unlikely that they would switch.

The FTC considered the variety of ways in which postmerger Illumina could have the *ability* to foreclose its rivals. The firm could do so directly by refusing to sell its NGS equipment and reagents to its rivals or making them prohibitively expensive. Illumina could also delay or foreclose its rivals' access to new technological developments and technical assistance that would be necessary for developing cutting-edge tests. Finally, Illumina could impede its rivals' ability to get FDA clearance for their tests. The FDA requires an in vitro diagnostic agreement between the test developer and the NGS platform provider to ensure quality before granting FDA approval for the test. Without it, MCED test makers would be severely limited in marketing their products to the broader market. Clearly, Illumina could cut off its downstream rivals from a vital input, but it would only do so if it were profitable.

Next, the Agencies determined whether Illumina would have the *incentive* to foreclose its rivals – whether foreclosure would increase profits. GRAIL is likely to be the dominant player in the MCED test market, which is estimated to be worth tens of billions of dollars annually by 2035. Thus, capturing downstream market share would be quite lucrative. The Agencies concluded that Illumina would be able to make up any loss in sales of sequencing instruments and consumables to its rivals with increased market share in the downstream market.

The Agencies claimed that Illumina and GRAIL did not point to merger-specific procompetitive efficiencies that would save the merger. Although the elimination of double marginalization may provide benefits, they claimed that it would fall short of compensating for the anticompetitive harm of foreclosure. In their view, therefore, social welfare would decrease and consumers would be harmed if the merger were consummated.

Meanwhile, Illumina took the following steps to assuage the Agencies' fear of foreclosure. The firm (1) provided contractual guarantees to its clinical oncology customers that they would receive fair and equal access to its sequencing products, (2) committed to price decreases of 40 percent by 2025, and (3) pointed out various procompetitive efficiencies of the merger. By merging, Illumina could "leverage its global scale of manufacturing and clinical capabilities, as well as its global regulatory and reimbursement expertise" to accelerate the launch of Galleri and bring production up to scale.[22] Patients would receive MCED tests earlier than estimated. The test could potentially be more affordable since Illumina would be able to quickly take advantage of economies of scale and scope.

Although not specifically mentioned by Illumina, the merger may lead to other procompetitive efficiencies. First, the merger would likely lead to EDM. Galleri is poised to be the first MCED test on the market, which would make GRAIL a monopolist for some period of time and lead to a successive monopoly.[23] If other firms entered the downstream market, double marginalization could continue to exist if the firms collude or act as Cournot oligopolists. Vertical integration would serve to mitigate the welfare loss. Additionally, the idea for MCED tests originated from Illumina's research. It is likely that joining the two companies could lead to increased synergies in research, which could launch new technology in the MCED market.

We would caution the Agencies to avoid jumping to conclusions, especially when the MCED market is currently being

---

[22] Illumina (2021).

[23] EDM can also be achieved through a vertical contract. Given that Illumina owns 12 percent of GRAIL, Illumina could more easily set up such a contract, making EDM less likely to be a merger-specific benefit.

developed. Although Illumina has the ability to foreclose its rivals, it may not have the incentive to do so. Complete ownership could change Illumina's incentives, making foreclosure more likely, but not necessarily so. Illumina already holds an upstream monopoly, making it likely that it could extract much of the downstream profit without vertical integration. Vertical integration, therefore, must present some increased benefit to the firm, perhaps in the form of efficiencies.[24] Finally, the Agencies seemed to discount the possible procompetitive efficiencies.

Illumina closed its deal with GRAIL in August 2021 while it was still being investigated by the European Union. The FTC filed suit against Illumina with a trial by administrative law judge.[25] Closing arguments were submitted on June 8, 2022.[26]

20.5 THE MERGER OF A HEALTH INSURER AND A PHYSICIAN GROUP: UNITEDHEALTHCARE/DAVITA

UnitedHealth Group Inc. operates a number of subsidiaries, two of which are UnitedHealthcare and Optum. UnitedHealthcare is one of the largest health insurers in the US market. Additionally, it holds the dominant share of Medicare Advantage plans in the Colorado Springs area. Optum, meanwhile, owns a number of medical groups, independent physician associations, ambulatory surgery centers, and urgent care centers.[27]

---

[24] Angerhofer and Blair (2021) argue that a monopolist in an upstream market would have no incentive to merge with a downstream firm to prevent downstream entry. In some cases, downstream entry increases the monopolist's profits due to an increase in bargaining power and demand for its products (e.g., if the downstream firms act as Cournot oligopolists). There would be no incentive to merge unless significant efficiencies existed. Without knowing the market structure of the downstream market, the Agencies cannot make accurate predictions about the effects of vertical integration.

[25] McLaughlin (2021).

[26] See www.ftc.gov/legal-library/browse/cases-proceedings/201-0144-illumina-inc-grail-inc-matter for updates on the suit.

[27] *Colorado v. UnitedHealth Group* (D.C. Col. 2019), Complaint.

DaVita Medical Group (DaVita) was a for-profit managed care group that operated in six states. Managed care organizations employ a number of primary care physicians and specialists, which allows them to effectively coordinate patient care. DaVita operated Colorado Springs Health Partners and Mountain View Medical Group in the Colorado Springs area, which together made up the largest managed care physician organization in the area.[28]

UnitedHealth Group entered into an agreement to acquire DaVita Medical Group for $4.3 billion in December 2017.[29] Since the merger exceeded the HSR threshold, it was subject to Agency approval and the FTC took on the case. Although the FTC largely focused on horizontal aspects of the merger, it also considered vertical effects of the merger in El Paso and Teller counties in Colorado ("Colorado Springs area"). Ultimately, the FTC commissioners found that vertical effects were too ambiguous to pursue and allowed the merger to proceed.[30] The Colorado attorney general, however, picked up where the FTC left off and challenged the merger based on vertical anticompetitive effects that would harm consumers of Medicare Advantage plans.[31]

Antitrust Analysis

The proposed merger between UnitedHealth Group and DaVita is vertical because it involves a health insurer purchasing an input producer of medical services that it offered in its plans.[32] The Colorado Attorney General (AG) Complaint argued that the merger of UnitedHealth Group and DaVita would have considerable

---

[28] *Colorado* v. *UnitedHealth Group* (D.C. Col. 2019), Complaint.

[29] The original price tag for the acquisition was approximately $4.9 billion. The price changed to $4.3 billion after further negotiations a year later.

[30] Morse (2019). The FTC required divestiture of DaVita Medical Group's healthcare provider organization in the Las Vegas area. However, it imposed no requirements on the Colorado market.

[31] *Colorado* v. *UnitedHealth Group* (D.C. Col. 2019), Complaint.

[32] Much of this analysis comes from *Colorado* v. *UnitedHealth Group* (D.C. Col. 2019), Complaint.

anticompetitive effects in the relevant product market, which constitutes Medicare Advantage plans.[33] As outlined in the VMGs, the Colorado AG needed to consider both the anticompetitive and procompetitive effects of the merger.

First, the Complaint sought to demonstrate that the merged firm had the *ability* and *incentive* to harm its rivals through foreclosure. Per the Complaint, foreclosure would take the form of increasing the prices of DaVita's health services to other insurers that operated Medicare Advantage plans. Since DaVita was one of the largest managed health care organizations in the area, its increased prices would substantially increase the amount that other insurers would need to pay to cover their policyholders. In turn, the insurers would likely increase their premiums for their Medicare Advantage plans to cover the increase in costs. UnitedHealthcare also had an exclusive agreement with Centura Health, which operates two hospitals in the Colorado Springs area. The agreement prevented other Medicare Advantage HMO health insurers from including Centura's hospitals in their networks, further limiting rivals' access to health care services for their policyholders. So UnitedHealthcare clearly would have the ability to raise the costs of its rivals.

Next, the Complaint considered the merged entity's *incentive* to foreclose rivals. Specifically, the Complaint considered whether UnitedHealth Group would be able to recoup its losses from increasing the prices of health services to insurers by gaining market share in the Medicare Advantage plan market. But such a conjecture is difficult to substantiate.

Next, the Colorado AG considered possible procompetitive benefits of the merger. The Colorado Complaint alleged that most of the procompetitive efficiencies suggested by the defendants were neither merger specific nor substantiated. However, it is likely that

---

[33] Patients who qualify for Medicare benefits from the government can opt for a Medicare Advantage plan, which is managed by a private insurer. The government pays the private insurer.

EDM could contribute significant cost savings.[34] Since both DaVita and UnitedHealthcare held significant market power in their respective markets, it stands to reason that some double marginalization occurred that would be reduced after the merger. The merger could also lead to more integrated care, which could increase the quality of care.

Although both anticompetitive and procompetitive effects could occur, it is difficult to determine which effect would dominate. Colorado eventually settled with the defendants, and the merger was allowed on the conditions that (1) UnitedHealthcare ended its exclusive agreement with Centura Health for at least 3.5 years and (2) DaVita Medical Group would continue its agreements with rival insurers until 2020.[35] In this way, the settlement reduced the ability of UnitedHealthcare to foreclose its rivals.

As UnitedHealth Group continues to acquire providers of health care, it has an incentive to steer its patients toward its own health care services rather than those offered by other groups – in other words, foreclosure. So far, no foreclosure complaints have been filed against the merged entity in the Colorado Springs area. But UnitedHealth Group has not escaped such allegations in other parts of the country. A new complaint by an anesthesiology group, US Anesthesia Partners, alleged that UnitedHealthcare forced its doctors out of network in order to give UnitedHealth Group's anesthesiologists more business.[36] This may indicate that the Colorado AG's original foreclosure argument had some merit.

20.6 THE MERGER OF A HOSPITAL SYSTEM AND A PHYSICIAN GROUP: ST. LUKE'S/SALTZER

Hospital acquisitions of physician groups are becoming more common. Between July 2012 and January 2018, the number of

---

[34] Phillips and Wilson (2019).   [35] Weiser (2019).

[36] *US Anesthesia Partners of Colorado Inc.* v. *UnitedHealthcare Insurance Company et al.*, No. 2021-cv-31061 (D.C. Denver 2021). For additional information, see Abelson (2021).

hospital-owned physician practices in the United States increased from 35,700 to 80,000.[37] Since physician groups rarely – if ever – have enough assets to trigger the HSR threshold, many of these mergers have fallen through the cracks without Agency review. Often, hospitals purchase a number of small physician practices over time, allowing them to accumulate market power to possibly harmful levels. Such was the case in Idaho, where the St. Luke's hospital system acquired more than 70 physician practice groups between 2004 and 2012.[38] In 2012, St. Luke's Health System Ltd. (St. Luke's) acquired a dominant physician group, Saltzer Medical Group, PA (Saltzer), in Nampa and Caldwell, Idaho (Nampa area), which supply complementary services.

St. Luke's is a large not-for-profit hospital system in Idaho. At the time of the merger, it owned six hospitals, an emergency care center, a children's hospital, a cancer referral center, and more than 100 clinics spread over central and southwest Idaho and eastern Oregon. Before its merger with Saltzer, St. Luke's had already acquired 16 other physician groups in the Nampa area, which gave it an 18 percent share of the adult primary care market.

At the time of the merger, Saltzer was the largest and oldest independent multi-specialty physician group in Idaho. It provided services for about 38 percent of the adult primary care market. Its merger with St. Luke's increased St. Luke's market share of the primary care market to 56 percent.[39]

A competing hospital and the FTC later filed complaints in 2012 that were successful in breaking up the merger of St. Luke's and Saltzer. These complaints focused on horizontal aspects of the mergers because St. Luke's already owned a number of physician

---

[37] Rodriguez (2019).

[38] *Federal Trade Commission and State of Idaho* v. *St. Luke's Health System, Ltd. and Saltzer Medical Group*, No. 13-cv-116-BLW (D. Idaho 2013), Complaint for Permanent Injunction.

[39] *Federal Trade Commission and State of Idaho* v. *St. Luke's Health System, Ltd. and Saltzer Medical Group*, No. 13-cv-116-BLW (D. Idaho 2013), Complaint for Permanent Injunction.

groups in the Nampa area. In what follows, we analyze the merger of the hospital system and the physician group.

Antitrust Analysis

The first round of mergers between a hospital and a physician group may seem innocuous, especially since they can increase integration of care and produce procompetitive efficiencies. An integrated hospital and physician group can better coordinate care for patients and can improve the transfer of medical documents and other administrative tasks. But many hospital systems do not stop at acquiring one group.

Further mergers can increase horizontal market power in the physician group market, giving the merged firm substantial market share in at least one of the complementary markets in which it operates. For example, St. Luke's acquired 16 physician groups along with Saltzer to obtain a 56 percent share of the primary care market.[40] This additional market power may allow a hospital to take advantage of bundling and tying to force health insurers to increase their reimbursement rates. Insurers are likely to pass on the higher costs to their policyholders and thereby harm consumers.

In order to offer attractive plans to employers and individuals, insurers need to offer comprehensive care by including in-network services of both hospitals and physician groups. With St. Luke's control of the hospital and the primary care market, health insurers in the Nampa area had no choice but to interact with St. Luke's and buy a bundle of hospital and physician services. Implicitly, by offering St. Luke's physician services through their insurance plans, insurers would also need to include St. Luke's hospital services since St. Luke's physicians would generally refer patients to St. Luke's hospitals. Therefore, if insurers wanted to include any of St. Luke's physician groups in their policies, they would also need to include

---

[40] Another source claims St. Luke's market share would have been 80 percent with the merger. See *Saint Alphonsus Medical Center – Nampa, Inc. et al.* v. *St. Luke's Health System, Ltd.*, No. 1:12-cv-00560-BLW (D. Idaho 2012), Findings of Fact and Conclusions of Law.

St. Luke's hospitals. This translated into much higher reimbursement rates for the services that St. Luke's provided.[41] For example, the cost of treating a superficial wound was 274 percent higher at St. Luke's than at other nonaffiliated clinics in the area.[42] Insurers, meanwhile, increased the price of their policies to cover the increase in costs, which also harmed consumers. By controlling two important complementary inputs of health insurance plans, St. Luke's was able to leverage its bargaining power and increase its reimbursement rates to anticompetitive levels.

Integrating with physician groups can also be profitable for hospitals due to referrals. When a patient requires more intensive treatment or an operation, his or her primary care physician will recommend an experienced doctor. Without affiliation, the physician will generally advise patients to do what is best for them. When a hospital acquires a physician group, however, the hospital will have an incentive to keep referrals in-house. Then primary care physicians may provide referrals to physicians who are affiliated with the acquiring hospital. This increase in demand for in-network services allows the acquiring hospital to increase its prices and/or reduce quality. Baker, Bundorf, and Kessler (2016) indicated that a (Medicare) patient is more likely to choose a high-cost, low-quality hospital when their physician is affiliated with that hospital.

In a world of perfect information, patients would know which doctors provide the highest quality care and would choose which services to buy based on their own internal cost–quality trade-off. The health care industry, however, is rife with asymmetric information. Most patients trust their doctors for referrals since they have neither the time nor the expertise to determine the best-value services to buy. By acquiring physician groups, hospitals can capitalize on this

---

[41] Horizontal aspects of the merger were also important. With 56 percent of the primary care market, St. Luke's also had significant bargaining power.

[42] *Federal Trade Commission and State of Idaho* v. *St. Luke's Health System, Ltd. and Saltzer Medical Group*, No. 13-cv-116-BLW (D. Idaho 2013), Complaint for Permanent Injunction.

asymmetric information and increase their profits at the expense of patients.

Many studies show that hospital acquisitions of physician groups increase prices and lower the quality of health care services for patients.[43] Mergers of suppliers of complementary products can often be procompetitive. But when a merged firm attains a high level of market power in one input market, some analysts suspect that it can lead to anticompetitive effects of bundling or tying. The prevalence of asymmetric information exacerbates the anticompetitive effects in hospital–physician group acquisitions.

20.7 CONCLUDING REMARKS

It can be difficult to determine the likely effects of a merger when both anticompetitive and procompetitive effects exist. On the one hand, vertical mergers can lead to foreclosure and raising rivals' cost, whereas mergers of complementary input suppliers can lead to anticompetitive bundling or tying. On the other hand, vertical mergers can eliminate transaction costs and double marginalization, and mergers of complementary input suppliers can internalize price externalities and eliminate transaction costs. It is difficult to quantify each of these effects when a merger between two firms has not been consummated. This difficulty has allowed mergers to be consummated even though they harm consumers.

Recently, the Agencies have viewed merger proposals with a great deal of skepticism. But still too little is known about the risk factors of vertical mergers and mergers of complementary input suppliers. More research and empirical studies are needed to allow the Agencies to accurately separate the wheat from the chaff. Fortunately, such efforts have already begun.[44]

---

[43] See, for example, Capps, Dranove, and Ody (2018), Neprash et al. (2015), and Robinson and Miller (2014).

[44] For example, the FTC has launched a study of hospital–physician group mergers. See Federal Trade Commission (2021).

REFERENCES

Abelson, Reed. (2021). Doctors Accuse UnitedHealthcare of Stifling Competition. *New York Times.* www.nytimes.com/2021/04/01/health/unitedhealthcare-lawsuit.html.

Angerhofer, Tirza J., and Roger D. Blair. (2021). Successive Monopoly, Bilateral Monopoly, and Vertical Integration. *Review of Industrial Organization* 59: 343–361.

Baker, Laurence C., M. Kate Bundorf, and Daniel P. Kessler. (2016). The Effect of Hospital/Physician Integration on Hospital Choice. *Journal of Health Economics* 50: 1–8.

Blair, Roger D., and David L. Kaserman. (2009). *Antitrust Economics.* 2d ed. New York: Oxford University Press.

Capps, Cory, David Dranove, and Christopher Ody. (2018). The Effect of Hospital Acquisitions of Physician Practices on Prices and Spending. *Journal of Health Economics* 59: 139–152.

Department of Justice and Federal Trade Commission. (2020). Vertical Merger Guidelines. www.ftc.gov/system/files/documents/reports/us-department-just ice-federal-trade-commission-vertical-merger-guidelines/vertical_merger_guide lines_6-30-20.pdf.

Federal Trade Commission. (2021). FTC to Study the Impact of Physician Group and Healthcare Facility Mergers. www.ftc.gov/news-events/press-releases/ 2021/01/ftc-study-impact-physician-group-healthcare-facility-mergers.

Herper, Matthew. (2017). Company Will Raise $1 Billion to Create Blood Test to Detect Cancer. *Forbes.* www.forbes.com/sites/matthewherper/2017/01/05/ grail-which-aims-to-invent-blood-test-to-detect-cancer-to-raise-1-billion/?sh= 2483a1493792.

Illumina. (2020). Form 10-K. https://s24.q4cdn.com/526396163/files/doc_finan cials/2020/q4/13eff379-c1ce-48fe-a760-8ff5147866b2.pdf.

Illumina. (2021). Illumina Committed to Pursuing GRAIL Acquisition to Accelerate Access to Breakthrough Multi-Cancer Early Detection Blood Test. Illumina Press Release. www.illumina.com/company/news-center/press-releases/2021/32156cec-c392-4d23-be23-66d7729892db.html.

McLaughlin, David. (2021). *Illumina Fights US Bid to Unwind $8 Billion Grail Takeover.* Bloomberg Law. https://news.bloomberglaw.com/antitrust/illumina-fights-u-s-bid-to-unwind-8-billion-grail-takeover.

Morse, Susan. (2019). *FTC Approves UnitedHealth Group $4.3 Billion Acquisition of DaVita, with Conditions.* Healthcare Finance. www.healthcarefinancenews.com/ news/ftc-approves-unitedhealth-group-43-billion-acquisition-davita-conditions.

Neprash, Hannah T., Michael E. Chernew, Andrew L. Hicks, Teresa Gibson, and Michael McWilliams. (2015). Association of Financial Integration between Physicians and Hospitals with Commercial Health Care Prices. *Journal of the American Medical Association* 175: 1932–1939.

Phillips, Noah Joshua, and Christine S. Wilson. (2019). *Statement of Commissioner Noah Joshua Phillips and Commissioner Christine S. Wilson: In the Matter of UnitedHealth Group and DaVita.* Federal Trade Commission. www.ftc.gov/system/files/documents/public_statements/1529366/181_0057_united_davita_statement_of_cmmrs_p_and_w.pdf.

Premerger Notification Office Staff. (2021). *HSR Threshold Adjustments and Reportability for 2021.* Federal Trade Commission. www.ftc.gov/news-events/blogs/competition-matters/2021/02/hsr-threshold-adjustments-reportability-2021.

Robinson, James C., and Kelly Miller. (2014). Total Expenditures per Patient in Hospital-Owned and Physician-Owned Physician Organizations in California. *Journal of the American Medical Association* 312: 1663–1669.

Rodriguez, Carmen Heredia. (2019). *Hospitals Chafe under a Medicare Rule That Reduces Payments to Far-Flung Clinics.* NPR. www.npr.org/sections/health-shots/2019/04/23/716110288/hospitals-chafe-under-a-medicare-rule-that-reduces-payments-to-far-flung-clinics.

Weiser, Phil. (2019). Antitrust Challenge and Settlement to the UnitedHealth Group and DaVita merger Will Safeguard Competition, Cost, and Quality of Healthcare for Seniors in the Colorado Springs Area. Colorado Attorney General Press Release. https://coag.gov/press-releases/06-19-19/.

21 Concluding Remarks

For the most part, those who participate in our health care system are well intentioned. Acute care hospitals and physicians provide medical care to their patients in an effort to restore good health. Pharmaceutical firms produce a wide assortment of drugs that treat various illnesses. Medical equipment companies develop and supply advanced imaging equipment, artificial joints, hospital beds, retractable needles, and a host of other devices and supplies that are essential for health care. Dental suppliers and eye care providers similarly promote good health for US citizens.

While we recognize and applaud the efforts of these participants in the provision of health care, we must also recognize that they are businesses. Individuals are concerned with their incomes, and firms are concerned with their profits. There is an incentive among firms to reduce competition in the pursuit of higher income or greater profit. But efforts to reduce competition impose economic harm on patients. This is where antitrust enforcement can step in to promote competition.

We began this book by describing the antitrust statutes and the economic rationale for their existence. Public and private enforcement of the antitrust laws aid in controlling the adverse economic consequences of monopoly, monopsony, and collusion among ostensible competitors, which enrich firms while harming society. In addition, we have reviewed mergers and their potential for increasing concentration to anticompetitive levels. Although antitrust laws prohibit competitively unreasonable behavior that tends to create monopolies or monopsonies and directly criminalize actions to form cartels, there have been numerous examples of this kind of behavior in health care settings. The lure of greater profits appears to be irresistible. In some instances, firms can find refuge in patent laws. In other instances, firms rely on secrecy. Existing public policy cannot do much about how the patent system protects firms. However, antitrust policy can mitigate the misuse of patents. It can also be used to challenge firms that engage in anticompetitive, monopolizing behavior or collusion. Worryingly, firms will continue to find ways to engage in anticompetitive behavior when they think they can do so without punishment. Our hope is that by explaining the underlying mechanisms of markets, we can equip our readers with the ability to recognize anticompetitive behavior and to understand the available antitrust remedies that mitigate anticompetitive harm.

We cannot emphasize strongly enough that competitive markets should be protected because they provide the largest welfare payoff to society. For this reason, the antitrust laws were created to deter and punish the monopolistic, monopsonistic, and collusive behavior of firms. Making health care markets more competitive will require a twofold process. First, the antitrust laws should be used to punish firms that are currently practicing anticompetitive behavior in hopes of stopping such behavior in the present and future. The antitrust Agencies and private parties should use their authority to sue and recover damages to compensate those who have been harmed and also to make the underlying behavior less profitable.

Second, policymakers should deter future anticompetitive behavior. This can be done in two ways. Sanctions and monitoring should be increased, which will make punishment harsher and more likely. Currently, sanctions appear to be quite high, but settlements often allow firms to mitigate those sanctions. Then punishment is merely a slap on the wrist that equates to the cost of doing business. Increasing sanctions will disincentivize firms from engaging in anticompetitive behavior for fear of the consequences. Increasing monitoring and enforcement actions will make it more difficult for firms to act anticompetitively without detection. Second, the antitrust Agencies should challenge anticompetitive mergers since they can increase concentration, which facilitates the ability of firms to act anticompetitively. In the past few years, merger frequency in health care markets has increased dramatically. Often, the antitrust Agencies ignore these mergers because they are too small to attract their notice. Allowing state attorneys general to evaluate smaller local mergers may be helpful in addressing harmful concentration in local markets.

Some critics have examined the burgeoning costs of health care in the United States and have called for massive changes to the system. But reforming the current system with increased government involvement is not our focus. Instead, conditional on our current health care system, we propose vigorous antitrust enforcement to protect and promote competition whenever feasible. In this book, we have identified many examples of impaired competition: abuses of both monopoly and monopsony power, collusion among buyers and sellers, and mergers that lead to increased market power. In most health care markets, we have observed antitrust enforcement and applaud these efforts. Our hope is that unrelenting antitrust enforcement will improve the functioning of health care markets and thereby save patients, health insurers, and the government billions of dollars while increasing the accessibility of lifesaving care.

Index